ACP | MKSAP 17

Board Basics®

An Enhancement to MKSAP 17®

ACP American College of Physicians®
Leading Internal Medicine, Improving Lives

Your Last Stop before the Boards

For the fourth consecutive edition of MKSAP, we bring you Board Basics, the only publication that compiles the essential facts and strategies for passing the Internal Medicine Certification and Maintenance of Certification (MOC) Exam into one print book and e-book. We are confident that this volume will continue to meet your needs. A total of 83% of surveyed Board Basics users told us that the previous edition of Board Basics effectively helped them prepare for the Certification or MOC exams. Nearly all respondents found this resource to be user-friendly and an overwhelming majority—84%—said they would recommend it to a colleague.

How to Use Board Basics

The goal of Board Basics is to prepare you for the Boards after you have completed a systematic review of MKSAP 17 and its more than 1200 multiple-choice questions. Once again, we have combed through volumes to produce a concise compilation of only the information that you will most likely see in the exam. And, with this fourth edition, we have reorganized the sections of Board Basics to mirror those of MKSAP, making it easier for you to locate information within the 11 MKSAP subspecialty sections to further your learning on specific topics as you need. Board Basics is not a concise guide to patient care but, rather, an exam preparation tool to help you quickly recognize the most likely answers on a multiple-choice exam. Drug dosages are not included since they are rarely, if ever, tested. You will also see many sections where information has been omitted because it is difficult to test or is otherwise unlikely to appear on the exam.

Broad differential diagnoses are not provided for most problems. Instead, Board Basics focuses on the entities that have the highest probability of appearing on the exam as the "correct answers." Critical points that appear on the exam are often presented here in isolation, stripped of context that is not relevant to answering a multiple-choice question. If you review these points shortly before your exam, you will have the best chance of remembering what you need to know to do well. Knowing that most Board questions are prefaced with the words "most likely," we have tried to be very directive, skipping important steps in the patient evaluation. When you see the words "select" or "choose," think in terms of *selecting or choosing a particular answer*, not an

intervention in the practice of medicine. Remember that Board Basics is *not* a patient care resource.

Content Organization

Abbreviations, spelled out in a convenient list at the back of the book, are used frequently to increase reading efficiency. Content is organized by topic and in consistent categories, such as Prevention, Screening, Diagnosis, Therapy, and Follow-up. Special components have been designed to enhance learning and recall. Look for:

- *Don't Be Tricked*: Incorrect answers that may masquerade as correct choices.
- *Test Yourself*: Abbreviated case histories and answers found in Board exam questions.
- *Study Tables*: Key concepts to prepare you for specific types of questions.
- *Yellow highlighting*: We applied our own "marker" to call your attention to important phrases.

Why This Text Makes Sense

For this edition of Board Basics, MKSAP 17 authors reviewed the latest literature and produced 11 concise text sections and 1200 Board-like multiple-choice questions. Next, the content was turned over to 13 carefully selected program directors, instructors, and professors of medicine with expertise in Board preparation and the subspecialties of internal medicine. These physicians culled the essential points from MKSAP 17 and added their insights to update the content of Board Basics.

Patrick Alguire, MD, FACP, Senior Vice President of the Medical Education Division of the American College of Physicians, served as Editor-in-Chief, reviewing and distilling the MKSAP 17 text by eliminating overlap and excessive material to focus the text as sharply as possible. The end product is what you have in your hands—the best Board prep tool that you will find anywhere. We hope you enjoy it and benefit from your study. Best wishes on your exam.

Douglas S. Paauw, MD, MACP
Editor
Board Basics

Board Basics

Ted Wun, MD[2]
Professor and Associate Dean (Research)
Chief, Division of Hematology Oncology
UC Davis School of Medicine
Sacramento, California

Board Basics ACP Editorial Staff

Susan Galeone[1], Staff Editor
Margaret Wells[1], Director, Self-Assessment and Educational
   Programs
Becky Krumm[1], Managing Editor

ACP Principal Staff

Patrick C. Alguire, MD, FACP[2]
Senior Vice President, Medical Education

Sean McKinney[1]
Vice President, Medical Education

Margaret Wells[1]
Director, Self-Assessment and Educational Programs

Philip A. Masters, MD, FACP[1]
Director, Clinical Content Development
Senior Physician Educator

Cynthia D. Smith, MD, FACP[2]
Director, Clinical Program Development
Senior Physician Educator

Becky Krumm[1]
Managing Editor

Katie Idell[1]
Manager, Clinical Skills and Digital Programs

Valerie A. Dangovetsky[1]
Administrator

Ellen McDonald, PhD[1]
Senior Staff Editor

Megan Zborowski[1]
Senior Staff Editor

Randy Hendrickson[1]
Production Administrator/Editor

Linnea Donnarumma[1]
Staff Editor

Susan Galeone[1]
Staff Editor

Jackie Twomey[1]
Staff Editor

Julia Nawrocki[1]
Staff Editor

Kimberly Kerns[1]
Administrative Coordinator

Rosemarie Houton[1]
Administrative Representative

Disclosure of Relationships with any entity producing, marketing, reselling, or distributing health care goods or services consumed by, or used on, patients.

Patrick C. Alguire, MD, FACP
Consultantship
National Board of Medical Examiners
Royalties
UpToDate
Stock Options/Holdings
Amgen, Bristol-Myers Squibb, GlaxoSmithKline, Stryker
   Corporation, Zimmer, Teva Pharmaceutical Industries,
   Medtronic, Covidien, Express Scripts

Aaron J. Calderon, MD, FACP
Speakers Bureau
MedStudy
Stock Options/Holdings
Pfizer, Merck, Abbott, Medtronic

John Flaherty, MD
Board Member
Alliance of Academic Internal Medicine
Consultantship
CVS Caremark

Brian Porter, MD
Employment
University of Washington

Cynthia D. Smith, MD, FACP
Stock Options/Holdings
Merck and Co.; spousal employment at Merck

Ted Wun, MD
Other
Committee Memberships: Alliance for Academic Internal
   Medicine, American Society of Hematology, Sickle Cell
   Adult Provider Network
Advisory Boards and Steering Committees
CALLISTO Program (Janssen, Inc.), RESET Study (Pfizer,
   Inc.)

Acknowledgments

The American College of Physicians (ACP) gratefully acknowledges the special contributions to the development and production of the 17th edition of the Medical Knowledge Self-Assessment Program® (MKSAP® 17) made by the following people:

Graphic Design: Michael Ripca (Graphics Technical Administrator) and WFGD Studio (Graphic Designers).

Production/Systems: Dan Hoffmann (Director, Web Services & Systems Development), Neil Kohl (Senior Architect), Chris Patterson (Senior Architect), and Scott Hurd (Manager, Web Projects & CMS Services).

MKSAP 17 Digital: Under the direction of Steven Spadt, Vice President, Digital Products & Services, the digital version of MKSAP 17 was developed within the ACP's Digital Product Development Department, led by Brian Sweigard (Director). Other members of the team included Dan Barron (Senior Web Application Developer/Architect), Chris Forrest (Senior Software Developer/Design Lead), Kara Kronenwetter (Senior Web Developer), Brad Lord (Senior Web Application Developer), John McKnight (Senior Web Developer), and Nate Pershall (Senior Web Developer).

The College also wishes to acknowledge that many other persons, too numerous to mention, have contributed to the production of this program. Without their dedicated efforts, this program would not have been possible.

MKSAP Resource Site (mksap.acponline.org)

The MKSAP Resource Site (mksap.acponline.org) is a continually updated site that provides links to MKSAP 17 online answer sheets for print subscribers; the latest details on Continuing Medical Education (CME) and Maintenance of Certification (MOC) in the United States, Canada, and Australia; errata; and other new information.

Disclosure Policy

It is the policy of the American College of Physicians (ACP) to ensure balance, independence, objectivity, and scientific rigor in all of its educational activities. To this end, and consistent with the policies of the ACP and the Accreditation Council for Continuing Medical Education (ACCME), contributors to all ACP continuing medical education activities are required to disclose all relevant financial relationships with any entity producing, marketing, re-selling, or distributing health care goods or services consumed by, or used on, patients. Contributors are required to use generic names in the discussion of therapeutic options and are required to identify any unapproved, off-label, or investigative use of commercial products or devices. Where a trade name is used, all available trade names for the same product type are also included. If trade-name products manufactured by companies with whom contributors have relationships are discussed, contributors are asked to provide evidence-based citations in support of the discussion. The information is reviewed by the committee responsible for producing this text. If necessary, adjustments to topics or contributors' roles in content development are made to balance the discussion. Further, all readers of this text are asked to evaluate the content for evidence of commercial bias and send any relevant comments to mksap_editors@acponline.org so that future decisions about content and contributors can be made in light of this information.

Resolution of Conflicts

To resolve all conflicts of interest and influences of vested interests, the ACP precluded members of the content-creation committee from deciding on any content issues that involved generic or trade-name products associated with proprietary entities with which these committee members had relationships. In addition, content was based on best evidence and updated clinical care guidelines, when such evidence and guidelines were available. Contributors' disclosure information can be found with the list of contributors' names and those of ACP principal staff listed in the beginning of this book.

Educational Disclaimer

The editors and publisher of MKSAP 17 recognize that the development of new material offers many opportunities for error. Despite our best efforts, some errors may persist in print. Drug dosage schedules are, we believe, accurate and in accordance with current standards. Readers are advised, however, to ensure that the recommended dosages in MKSAP 17 concur with the information provided in the product information material. This is especially important in cases of new, infrequently used, or highly toxic drugs. Application of the information in MKSAP 17 remains the professional responsibility of the practitioner.

The primary purpose of MKSAP 17 is educational. Information presented, as well as publications, technologies, products, and/or services discussed, is intended to inform subscribers about the knowledge, techniques, and experiences of the contributors. A diversity of professional opinion exists, and the views of the contributors are their own and not those of the ACP. Inclusion of any material in the program does not constitute endorsement or recommendation by the ACP. The ACP does not warrant the safety, reliability, accuracy, completeness, or usefulness of and disclaims any and all liability for damages and claims that may result from the use of information, publications, technologies, products, and/or services discussed in this program.

Publisher's Information

Unauthorized Use of This Book Is Against the Law

The ACP will consider granting an individual permission to reproduce only limited portions of this publication for his or her own exclusive use. Send requests in writing to MKSAP® Permissions, American College of Physicians, 190 N. Independence Mall West, Philadelphia, PA 19106-1572, or email your request to mksap_editors@acponline.org.

MKSAP 17 ISBN: 978-1-938245-18-3
(Board Basics) ISBN: 978-1-938245-44-2

Printed in the United States of America.

For order information in the U.S. or Canada call 800-523-1546, extension 2600. All other countries call 215-351-2600, (M-F, 9 AM – 5 PM ET). Fax inquiries to 215-351-2799 or email to custserv@acponline.org.

Errata

Errata for MKSAP 17 will be available through the MKSAP Resource Site at mksap.acponline.org as new information becomes known to the editors.

Table of Contents

Gastroenterology and Hepatology

General Internal Medicine

Hematology

Infectious Disease

Cardiovascular Medicine

Acute Coronary Syndromes

Diagnosis

Classic anginal symptoms include substernal chest pain with exertion, and relief with rest or nitroglycerin. Anginal equivalents are most commonly found in patients with diabetes and in women and include exertional dyspnea, fatigue, nausea, and vomiting.

Signs of cardiac ischemia include new MR murmur and S_3 and S_4 gallops.

The 12-lead ECG and serum biomarkers distinguish three types of ACS:

STUDY TABLE: Acute Coronary Syndromes	
Syndrome	**Description**
Unstable angina	Normal cardiac biomarkers (troponin, CK-MB)
	No characteristic ECG changes
NSTEMI	Positive biomarkers without ST elevations or ST-elevation equivalents
	ST depression and nonspecific changes may be seen
STEMI	Positive biomarkers and ST-segment elevation in ≥2 contiguous leads
	ST-elevation equivalents include new LBBB or posterior MI (tall R waves and ST depressions in V_1-V_3)

Echocardiogram may show regional wall motion abnormalities in ACS. This may be especially useful in patients with LBBB.

STUDY TABLE: ECG Localization of Acute MI		
Anatomic Location	**ST-Segment Change**	**Indicative ECG Leads**
Inferior	Elevation	II, III, aVF
Anteroseptal	Elevation	V_1-V_3
Lateral and apical	Elevation	V_4-V_6, possibly I and aVL
Posterior wall*	Depression	Tall R waves in V_1-V_3
Right ventricle*	Elevation	V_4R-V_6R; tall R waves in V_1-V_3

*Often associated with inferior and/or lateral ST-elevation infarctions.

The Thrombolysis in Myocardial Infarction (TIMI) risk score is a seven-point score for estimating risk in patients with unstable angina/NSTEMI and is used to guide therapy in these conditions. The rate of death for MI significantly increases with a higher TIMI risk score. One point is awarded for each of the following prognostic factors:

- age ≥65 years
- ≥3 traditional CAD risk factors
- prior coronary obstruction ≥50%
- ST-segment deviation
- ≥2 episodes of angina in the past 24 hours
- aspirin use in the past week
- elevated biomarkers

Do not attempt to memorize the scoring system but understand the difference in approach for a patient with a low-risk score (0-2) and higher score (3-7).

STUDY TABLE: Unstable Angina or NSTEMI Risk Stratification	
TIMI Risk Score	**Strategy**
3-7	Begin aspirin, β-blocker, nitrates, heparin, statin, GP IIb/IIIa inhibitor, clopidogrel, and early angiography
0-2	Begin aspirin, β-blocker, nitrates, heparin, statin, clopidogrel. Predischarge stress testing and angiography if testing reveals significant myocardial ischemia

Immediate angiography is also indicated if any of the following are present:

- hemodynamic instability
- HF
- recurrent rest angina despite therapy
- new or worsening MR murmur
- sustained VT

◆ DON'T BE TRICKED

- **STEMI is not the only cause of ST-segment elevations. Consider acute pericarditis, LV aneurysm, takotsubo (stress) cardiomyopathy, coronary vasospasm (Prinzmetal angina), or normal variant.**

STUDY TABLE: Other Causes of Acute Chest Pain		
Vignette	**Consider**	**Test/Therapy**
Young woman with history of migraines, acute chest pain, and ST-segment elevation	Coronary vasospasm (Prinzmetal angina, variant angina)	Calcium channel blocker
Young person with chest pain following a party	Cocaine	Calcium channel blocker (avoid β-blockers)
A tall, thin person with long arms with acute chest and back pain, a normal ECG, and an aortic diastolic murmur	Marfan syndrome and aortic dissection	MRI, contrast CT, or TEE. Immediate surgery for type A dissection
A patient who recently traveled or with immobility, sharp or pleuritic chest pain, and nondiagnostic ECG	PE	UFH or LMWH; CTA
A tall, thin young man who smokes with sudden pleuritic chest pain and dyspnea	Spontaneous pneumothorax	Chest x-ray
A postmenopausal woman with substernal chest pain following severe emotional/physical stress has ST-segment elevation in the anterior precordial leads, troponin elevation, and unremarkable coronary angiography	Stress-induced (takotsubo) cardiomyopathy. Look for characteristic apical ballooning on ventriculogram.	β-blocker
A young man with substernal chest pain, deep T-wave inversions in V_2-V_4, and a harsh systolic murmur that increases with Valsalva maneuver	HCM	Echocardiography, β-blocker

Therapy

In STEMI, percutaneous coronary intervention (PCI) is the preferred strategy and should be performed as soon as possible, with first medical contact to PCI time ≤90 minutes in PCI-capable hospital and ≤120 minutes if transferred from a non–PCI-capable hospital to a PCI-capable hospital.

Other indications for PCI are:

- failure of thrombolytic therapy (continued chest pain, persistent ST elevations on ECG)
- fibrinolytic therapy is contraindicated
- STEMI with continued chest pain or ST-segment elevation 12-24 hours after onset
- new HF or cardiogenic shock

Administer thrombolytic agents when PCI is not available. The most commonly encountered contraindications include active bleeding or high risk for bleeding (recent major surgery) and BP >180/110 mm Hg on presentation.

CABG surgery is indicated acutely for STEMI in the presence of:

- failure of thrombolysis or PCI
- important mechanical complications (papillary muscle rupture, VSD, free wall rupture)

Patients with an RV/posterior MI may present with hypotension or may develop hypotension following the administration of nitroglycerin or morphine; treat these patients with IV fluids. Look for elevated CVP with clear lungs, hypotension, and tachycardia. The most predictive ECG finding is ST-segment elevation on right-sided ECG lead V_4R.

Place an intra-aortic balloon pump for patients with cardiogenic shock, acute MR or VSD, intractable VT, or refractory angina.

◆ DON'T BE TRICKED

- Choose transfer for PCI instead of thrombolytic therapy for STEMI only if transfer and PCI can be done ideally in ≤120 minutes.
- Do not choose thrombolytic therapy for patients with NSTEMI or for asymptomatic patients with onset of pain >24 hours ago.
- Reperfusion arrhythmias following thrombolytic therapy, typically manifested as a transient accelerated idioventricular arrhythmia, do not require additional antiarrhythmic therapy.

STUDY TABLE: Drug Therapy for MI	
Drug	**Indication**
Aspirin	ASAP for all patients with ACS
	Continue indefinitely as secondary prevention
P2Y$_{12}$ inhibitor (clopidogrel, ticagrelor, prasugrel)	ASAP for all patients with ACS
	Continue for 1 year following MI
Anticoagulant (UFH, LMWH, bivalirudin)	ASAP for definite or likely ACS
GP IIb/IIIa antagonists (abciximab, eptifibatide, tirofiban)	ASAP for high-risk NSTEMI
	Administer prior to PCI
β-Blockers (metoprolol, carvedilol)	Administer within 24 hours
	Continue indefinitely as secondary prevention
Calcium channel blockers (not nifedipine)	Use if β-blocker is contraindicated
ACE inhibitors	Administer within 24 hours
	Continue indefinitely in patients with reduced LVEF or clinical HF
ARB	Administer if intolerant of ACE inhibitor
Nitroglycerin	Administer in presence of ongoing chest pain or HF
Statin	Administer high-intensity statin early
	Continue indefinitely as secondary prevention
Eplerenone	Administer 3 to 14 days after MI when LVEF ≤40% and clinical HF or diabetes

Stent thrombosis may occur 24 hours to 1 year after placement and often presents as recurrent angina, sudden death, or MI, usually with ST-segment elevation. Prevent stent thrombosis with dural antiplatelet therapy.

STUDY TABLE: Indication and Duration of Dual Antiplatelet Therapy			
Condition	**No Stent**	**Bare-Metal Stent**	**Drug-Eluting Stent**
Stable angina pectoris	Clopidogrel, only if aspirin is contraindicated	Clopidogrel	Clopidogrel
		1 month and continue aspirin thereafter	1 year and continue aspirin thereafter

(Continued on next page)

STUDY TABLE: Indication and Duration of Dual Antiplatelet Therapy (Continued)			
Condition	**No Stent**	**Bare-Metal Stent**	**Drug-Eluting Stent**
Unstable angina/NSTEMI	Clopidogrel or ticagrelor 1 year and continue aspirin thereafter	Clopidogrel, prasugrel, or ticagrelor At least 4 weeks, up to 1 year and continue aspirin thereafter	Clopidogrel, prasugrel, or ticagrelor 1 year and continue aspirin thereafter
STEMI	Clopidogrel or ticagrelor 1 year and continue aspirin thereafter	Clopidogrel, prasugrel, or ticagrelor At least 4 weeks, up to 1 year and continue aspirin thereafter	Clopidogrel, prasugrel, or ticagrelor 1 year and continue aspirin thereafter

◆ DON'T BE TRICKED

- Do not select spironolactone, because its effectiveness in patients with acute MI is unknown.

Recommendations for temporary pacing in the setting of acute MI are:

- asystole
- symptomatic bradycardia (including complete heart block)
- alternating LBBB and RBBB
- new or indeterminate-age bifascicular block with first-degree AV block

Mechanical complications (VSD, papillary muscle rupture, and LV free wall rupture) may occur 2 to 7 days after an MI. Emergency echocardiography is the initial diagnostic study.

- Patients with VSD or papillary muscle rupture develop abrupt pulmonary edema or hypotension and a loud holosystolic murmur and thrill.
- LV free wall rupture causes sudden hypotension or cardiac death associated with pulseless electrical activity.

Mortality rate is high for mechanical complications and aggressive intervention is indicated:

- Stabilize patients with papillary muscle rupture and VSD with an intra-aortic balloon pump, afterload reduction with sodium nitroprusside, diuretics, and then emergent surgical intervention.
- Treat free wall rupture with emergent pericardiocentesis and surgery.

Cardiac catheterization is indicated for patients with postinfarction angina or the following post-MI stress test results:

- exercise-induced ST-segment depression or elevation
- inability to achieve 5 METs during testing
- inability to increase SBP by 10 to 30 mm Hg
- inability to exercise (arthritis)

ICDs are indicated in patients meeting the following criteria:

- >40 days since MI
- >3 months since PCI or CABG
- EF <35%
- History of hemodynamically significant ventricular arrhythmia or cardiac arrest (secondary prevention)

All post-MI patients should be screened for depression, because it is associated with increased hospitalization and death.

A 56-year-old woman has a 3-hour history of chest pain. BP is 80/60 mm Hg, respiration rate is 30/min, and pulse rate is 120/min. Physical examination shows jugular venous distention, inspiratory crackles, and an S_3 gallop. ECG shows ST-segment elevation in leads V_2-V_6.

ANSWER: The diagnosis is STEMI and cardiogenic shock. Choose cardiac catheterization and PCI.

A 58-year-old man with acute chest pain has ST-segment elevation in leads II, III, and aVF. BP is 82/52 mm Hg and pulse rate is 54/min. Physical examination shows jugular venous distention, clear lungs, and no murmur or S_3.

ANSWER: Choose IV fluids to treat RV MI. Obtain ECG lead V_4R tracing.

A 34-year-old woman has exertional chest pain and nausea. Medical history is remarkable for Hodgkin lymphoma treated with mantle radiation.

ANSWER: ACS due to premature CAD from ionizing radiation.

ST-Elevation Myocardial Infarction: The ECG shows abnormal Q waves in leads V_3-V_5 and ST-segment elevation in leads V_2-V_5. The T waves are beginning to invert in leads V_3-V_6. This pattern is most consistent with a recent anterolateral MI.

Follow-up

Arrange for an exercise program in cardiac rehabilitation. Medications upon discharge from the hospital should include those important for risk reduction, including antiplatelet drugs, a β-blocker, a statin, and possibly an ACE inhibitor or an ARB.

Chronic Stable Angina

Diagnosis

Typical anginal chest pain has three components:

- substernal chest pain or discomfort
- provoked by exertion or emotional stress
- relieved by rest and/or nitroglycerin

Atypical chest pain has two of the three components for typical chest pain. Nonanginal chest pain has one or none of the components for typical chest pain. The probability of ischemic heart disease increases with age, with male gender, and with category of chest pain (typical angina > nonanginal chest pain > atypical angina).

Consider non–coronary artery causes of angina, especially AS and HCM.

Choose the proper stress test for patients with intermediate probability (10%-90%) of CAD.

STUDY TABLE: Selecting the Correct Stress Test	
Stress Test	**Indications**
Exercise ECG without imaging	Patients who can exercise
	Normal or nonspecific baseline ECG changes (e.g., <1 mm ST depression)
	Complete RBBB
Exercise ECG with myocardial perfusion imaging or exercise echocardiography	Pre-excitation (WPW)
	>1 mm ST depression
	Previous CABG or PCI
	LBBB (exercise echo)
	Intermediate risk result following exercise ECG
Pharmacologic stress myocardial perfusion imaging or dobutamine echocardiography	Unable to exercise
	Electrically paced ventricular rhythm
	LBBB

Select coronary angiography for patients with high pretest probability of disease or:

- LV dysfunction
- class III or IV angina despite therapy
- highly positive stress or imaging test
- high pretest probability of left main or three-vessel CAD (a Duke treadmill score ≤-11)
- uncertain diagnosis after noninvasive testing
- history of surviving sudden cardiac death
- suspected coronary spasm

Therapy

Intensive lifestyle modification is appropriate for all patients (smoking cessation, regular physical activity, "heart healthy" diet). Treatment is indicated to achieve the following goals: BP <140/90 mm Hg, and hemoglobin A_{1c} <7%.

The three major classes of antianginal medications for stable angina are β-blockers, nitrates, and calcium channel blockers. Most patients with stable angina will require combination therapy.

Cardioselective β-blockers are first-line therapy in patients with chronic stable angina. Dosage should be adjusted to achieve a resting HR of approximately 60/min. Absolute contraindications to β-blockers include severe bradycardia, advanced AV block, decompensated HF, and severe reactive airways disease.

Nitrates are as effective as β-blockers and calcium channel blockers in reducing angina. Prevent nitrate tachyphylaxis by establishing a nitrate-free period of 8 to 12 hours per day (typically overnight), during which nitrates are not used. For patients using nitrates, sildenafil, vardenafil, and tadalafil are contraindicated.

For patients with absolute contraindications to β-blockers, calcium channel blockers should be initiated as first-line therapy. In the setting of continued angina despite optimal doses of β-blockers and nitrates, calcium channel blockers can be added. Avoid short-acting calcium channel blockers. Bradycardia and heart block can occur in patients with significant conduction system disease.

Ranolazine should be considered in patients who remain symptomatic despite optimal doses of β-blockers, calcium channel blockers, and nitrates.

Cardioprotective drugs reduce the progression of atherosclerosis and subsequent cardiovascular events.

- Aspirin reduces the risk of stroke, MI, and vascular death in patients with CAD.
- ACE inhibitors reduce risk of cardiovascular and all-cause mortality for most patients.
- High-intensity statins reduce cardiovascular events, including MI and death.

Revascularization therapy with PCI or CABG may be considered in patients with persistent symptoms despite maximal medical therapy. Revascularization does not confer additional protection from cardiovascular events except for those with left-main CAD or triple-vessel disease with LV dysfunction.

◆ DON'T BE TRICKED

- Do not select PCI or CABG as a treatment for chronic stable angina in the absence of high-risk features for early mortality or unresponsiveness to medical therapy.
- Do not select hormone replacement therapy (in women), antioxidant vitamins (vitamin E), or treatment of elevated serum homocysteine levels with folic acid or vitamin B_{12}.

❖ Test Yourself

A 69-year-old man has burning retrosternal discomfort related to exertion. His father died of an acute MI at 61 years of age. Physical examination is unremarkable, and the resting ECG is normal.

ANSWER: Prescribe aspirin, sublingual nitroglycerin, and a β-blocker, and follow up with an exercise stress test.

Heart Failure

Diagnosis

One half of patients with HF have LV dysfunction, known as HF with reduced ejection fraction (HFrEF); the remainder has diastolic dysfunction, or HF with preserved ejection fraction (HFpEF). Patients with HFrEF often have dilated ventricles and patients with HFpEF have normal systolic contraction and normal size ventricles. Symptoms are the same for HFrEF and HFpEF.

Features that increase the likelihood of HF include:

- paroxysmal nocturnal dyspnea (>2-fold likelihood)
- an S_3 (11-fold likelihood)

The likelihood of HF is decreased 50% by:

- absence of dyspnea on exertion
- absence of crackles on pulmonary auscultation

Elevated CVP and an S_3 are independently associated with adverse outcomes, including progression of HF.

A BNP level >500 pg/mL is compatible with HF, and a level <100 pg/mL effectively excludes HF as a cause of acute dyspnea.

The ECG may show a previous MI, ventricular hypertrophy, arrhythmias, or conduction abnormalities. Chest x-rays may show cardiomegaly, pulmonary edema, or pleural effusion. Echocardiography will estimate EF and may detect valvular heart disease, HCM, and regional wall abnormalities suggesting CAD.

Other studies include stress testing to detect myocardial ischemia, coronary angiography in patients with symptoms or risk factors for CAD, and measurement of serum TSH levels. In the presence of suggestive symptoms, evaluate for sleep apnea.

Endomyocardial biopsy is rarely indicated. Endomyocardial biopsy can assist in the diagnosis of giant cell myocarditis, amyloidosis, and hemochromatosis.

◆ DON'T BE TRICKED

- Routine evaluation for unusual causes of HF, including hemochromatosis, Wilson disease, multiple myeloma, and myocarditis, should not be performed.
- BNP cannot be used to differentiate between HFrEF and HFpEF.
- Don't order BNP to monitor HF.
- Kidney failure, older age, and female sex all increase BNP; obesity reduces BNP.

Therapy

For making treatment decisions, disease classification systems have been developed.

STUDY TABLE: NYHA Classification of Heart Failure
NYHA Functional Class
I (structural disease but no symptoms)
II (symptomatic; slight limitation of physical activity)
III (symptomatic; marked limitation of physical activity)
IV (inability to perform any physical activity without symptoms)

Pharmacologic agents for HF:

- ACE inhibitors for all stages of HF to reduce mortality. If a patient cannot tolerate ACE inhibitors, ARBs are an acceptable alternative.
- Hydralazine plus nitrates, in addition to standard therapy, for NYHA class III-IV to reduce mortality in patients who are black and in patients who cannot tolerate ACE inhibitors or ARBs.
- β-Blockers (only metoprolol succinate, carvedilol, and bisoprolol) for NYHA classes I-IV to reduce mortality.
- Spironolactone for NYHA class II-IV HF to reduce mortality. If a patient cannot tolerate spironolactone, eplerenone is an alternative.
- Digitalis for NYHA class III-IV HF to reduce symptoms and length of hospitalization.
- Diuretics to improve symptoms of volume overload.
- ICD for ischemic and nonischemic cardiomyopathy with an EF ≤35%.
- Biventricular pacing for NYHA class II-IV HF, LVEF ≤35%, and LBBB with QRS duration >150 ms.
- Cardiac transplantation for patients with refractory HF symptoms.

◆ **DON'T BE TRICKED**

- Do not begin β-blocker therapy in patients with decompensated HF.
- Generally, continue β-blockers during decompensated states of HF if the patient was previously stable while using β-blocker therapy.
- There is no advantage to a continuous IV infusion of furosemide vs. bolus therapy in decompensated HF.
- Do not prescribe or continue NSAIDs or thiazolidinediones because they worsen HF.
- Calcium channel blockers have no direct role in the treatment of systolic HF.
- Dihydropyridine calcium channel blockers (diltiazem or verapamil) may be harmful to patients with HF.
- Avoid digoxin in patients with changing kidney status or CKD.

❖ **Test Yourself**

A 64-year-old woman with previously stable HF now has increasing orthopnea. Medications are lisinopril 5 mg BID and furosemide 20 mg/d. BP is 140/68 mm Hg and HR is 102/min. Pulmonary crackles and increased jugular venous distention are present.

ANSWER: Increase the furosemide and lisinopril dosages and add a β-blocker when the patient is stable.

Heart Failure with Preserved Ejection Fraction

Diagnosis

Diagnose HFpEF (also known as diastolic HF) when signs and symptoms of HF are present but the echocardiogram reveals EF >50% and significant valvular abnormalities are absent.

Therapy

The primary treatment goals in HFpEF are to treat the underlying etiology (hypertension, AF), to manage potentially exacerbating factors (e.g., tachycardia), and to optimize diastolic filling (control HR and avoid decreased effective circulating blood volume).

Dilated Cardiomyopathy

Diagnosis

Dilated cardiomyopathy is characterized by dilation and reduced function of one or both ventricles manifesting as HF, arrhythmias, and sudden death. The most common cause is idiopathic dilated cardiomyopathy (50%), but the differential diagnosis is broad.

STUDY TABLE: Differential Diagnoses of Dilated Cardiomyopathy	
Condition	**Distinguishing Characteristics**
Acute myocarditis	Associated with bacterial, viral, and parasitic infections and autoimmune disorders. Cardiac troponin levels are typically elevated; ventricular dysfunction may be global or regional. Can cause cardiogenic shock and ventricular arrhythmias. Choose supportive care in the acute phase, then standard HF therapy.
Alcoholic cardiomyopathy	Associated with chronic heavy alcohol ingestion, but other manifestations of chronic alcohol abuse may be absent. Typically, the LV (and frequently both ventricles) is dilated and hypokinetic. Choose standard HF therapy and total abstinence from alcohol.

(Continued on next page)

STUDY TABLE: Differential Diagnoses of Dilated Cardiomyopathy (*Continued*)	
Condition	**Distinguishing Characteristics**
Arrhythmogenic RV dysplasia	Characterized by pathologic fibrofatty infiltration of the RV evident on biopsy or by MRI. Manifests as significant RV enlargement and dysfunction out of proportion to preserved LV function or as VT and sudden death.
Drug-induced cardiomyopathy	Illicit use of cocaine and amphetamines has been associated with myocarditis and dilated cardiomyopathy, as well as MI, arrhythmia, and sudden death. Choose standard HF treatment. In patients with stimulant-induced acute myocardial ischemia, β-blockers may exacerbate coronary vasoconstriction; labetalol is preferred.
Giant cell myocarditis	Rare disease characterized by biventricular enlargement, refractory ventricular arrhythmias, and rapid progression to cardiogenic shock in young to middle-aged adults. Histologic examination demonstrates the presence of multinucleated giant cells in the myocardium. Choose immunosuppressant treatment and/or cardiac transplantation.
Stress-induced (takotsubo) cardiomyopathy	Characterized by acute LV dysfunction in the setting of intense emotional or physiologic stress. May mimic acute MI with ST-segment elevation and elevated biomarkers. Dilation and akinesis of the LV apex occur in the absence of CAD. Resolves in days to weeks with supportive care.
Tachycardia-mediated cardiomyopathy	Occurs when myocardial dysfunction develops as a result of chronic tachycardia. Primary treatment is to slow or eliminate the arrhythmia.

Therapy

In addition to reversal of the underlying cause, if possible (alcohol, drug, and tachycardia-mediated cardiomyopathies), choose the standard medical therapy for HF.

❖ **Test Yourself**

A 35-year-old man develops abdominal discomfort and swelling in both legs. He has an 18-pack-year smoking history and drinks a six-pack of beer daily but has no other significant medical history. Physical examination shows an elevated CVP, a displaced apical impulse, distant heart sounds, a grade 2/6 apical holosystolic murmur, an enlarged and tender liver, and peripheral edema.

ANSWER: The diagnosis is alcoholic cardiomyopathy. Choose echocardiography and alcohol cessation.

Peripartum Cardiomyopathy

Diagnosis

Peripartum cardiomyopathy is the presence of HF with an LVEF <45% diagnosed between 1 month before and 5 months after delivery.

Therapy

Management includes early delivery (when peripartum cardiomyopathy is identified before parturition) and HF treatment similar to that in nonpregnant women, except that ACE inhibitors, ARBs, and aldosterone antagonists (e.g., eplerenone) should be avoided (teratogenicity) during pregnancy. Anticoagulation with warfarin is recommended for women with peripartum cardiomyopathy with LVEF <35%. In women with acute severe peripartum cardiomyopathy, bromocriptine improves LVEF and clinical outcome when added to peripartum-related HF therapy.

Follow-up

Women with persistent LV dysfunction should avoid subsequent pregnancy because another pregnancy is often associated with recurrent or further reduction of LV function.

Hypertrophic Cardiomyopathy

Screening

All first-degree relatives of patients with HCM should have echocardiographic screening. Ongoing screening is recommended throughout adulthood starting at age 12 years because of the possibility of disease expression at any age.

Diagnosis

HCM is an uncommon primary cardiac disease characterized by diffuse or focal myocardial hypertrophy. The disease is genetically inherited in an autosomal dominant pattern in approximately 50% of patients. Symptoms of HCM are caused by a combination of diastolic dysfunction, ischemia, arrhythmias, and outflow obstruction. Patients may present with syncope (often arrhythmogenic), chest pain, and sudden cardiac death. Patients may present with exertional syncope or syncope associated with volume depletion.

◆ DON'T BE TRICKED

- All patients with HCM should receive genetic counseling.

STUDY TABLE: Distinguishing HCM from AS		
Assessment/Finding	**HCM**	**AS**
Carotid pulse	Rises briskly, then declines, followed by a second rise (pulsus bisferiens)	Rises slowly and has low volume (pulsus parvus et tardus)
Ejection sound	None	Present
Aortic regurgitation	None	May be present
Valsalva maneuver	Increased murmur intensity	Decreased murmur intensity
Squatting to standing position	Increased murmur intensity	Decreased murmur intensity
Standing to squatting position	Decreased murmur intensity	Increased murmur intensity
Carotid radiation	None	Usually present
Apex beat	"Triple ripple"	Sustained single

The ECG shows LV hypertrophy and left atrial enlargement. Deeply inverted, symmetric T waves in leads V_3-V_6 are present in the apical hypertrophic form of the disease (mimics ischemia). Echocardiography is the diagnostic technique of choice.

Therapy

Patients with HCM should avoid strenuous exercise, including competitive sports and intense isometric exercise. β-Blockers are first-line agents for patients with an EF ≥50%, dyspnea, and/or chest pain. Calcium channel blockers (verapamil) may be substituted for β-blockers. Disopyramide (third-line agent) may be added if symptoms and a significant outflow gradient persist. ACE inhibitors are used only if systolic dysfunction is present. Treat all patients with HCM and AF with warfarin regardless of $CHADS_2$ score. Surgery or septal ablation is indicated for patients with an outflow tract gradient of >50 mm Hg and continuing symptoms despite maximal drug therapy.

STUDY TABLE: Sudden Death Risk Factors in HCM
Major Risk Factors
Previous cardiac arrest
Spontaneous sustained VT
Family history of sudden death (first-degree relative)
Unexplained syncope
LV wall thickness ≥30 mm
Blunted increase or decrease in SBP with exercise
Nonsustained spontaneous VT
HF that has progressed to dilated cardiomyopathy and LVEF ≤30%

Patients at high risk for sudden death (one or more major risk factors) are candidates for an ICD.

The absence of any risk factors has a high negative predictive value (>90%) for sudden death.

◆ DON'T BE TRICKED

- Electrophysiologic studies are not useful in predicting sudden cardiac death.
- Do not prescribe digoxin, vasodilators, or diuretics, which increase LV outflow obstruction.

Athlete's heart is a syndrome of myocardial hypertrophy that can be difficult to differentiate from HCM.

STUDY TABLE: Clinical Features Distinguishing HCM from Athlete's Heart		
Feature	**Hypertrophic Cardiomyopathy**	**Athlete's Heart**
Family history	Positive	Negative
ECG	Pathologic Q waves, T-wave inversions, conduction defects	Absence of these features
Doppler echocardiography	Diastolic filling abnormalities	Normal diastolic filling
Extent of hypertrophy	>15 mm	≤12 mm
Pattern of hypertrophy	Asymmetric, concentric, or eccentric	Concentric
LV end-diastolic dimension	<45 mm	>55 mm
Genetic testing	Positive	Negative

❖ Test Yourself

An 18-year-old high school basketball player is evaluated after he collapsed during practice and was resuscitated.

ANSWER: HCM is the most likely diagnosis in almost every young person who collapses during an athletic event.

Hypertrophic Cardiomyopathy: The ECG shows ST-segment depression and deeply inverted T waves (*arrows*) in the precordial leads consistent with marked apical hypertrophy.

Restrictive Cardiomyopathy

Diagnosis

Although the cause of restrictive cardiomyopathy is often unknown, be alert for the following:

- infiltrative diseases (amyloidosis, sarcoidosis, hemochromatosis)
- lysosomal storage diseases (e.g., Fabry disease)
- endomyocardial processes (endomyocardial fibrosis, HES, carcinoid, radiation therapy, anthracycline toxicity)
- noninfiltrative diseases (scleroderma)

In restrictive cardiomyopathy, abnormally rigid ventricular walls cause diastolic dysfunction in the absence of systolic dysfunction, manifesting as impaired ventricular filling and elevated diastolic ventricular pressures. Pulmonary venous congestion, PH, and right-sided HF ensue. Jugular veins may engorge with inspiration (Kussmaul sign). Cardiac catheterization shows elevated LV and RV end-diastolic pressures and a characteristic early ventricular diastolic dip and plateau. Systolic function is normal in many patients.

STUDY TABLE: Clues to Underlying Systemic Diseases Causing Restrictive Cardiomyopathy	
Disease	**Clues**
Amyloidosis	Neuropathy, proteinuria, hepatomegaly, periorbital ecchymosis, bruising, low-voltage ECG. Diagnosis can be confirmed with abdominal fat pad aspiration.
Sarcoidosis	Bilateral hilar lymphadenopathy; possible pulmonary reticular opacities; and skin, joint, or eye lesions. Cardiac involvement is suggested by the presence of arrhythmias, conduction blocks, or HF. Diagnosis is supported by CMR imaging with gadolinium.
Hemochromatosis	Abnormal aminotransferase levels, OA, diabetes, erectile dysfunction, and HF; elevated serum ferritin and transferrin saturation level.
Fabry Disease	X-linked recessive disorder. Consider in males with HF, urinary concentrating defects, proteinuria, CKD, premature CAD, painful neuropathy, angiokeratomas. Low α-galactosidase A level confirms diagnosis.

Restrictive cardiomyopathy must be differentiated from constrictive pericarditis.

Therapy

Treat any underlying disease that affects diastolic function (hypertension, diabetes, ischemic heart disease, amyloidosis). Loop diuretics are used to treat dyspnea and peripheral edema. β-Blockers and/or nondihydropyridine calcium channel antagonists enhance diastolic function and should be considered if diuretic therapy is not effective or in the presence of atrial tachyarrhythmias. ACE inhibitors and ARBs improve diastolic filling and may be beneficial in patients with diastolic dysfunction.

❖ Test Yourself

A 63-year-old man develops dyspnea and fatigue. Physical examination shows jugular venous distention, a prominent jugular a wave, a prominent S_4, and a grade 2/6 holosystolic murmur at the left sternal border. The lungs are clear. Other findings include an enlarged, tender liver; petechiae over the feet; and periorbital ecchymoses.

ANSWER: The diagnosis is amyloid cardiomyopathy, indicated by the noncardiac symptoms and signs.

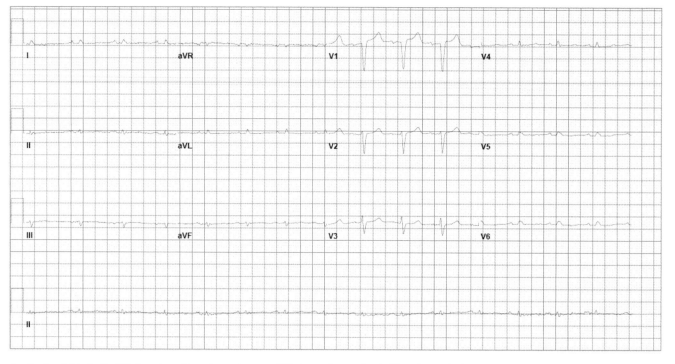

Cardiac Amyloidosis: The ECG shows low voltage, the most common ECG abnormality associated with cardiac amyloidosis.

Palpitations and Syncope

In a patient with palpitations and syncope, the key diagnostic test is an ECG recorded during the clinical event. Several approaches are available for recording an intermittent arrhythmia; the most appropriate test is based on the frequency and duration of symptoms. Obtain an echocardiogram in patients with suspected structural heart disease.

STUDY TABLE: Diagnostic Studies for Suspected Arrhythmias

Diagnostic Test	Utility	Advantages	Limitations
Resting ECG	Initial diagnostic test in all patients	Diagnostic if recorded during the arrhythmia	Most arrhythmias are intermittent and not recorded on a resting ECG
Ambulatory (24-hour) ECG	Indicated for frequent (at least daily) arrhythmias	Records every heart beat during a 24-hour period	Not helpful if arrhythmia is infrequent
Exercise ECG	Indicated for arrhythmias provoked by exercise	Allows diagnosis of exercise-related arrhythmias	Physician supervision required
Event monitor	Indicated for infrequent arrhythmias >1-2 min in duration	Small recorder is held to the chest when symptoms are present	Limited to symptomatic arrhythmias that persist long enough for patient to activate the device. Not a viable choice for patients with syncope
Loop recorder	Indicated for infrequent symptomatic brief arrhythmias	Saves previous 30 s to 2 min ECG signal when patient activates the recorder. Can be activated following syncopal event to capture arrhythmia	ECG leads limit patient activities
Implanted recorder	Indicated for very infrequent arrhythmias	Long-term continuous ECG monitoring	Invasive procedure with some risk
Electrophysiology study	Indicated for treatment (e.g., catheter ablation), not for diagnosis	The origin and mechanism of an arrhythmia can be precisely defined	Invasive procedure with some risk

Heart Block

Diagnosis

AV nodal block results from functional or structural abnormalities at the AV node or in the His-Purkinje system. Half the cases are due to fibrosis of the conduction system.

STUDY TABLE: Heart Block	
Type	**Diagnostic Criteria**
First-degree block	PR interval >0.2 s without alterations in HR
Second-degree block	Intermittent P waves not followed by a ventricular complex; further classified as Mobitz type 1 or type 2
Third-degree block (complete heart block)	Complete absence of conducted P waves (P-wave and QRS complex rates differ, and the PR interval differs for every QRS complex) and an atrial rate that is faster than ventricular rate. It is the most common cause of ventricular rates 30 to 50/min
LBBB	Absent Q waves in leads I, aVL, and V_6; large, wide, and positive R waves in leads I, aVL, and V_6; QRS >0.12 s
RBBB	rsR' pattern in lead V_1 ("rabbit ears"), wide negative S wave in lead V_6, QRS >0.12 s
Bifascicular block	Right bundle branch and one of the fascicles of the left bundle branch are involved
Trifascicular block	Characterized by bifascicular block and prolongation of the PR interval
Left anterior hemiblock	Left axis usually –60°, upright QRS complex in lead I, negative QRS complex in aVF, and normal QRS duration
Left posterior hemiblock	Right axis usually +120°, negative QRS complex in lead I, positive QRS complex in lead aVF, and normal QRS duration

STUDY TABLE: Second-Degree AV Block: Mobitz Type 1 and Type 2		
Type	**Characteristics**	**Significance**
Mobitz type 1 (Wenckebach block)	Constant P-P interval with progressively increased PR interval until the dropped beat	Rarely progresses to third-degree heart block
Mobitz type 2	Usually associated with RBBB or LBBB; constant PR interval in the conducted beats; R-R interval contains the nonconducted (dropped) beat equal to two P-P intervals	May precede third-degree heart block

Therapy

Initial therapy of AV block includes correcting reversible causes of impaired conduction such as ischemia, increased vagal tone, and elimination of drugs that alter electrical conduction (digitalis, calcium channel blockers, β-blockers).

Guidelines for permanent pacemaker implantation include:

- symptomatic bradycardia without reversible cause
- AF with 5-second pauses
- complete heart block
- Mobitz type 2 second-degree AV block
- alternating bundle branch block

Choose IV atropine and/or transcutaneous or transvenous pacing for symptoms of hemodynamic compromise caused by bradycardia or heart block.

◆ DON'T BE TRICKED

- Don't place a pacemaker for asymptomatic bradycardia in the absence of second- or third-degree heart block.

Mobitz Type 1 Heart Block: Rhythm strip shows progressive prolongation of the PR interval until the dropped beat.

Mobitz Type 2 Heart Block: Rhythm strip shows constant PR interval. The R-R interval containing the nonconducted beat is equal to two P-P intervals.

Complete Heart Block: Rhythm strip shows third-degree heart block with three nonconducted atrial impulses and a pause of 4.5 seconds.

Bifascicular Block: ECG shows RBBB and left anterior hemiblock characteristic of bifascicular block.

Atrial Fibrillation

Diagnosis

Findings of AF include an irregularly irregular ventricular rhythm at a rate of 80 to 170/min and absence of P waves in all ECG leads. The presence of deformed T waves or ST segments "hiding" P waves rules out AF. Do not confuse AF with:

- sinus tachycardia with premature atrial beats
- MAT in patients with COPD
- Mobitz type 1 second-degree AV block (Wenckebach) with characteristic group-beating
- arrhythmia due to digitalis toxicity (atrial tachycardia with block)

AF can appear as irregular, wide-complex tachycardia mimicking VF in the setting of underlying intraventricular conduction delay (RBBB) or in the presence of an accessory pathway.

Diagnostic studies include measurement of serum TSH and digoxin levels (if appropriate), pulse oximetry, and echocardiography.

Therapy

Almost all patients with AF need chronic anticoagulation. The risk of stroke in patients who have nonvalvular AF (see $CHADS_2$ mnemonic) plus one other risk factor exceeds the risk of hemorrhage from anticoagulation.

STUDY TABLE: $CHADS_2$ Mnemonic
Chronic HF
Hypertension
Age >75 years
Diabetes mellitus
Stroke or TIA (presence of either scores 2 points)

STUDY TABLE: Anticoagulation Goals in AF	
Condition	**Treatment Recommendation**
No heart disease or $CHADS_2$ score = 0	Aspirin
$CHADS_2$ score = 1	Individual assessment
$CHADS_2$ score ≥2	Warfarin; INR 2.0-3.0

The CHA$_2$DS2-VASc risk score is helpful to further discern between low and intermediate risk in patients with a $CHADS_2$ score of 0 or 1.

1 point each is given for:

- HF
- hypertension
- diabetes
- vascular disease (prior MI, PAD, aortic plaque)
- female sex
- age 65 to 74 years

2 points each are given for:

- previous stroke, TIA, or thromboembolic disease
- age ≥75 years

Provide anticoagulation for a score ≥2.

In the treatment of nonvalvular AF, direct thrombin inhibitors such as dabigatran may be used in place of warfarin as well as factor Xa inhibitors rivaroxaban and apixaban. These drugs do not require monitoring but all of the novel oral anticoagulants are cleared renally and require dose adjustment in patients with CKD (typically eGFR <30 mL/min/1.73 m^2) and are contraindicated in end-stage kidney disease. These agents as of yet have no antidote to reverse bleeding. Of the new oral anticoagulants, only dabigatran is dialyzable.

Because the daily risk of stroke in nonvalvular AF is low, most patients do not require bridging anticoagulation when the oral anticoagulants are interrupted for procedures.

Perform emergency electrical cardioversion for patients with hemodynamically unstable AF. Before elective cardioversion, patients who have been in AF for ≥48 hours or an unknown duration should receive 3 weeks of oral anticoagulation or undergo TEE to rule out a clot. All patients undergoing cardioversion should receive oral anticoagulation for at least 4 weeks after cardioversion (or chronically, depending on other risk factors).

No mortality benefit is evident from restoration of sinus rhythm ("rhythm control") compared with rate control. Older patients with chronic AF or AF of unknown duration should have rate control with diltiazem, verapamil, atenolol, or metoprolol. For older, asymptomatic patients, clinical outcomes are not improved with a ventricular resting rate <80/min compared with a more lenient target rate (<110/min).

Rhythm control is an appropriate management for younger patients with persistent symptomatic AF. Rhythm control may be achieved with medications, synchronized cardioversion, or both. If rhythm control is unsuccessful or not tolerated, catheter-based AF ablation is an option. A "maze" procedure may be useful for patients undergoing cardiac surgery for other reasons.

Patients with infrequent paroxysmal AF will benefit from the "pill-in-the-pocket" approach: flecainide or propafenone with a β-blocker or calcium channel blocker.

◆ DON'T BE TRICKED

- Only warfarin is indicated for AF secondary to valvular heart disease
- Do not begin digoxin as a single agent for rate control.
- Do not begin calcium channel blockers, β-blockers, or digoxin in patients with AF and WPW syndrome; use procainamide instead.

❖ Test Yourself

A 55-year-old woman has dyspnea and chest pain of 12 hours' duration. BP is 75/44 mm Hg, and bibasilar crackles are heard. ECG shows a wide-complex tachycardia of 160/min.

ANSWER: Cardioversion is always the answer in patients with any arrhythmia who are hemodynamically unstable.

Atrial Fibrillation: ECG rhythm strip (*bottom*) shows two sinus beats followed by AF. The AF rhythm is irregular, and fibrillatory waves are clearly seen. RBBB is also present.

Atrial Flutter

Diagnosis

Atrial flutter is a reentrant arrhythmia with atrial rates typically between 250 and 340/min. ECG typically shows a saw-tooth pattern on the inferior leads and a positive deflection in lead V_1. The ventricular response is often regular. Most patients have 2:1 conduction resulting in a ventricular response close to 150/min. Atrial flutter may be seen interspersed with AF or may follow treatment of AF. Atrial flutter is often the result of pulmonary disease exacerbation or pericarditis, or may occur after open heart surgery.

Therapy

Atrial flutter can be successfully eliminated with radiofrequency catheter ablation, which is superior to medical therapy. Guidelines for anticoagulation for atrial flutter are similar to those for AF.

Atrial Flutter: ECG shows a "saw-tooth" pattern in leads II and III characteristic of atrial flutter.

Supraventricular Tachycardia

Diagnosis

SVTs are a group of arrhythmias that arise in atrial tissue or the AV node. The most common SVTs, exclusive of AF and atrial flutter, are AVNRT, AVRT, and atrial tachycardia. The ECG usually reveals a narrow-complex tachycardia, although the QRS complexes can be wide (>120 ms) in the presence of bundle branch block, aberrancy, pacing, or anterograde accessory pathway conduction.

The most common paroxysmal SVT is AVNRT. Typical AVNRT often has a RP interval so short that the P wave is buried within the QRS complex, but it may be seen as a pseudo R in lead V_1 and a pseudo S wave in the inferior leads.

AVRT is a reentrant circuit that includes a bypass pathway and the AV node. If a bypass pathway conducts antegrade, a preexcitation pattern may be seen on the ECG. This includes a short PR interval (because the bypass pathway conducts rapidly and faster than the AV node) and a delta wave, which is a slurred initial segment of the QRS complex resulting from slow conduction through ventricular tissue instead of the His-Purkinje system. When this pattern is accompanied by a symptomatic tachycardia, it is termed WPW syndrome (see Wolff-Parkinson-White Syndrome).

Multifocal atrial tachycardia (MAT) is an irregular SVT that demonstrates three or more P waves of different morphologies and is often seen in end-stage COPD.

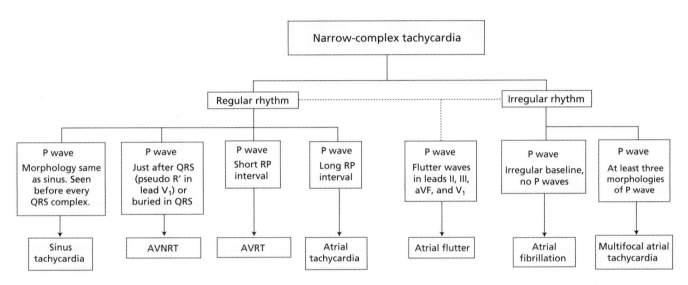

Classification of Narrow-Complex Tachycardia: AVNRT = atrioventricular nodal reentrant tachycardia; AVRT = atrioventricular reciprocating tachycardia.

Therapy

Episodes of SVT can often be terminated with Valsalva maneuvers, carotid sinus massage, or facial immersion in cold water.

Adenosine can be used to terminate SVT and to help diagnose the etiology. Termination with adenosine often suggests AV node dependence (AVNRT and AVRT), whereas continued atrial activity (P waves) during AV block can help identify atrial flutter and atrial tachycardia. Rate control for atrial tachycardia can be achieved with β-blockers or calcium channel blockers.

Use oral calcium channel blockers and β-blockers to prevent recurrent AVNRT. For recurrent AVNRT despite drug therapy or intolerance of drug therapy, select catheter ablation therapy.

Treatment of MAT is directed at correcting associated pulmonary and cardiac disease, hypokalemia, and hypomagnesemia. Drug therapy is indicated for patients who are symptomatic or experience complications such as HF or chest pain secondary to cardiac ischemia. Metoprolol is the drug of choice followed by verapamil in patients with bronchospastic disease.

◆ DON'T BE TRICKED

- Adenosine may induce bronchospasm in patients with reactive airways disease.
- Do not treat irregular wide-complex tachycardia or polymorphic tachycardia with adenosine.
- Catheter ablation, not medical therapy, is first-line therapy for symptomatic AVRT (WPW syndrome).

❖ Test Yourself

A 32-year-old woman has a 4-hour history of palpitations. BP is 80/50 mm Hg, and the HR is very rapid. An ECG shows regular, narrow-complex tachycardia of 180/min and normal QRS complex morphology. No P waves are seen.

ANSWER: The diagnosis is AVNRT. Choose the Valsalva maneuver, carotid sinus massage, verapamil, or IV adenosine.

AV-Nodal Reentrant Tachycardia: The ECG shows a narrow-complex tachycardia at 144/min and no visible P waves.

AV Reciprocating Tachycardia: ECG shows a narrow-complex tachycardia with the P wave buried in the ST segment.

Atrial Tachycardia: The ECG shows a narrow-complex tachycardia with P waves most clearly seen in lead V$_1$ and at the end of the T wave in other leads.

Multifocal Atrial Tachycardia: The ECG shows an irregular tachycardia with three distinct P wave morphologies characteristic of MAT (*arrows*).

Wolff-Parkinson-White Syndrome

Diagnosis

WPW syndrome is a symptomatic AVRT caused by an accessory AV conduction pathway that is:

- usually antegrade to the ventricles, resulting in the delta wave that indicates ventricular preexcitation (in this situation, WPW is described as "manifest")
- occasionally concealed or retrograde; ventricles are depolarized over the normal AV node–His-Purkinje network, resulting in a normal surface ECG (in this situation, WPW is described as "concealed")

ECG findings include a short PR interval, delta wave, and normal or prolonged QRS. AF associated with WPW syndrome is a risk factor for sudden death caused by degeneration into VF. Look for an irregular, wide-complex tachycardia.

Therapy

Begin procainamide or another class I or class III agent for patients with wide-complex tachycardia, especially when AF and preexcitation are present. Cardioversion is the preferred treatment for any unstable patient with WPW syndrome.

Ablation of the accessory bypass tract is first-line therapy for patients with preexcitation and symptoms. Antiarrhythmic agents are second-line therapy.

◆ **DON'T BE TRICKED**
- Asymptomatic WPW conduction without arrhythmia does not require investigation or treatment.
- Do not select calcium channel blockers, β-blockers, or digoxin for patients who have AF with WPW syndrome; such treatment may convert AF to VT or VF.

A 28-year-old woman has a 4-hour history of palpitations. Physical examination shows a BP of 132/80 mm Hg, an irregularly irregular HR of 140/min, and no other abnormal findings. The ECG shows AF with a ventricular rate of 180 to 270/min. QRS complexes are broad and bizarre.

ANSWER: The diagnosis is WPW syndrome. Begin IV procainamide.

A 30-year-old woman has an episode of palpitations and syncope. ECG shows WPW.

ANSWER: Refer for ablation of the accessory tract.

WPW Syndrome: WPW syndrome is diagnosed by a short PR interval, prolonged QRS, and a slurred onset of the QRS (*delta wave*).

Ventricular Tachycardia

Diagnosis

Premature ventricular complexes (PVCs) can be single, in pairs (couplets), or alternating with sinus beats. These beats are usually followed by a compensatory pause. In healthy adults, PVCs are benign.

Ventricular tachyarrhythmias consist of VT, VF, and torsades de pointes. Ventricular tachyarrhythmias are characterized by:

- QRS >0.12 s
- AV dissociation

In VT, the ventricular rate typically ranges from 140 to 250/min, VF rate is typically >300/min, and torsades de pointes is characterized by a ventricular rate of 200 to 300/min.

VT can be further classified as sustained or nonsustained. Nonsustained VT lasts <30 s.

VT is also categorized by the morphology of the QRS complexes:

- Monomorphic VT: QRS complexes in the same leads do not vary in contour.
- Polymorphic VT: QRS complexes in the same leads do vary in contour.

Differentiating VT from SVT with aberrant conduction is important because the treatment differs markedly. VT is more common than SVT with aberrancy, particularly in persons with structural heart disease. A key point is that any wide QRS tachycardia should be considered to be VT until proven otherwise. In the presence of known structural heart disease, especially a previous MI, the diagnosis of VT is almost certain.

Torsades de pointes is a specific form of polymorphic VT associated with long QT syndrome, which may be congenital or acquired (see Sudden Cardiac Death). Torsades de pointes episodes are typically short-lived and terminate spontaneously, but multiple successive episodes may result in syncope or VF.

Therapy

In otherwise healthy patients, suppression of PVCs with β-blockers is only indicated for disabling symptoms. Patients with nonsustained VT should be treated with β-blockers only if symptoms are present. The acute treatment of sustained VT depends on the degree of hemodynamic compromise.

- For unstable patients: immediate electrical cardioversion is indicated. Pulseless VT is treated in the same way as VF.
- For hemodynamically stable patients with impaired LV function: IV lidocaine or amiodarone is preferred. Procainamide and sotalol are additional therapeutic possibilities.

An ICD reduces sudden cardiac death in patients with VF or sustained VT associated with hemodynamic compromise.

◆ DON'T BE TRICKED

- **In patients with structural heart disease, therapy to suppress PVCs does not affect outcomes.**

❖ Test Yourself

A 65-year-old woman with chronic stable angina and a history of an anterior MI is evaluated in the emergency department for palpitations and lightheadedness. Vital signs are stable. ECG shows a wide-complex tachycardia with an RBBB pattern. No previous ECGs are immediately available.

ANSWER: The diagnosis is most likely sustained VT. The acute treatment is IV lidocaine or amiodarone.

Monomorphic VT: Approximately one quarter of the way into this ECG rhythm strip (*bottom*), monomorphic VT begins; it is associated with an abrupt change in the QRS axis.

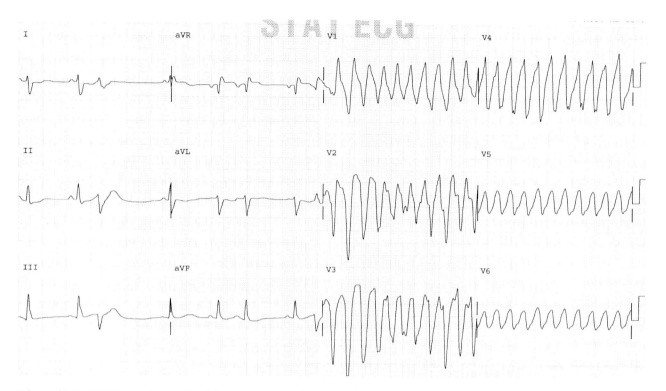

Polymorphic VT: This ECG shows degeneration of the sinus rhythm into polymorphic tachycardia.

Sudden Cardiac Death

Diagnosis

Sudden cardiac death is most often associated with structural heart disease, abnormal cardiac rhythms or conduction, HF, WPW syndrome, Brugada syndrome, and long QT syndrome.

Long QT syndrome may be inherited or acquired. Patients may experience syncope or sudden cardiac death as the result of torsades de pointes. Risk factors for acquired long QT syndrome include female sex, hypokalemia, hypomagnesemia, structural heart disease, and medications and drug interactions. In regards to medications and drug interactions, look specifically for:

- macrolide and fluoroquinolone antibiotics (especially moxifloxacin)
- terfenadine and astemizole antihistamines
- antipsychotic and antidepressant medications
- methadone
- antifungal medications
- Ia and class III antiarrhythmics

Risk is greatest with a QTc interval >500 ms.

Brugada syndrome is an inherited condition characterized by a structurally normal heart but abnormal electrical conduction associated with sudden cardiac death. Classic Brugada syndrome is recognized as an incomplete RBBB pattern with coved ST-segment elevation in leads V_1 and V_2. Other variations of this electrical pattern exist. The risk of sudden cardiac death is also increased in patients taking antiarrhythmic agents, using alcohol excessively, and taking illicit drugs.

Select echocardiography for survivors of sudden cardiac death to identify anatomic abnormalities, impaired ventricular function, and/or myopathic processes. Electrophysiologic studies are indicated for patients with suspected ventricular arrhythmias, episodes of impaired consciousness, and structurally abnormal hearts. Patients taking antiarrhythmic agents should have a serum drug level measurement and an ECG to look for long QT syndrome.

Therapy

Therapy includes pharmacologic treatment of underlying CAD and a revascularization procedure if anatomically possible. Inherited long QT syndrome may be treated with β-blockers.

Select an ICD in the following scenarios:

- for survivors of cardiac arrest due to VF or VT not explained by a reversible cause
- after sustained VT in the presence of structural heart disease
- after syncope and sustained VT/VF on electrophysiology study
- for ischemic and nonischemic cardiomyopathy with an EF <35%
- for Brugada syndrome
- for inherited long QT syndrome not responding to β-blockers
- after MI with an EF <30%
- for high-risk HCM (familial sudden death; multiple, repetitive nonsustained VT; extreme LVH; malignant genotype; and exercise hypotension)

STUDY TABLE: Inherited Arrhythmia Syndromes

Disorder	Characteristic Findings	Treatment
Long QT syndrome	Syncope, QTc interval usually >460 ms, torsades de pointes	β-blocker, ICD, exercise restriction
Short QT syndrome	Syncope, QT interval <340 ms, AF, VT, VF	ICD in all patients
Brugada syndrome	Syncope, VF, coved ST-segment elevation in early precordial leads (V$_1$-V$_3$)	ICD
Arrhythmogenic RV cardiomyopathy/ dysplasia	Syncope, T-wave inversions in V$_1$ to at least V$_3$, monomorphic VT, abnormal signal-averaged ECG, frequent PVCs, and abnormal RV size and function on echocardiography or CMR	ICD, β-blockers, antiarrhythmic medications, exercise abstinence

❖ Test Yourself

A 55-year-old man is evaluated 4 months after a large anterior MI. He has no symptoms, and his physical examination is normal. Follow-up echocardiography documents an LVEF of 28%.

ANSWER: This patient is at high risk for sudden cardiac death and should be considered for an ICD.

Prolonged QT syndrome: The ECG shows a prolonged QT interval of 590 ms.

Brugada Pattern on ECG: Incomplete RBBB pattern and elevation of the ST segments that gradually descends to an inverted T wave in leads V_1 and V_2 is characteristic of the classic variety of Brugada syndrome.

Acute Pericarditis

Diagnosis

The most common symptom is acute sharp or stabbing substernal chest pain that worsens with inspiration and when lying flat and is alleviated when sitting and leaning forward. Medical history may include:

- preceding viral symptoms
- cancer (current or in the past)
- recent trauma
- arthralgia, arthritis (suggesting systemic rheumatic disease)
- MI
- recent thoracic surgical procedures
- use of medications, including hydralazine, phenytoin, and minoxidil

A two- or three-component pericardial friction rub is characteristic. Pericardial tamponade (pulsus paradoxus ≥10 mm Hg) may be present. Typical ECG findings include diffuse ST-segment elevation with an upward concave movement (without the reciprocal ST-segment depression found in MI), PR-segment depression in limb leads, and PR-segment elevation in aVR. Electrical alternans (alternating high- and low-voltage QRS complexes) may be present in patients with large effusions.

An echocardiogram may show evidence of an effusion or of early tamponade.

STUDY TABLE: ECG Features Differentiating Acute Pericarditis from MI		
Feature	**Acute Pericarditis**	**Myocardial Ischemia**
ST-segment contour	Concave upwards	Convex upwards
ST-segment lead involvement	Diffuse	Localized
Reciprocal ST-T changes	No	Yes
PR-segment abnormalities	Yes	No
Pathologic Q waves	No	Yes

◆ **DON'T BE TRICKED**

- Cardiac enzyme values may be slightly elevated in patients with pericarditis (myopericarditis).
- Absence of a pericardial effusion on echocardiography does not rule out pericarditis.

Therapy

First-line treatment is aspirin (preferred after MI), NSAIDs, or NSAIDs and colchicine. NSAIDs and colchicine are associated with lower rates of treatment failure and recurrent pericarditis. Choose a 2- to 3-day course of glucocorticoids for pericarditis that does not respond to aspirin or NSAIDs or is related to an autoimmune process. Choose emergent pericardiocentesis for tamponade and hemodynamic instability.

❖ **Test Yourself**

A 57-year-old man has a 2-day history of chest pain that worsens when he lies flat. Cardiac examination shows a three-component friction rub.

ANSWER: The diagnosis is pericarditis. Look for diffuse ST-segment elevation and PR-segment depression. Ignore an elevated serum troponin level tempting you to answer "acute MI."

Acute Pericarditis: The ECG shows sinus rhythm with diffuse ST-segment elevation and PR-segment depression in lead II, characteristic of acute pericarditis.

Pericardial Tamponade and Constriction

Diagnosis

Patients with chronic cardiac tamponade present with dyspnea, fatigue, peripheral edema, hepatomegaly, hepatic dysfunction, and ascites in the absence of pulmonary congestion. The diagnosis may be suggested by risk factors for tamponade, including patients with:

- metastatic lung and breast cancer (most common cause)
- recent cardiac surgery
- dissecting aneurysm
- recent viral or bacterial pericarditis
- systemic rheumatic disease

Physical examination reveals jugular venous distention, pulsus paradoxus, tachycardia, reduced heart sounds, and/or hypotension. CVP may increase with inspiration (Kussmaul sign). Chest x-ray will show an enlarged silhouette ("water bottle sign"). Echocardiography can confirm an elevated intrapericardial pressure and presence of an effusion.

Absence of a pericardial effusion virtually excludes a diagnosis of cardiac tamponade.

Constrictive pericarditis is characterized by thickened, fibrotic, and adherent pericardium that restrains ventricular diastolic expansion, leading to impaired filling. Constrictive pericarditis is often a sequela of acute pericarditis. Other causes include post-radiation, previous cardiac surgery, and TB. Constrictive pericarditis is associated with a loud S_3 (pericardial knock), and a friction rub may be present. Long-standing constrictive pericarditis may be associated with liver failure and cirrhosis. Imaging findings that support the diagnosis include:

- calcified pericardium on x-ray (specific, but not sensitive)
- pericardial thickening on CT or MRI
- abnormal diastolic motion on echocardiography

Therapy

Acute management of cardiac tamponade includes maintenance of SBP with volume resuscitation and vasopressors. Pericardial fluid should be drained by percutaneous pericardiocentesis or surgery.

In patients with chronic constrictive pericarditis, cardiac output depends on a high preload; therefore, diuretics must be used cautiously, if at all. Pericardiectomy is the most effective treatment but is unnecessary in patients with early disease (NYHA functional class I) and is unwarranted in patients with advanced disease (NYHA functional class IV).

◆ **DON'T BE TRICKED**
- **In constrictive pericarditis, the echocardiogram will demonstrate shifting of the ventricular septum to and fro during diastole as a manifestation of the right and left ventricle competing for a confined space during filling; these findings are not seen in restrictive cardiomyopathy.**

❖ **Test Yourself**

A 44-year-old woman with a history of ovarian cancer presents with fatigue, dyspnea, and peripheral edema. Examination shows jugular venous distention that increases with inspiration, reduced heart sounds, BP of 94/50 mm Hg, and HR of 132/min. A 20 mm Hg pulsus paradoxus is present.

ANSWER: The diagnosis is acute pericardial tamponade probably secondary to metastatic disease. Order echocardiography, and support BP with fluids and vasopressors.

STUDY TABLE: Constrictive Pericarditis vs. Restrictive Cardiomyopathy		
Test	**Constrictive Pericarditis**	**Restrictive Cardiomyopathy**
Physical examination: pericardial knock	Supportive	Unusual but loud S_3 may be mistaken for pericardial knock
Physical examination: S_3	May be present	Supportive
ECG: LBBB or RBBB	Not helpful	Supportive
Chest x-ray: pericardial calcification	May be present	Absent
Echocardiography: LVH and atrial enlargement	Absent	Present
		(Continued on next page)

Test	Constrictive Pericarditis	Restrictive Cardiomyopathy
STUDY TABLE: Constrictive Pericarditis vs. Restrictive Cardiomyopathy *(Continued)*		
Echocardiography: accentuated drop in peak LV filling during inspiration	Present	Absent
MRI: increased pericardial thickness	Present	Absent
Right heart catheterization: elevated and equalized diastolic LV and RV pressures (within 5 mm Hg)	Present	Absent
BNP level	<100 pg/mL	>400 pg/mL

Heart Murmurs

Diagnosis

Right-sided heart murmurs increase in intensity during inspiration. Murmurs due to HCM increase in intensity during the Valsalva maneuver and on standing from a squatting position. The clicks due to MVP may move closer to S_1, and the murmur lengthens during the Valsalva maneuver and on standing from a squatting position.

Abnormal splitting of S_2 helps differentiate heart murmurs. Normally, a split S_2 is heard only during inspiration. Splitting during inspiration and expiration occurs in conditions that further delay RV ejection, including RBBB, pulmonary valve stenosis, VSD with left-to-right shunt, and ASD with left-to-right shunt. Reversed or expiratory splitting occurs in conditions that prolong LV ejection, including LBBB, AS, HCM, and ACS with LV dysfunction.

Innocent heart murmurs are typically midsystolic, located at the base of the heart, grade 1/6 to 2/6 without radiation, and associated with normal splitting of S_2. Signs of serious cardiac disease include an S_4, murmur grade ≥3/6 intensity, any diastolic murmur, continuous murmurs, and abnormal splitting of S_2. TTE is indicated in symptomatic patients, in those with a systolic murmur grade ≥3/6 intensity, and in those with any continuous murmur (a murmur that begins after S_1 and extends beyond S_2) or diastolic murmur.

◆ DON'T BE TRICKED

- An increased P_2, an S_3, and an early peaking systolic murmur over the upper left sternal border are normal findings during pregnancy.
- Innocent heart murmurs do not require echocardiographic confirmation.

❖ Test Yourself

A 19-year-old asymptomatic woman has a heart murmur first heard during a college sports physical examination. A non-radiating grade 2/6 midsystolic murmur is heard over the upper left sternal border. Physiologic splitting of S_2 is present, and a soft S_3 is heard at the cardiac apex.

ANSWER: The diagnosis is an innocent heart murmur.

Rheumatic Fever

Prevention

Give penicillin to patients with group A streptococcal infection (or erythromycin to patients with penicillin allergy). Patients with a history of RF require long-term prophylactic penicillin, and patients with rheumatic valvular disease should continue prophylaxis for at least 10 years after the last episode of RF or until at least 40 years of age (whichever is longer).

Diagnosis

RF is the most common cause of valvular heart disease in Africa, Asia, South America, and the Middle East. Mitral stenosis and regurgitation are common consequences of RF. The aortic valve is the second most likely affected valve.

STUDY TABLE: Jones Criteria for Diagnosis of Rheumatic Fever	
Manifestations*	
Major	Carditis, polyarthritis, chorea, subcutaneous nodules, erythema marginatum
Minor	Arthralgia, fever
Minor	Elevated ESR, elevated CRP, evidence of group A streptococcal infection, prolonged PR interval on ECG
*Note: two major manifestations or one major and two minor manifestations establish the diagnosis.	

Therapy

Antibiotic therapy is required even if the throat culture is negative for group A streptococci. Salicylates are the drug of choice; nonresponse to salicylates makes RF unlikely.

Aortic Stenosis

Diagnosis

The most common cause of AS is progressive calcific valve disease of a normal trileaflet valve that is usually diagnosed in patients ≥60 years of age. Aortic valve sclerosis, or valve thickening without outflow obstruction, is an earlier phase of calcific aortic valve disease present in more than 20% of persons >65 years. Patients with a congenital bicuspid aortic valve usually present at a younger age (40-60 years).

Cardinal symptoms of AS are HF, angina, and syncope. Findings include:

- midsystolic murmur at the upper right second intercostal space
- murmur that radiates to the carotid arteries
- decreased intensity of S_2
- delayed, low-amplitude carotid pulse (pulsus parvus et tardus)
- chest x-ray showing a boot-shaped cardiac silhouette and poststenotic aortic dilatation
- echocardiography showing left atrial enlargement and LVH, as well as calcified aortic valve leaflets with restricted motion
- severe AS associated with a valve area <1 cm² and a mean transvalvular gradient >40 mm Hg

Rarely, AS is diagnosed in the setting of GI bleeding in patients with Heyde syndrome. This disorder is associated with an acquired vWD, and the bleeding is thought to be caused by disruption of von Willebrand multimers during turbulent passage through the diseased aortic valve.

◆ DON'T BE TRICKED

- Echocardiography significantly underestimates the transvalvular gradient in patients with decreasing LV function.
- Do not select exercise stress testing for symptomatic patients with AS.

Therapy

In the absence of symptoms, patients have a low risk of death. Once symptoms develop, prognosis is poor without valve replacement. Surgical aortic valve replacement is the treatment of choice for most patients with symptomatic severe AS.

Transcatheter aortic valve replacement (TAVR) has a survival benefit similar to that of surgical replacement for high-risk patients and is superior to medical therapy in nonsurgical candidates. Contraindications to TAVR include a bicuspid aortic valve, significant AR, and mitral valve disease.

Medical therapy does not stall the progression of disease but is indicated for patients with symptoms and LV dysfunction who are awaiting valve repair or replacement. Treat these patients with diuretics, digoxin, and ACE inhibitors. Patients with severe AS may not tolerate nitrate preparations.

◆ DON'T BE TRICKED

- Do not select balloon valvuloplasty for adults with AS.
- Do not select β-blocker therapy in patients with AS and HF.
- Medical therapy with statins does not alter the natural history of AS.

Use serial echocardiography to evaluate the left aortic valve area, degree of ventricular hypertrophy, and LV function every year in asymptomatic patients with severe AS, every 1-2 years in patients with moderate AS, and every 3-5 years in those with mild AS.

◇ Test Yourself

A 71-year-old man is evaluated for symptoms of HF. On physical examination, the apical impulse is enlarged and displaced laterally, and a grade 2/6 midsystolic murmur is heard at the right upper sternal border that radiates to the carotid arteries. Echocardiography shows hypokinesis and an LVEF of 30%. The aortic valve cusp is calcified with diminished mobility, and the transvalvular mean gradient is 26 mm Hg.

ANSWER: The diagnosis is severe AS with cardiomyopathy despite the low transvalvular gradient (which is low because of severe LV dysfunction). Select cardiac catheterization and probable valve replacement.

Bicuspid Aortic Valve

Diagnosis

Bicuspid aortic valve disease is the most common congenital heart abnormality. Auscultatory findings include a systolic ejection click at the left lower sternal border and murmur of AS or AR in a young patient.

A bicuspid aortic valve may occur with other cardiovascular and systemic abnormalities:

- aortic coarctation
- aneurysm of the sinuses of Valsalva
- PDA
- aortic aneurysm and dissection

Therapy

Aortic valve replacement is first-line therapy for a stenotic bicuspid aortic valve and recommendations regarding when to intervene are the same as for tricuspid aortic valves.

For patients with a regurgitant bicuspid aortic valve, valve replacement is the treatment of choice when regurgitation is clinically significant, manifesting as symptomatic HF or asymptomatic LVEF <50%.

Surgery to repair the aortic root or replace the ascending aorta is indicated in patients with a bicuspid aortic valve when the aortic root diameter is >5 cm.

Follow-up

Asymptomatic patients with severe aortic valve stenosis or regurgitation require yearly echocardiography; those with mild stenosis or regurgitation require it every 3 to 5 years.

The ascending aortic diameter should be assessed annually by echocardiography if the aortic root or ascending aorta dimension is ≥4.0 cm and every 2 years if the dimension is <4.0 cm.

Aortic Regurgitation

Diagnosis

AR is classified as chronic or acute. Acute severe AR usually is caused by IE or aortic dissection. Chronic severe AR is most commonly associated with dilated ascending aorta from hypertension or primary aortic disease, calcific AS, bicuspid aortic valve, or rheumatic disease. Findings in chronic, severe AR include:

- angina, orthopnea, and exertional dyspnea
- widened pulse pressure
- soft S_1, soft or absent A_2, and loud S_3
- diastolic murmur immediately after A_2 along the left sternal border (primary aortic valvular disease) or right sternal border (secondary to aortic root dilatation)
- enhanced auscultation when leaning forward and exhaling
- left axis deviation and LVH on ECG
- cardiomegaly and aortic root dilatation and calcification on chest x-ray

Acute AR is associated with a short, soft, and sometimes inaudible diastolic murmur and normal heart size and pulse pressure. Severe acute AR causes early mitral valve closure and diastolic aortic flow reversal on echocardiography.

Therapy

Schedule immediate aortic valve replacement for patients with acute AR. Bridging medical therapy includes sodium nitroprusside and IV diuretics. Dobutamine or milrinone are also indicated if the BP is unacceptably low.

For chronic severe AR, valve replacement is indicated for symptomatic patients regardless of LV systolic function. Valve replacement also is indicated for asymptomatic patients with LVEF <50%. Combined aortic root replacement with aortic valve replacement is used when there is an associated aortic root aneurysm.

ACE inhibitors and nifedipine may be used in patients with chronic severe AR and HF pending valve replacement.

◆ DON'T BE TRICKED

- Do not select β-blockers or intra-aortic balloon pumps for patients with acute AR, because both may worsen the AR.
- Therapy with ACE inhibitors or calcium channel blockers does not delay the need for surgery in asymptomatic patients with chronic AR.

Follow-up

For patients with chronic AR who have no indications for valve replacement, perform clinical evaluation and echocardiography 2 to 3 months after diagnosis to exclude a rapidly progressive process, every 6 to 12 months in asymptomatic patients with LV dilatation, and every 2 to 3 years in asymptomatic patients with a normal left ventricle.

❖ Test Yourself

A 36-year-old man with aortic valve endocarditis is transferred to the ICU because of the abrupt onset of hypotension and hypoxemia. Physical examination findings include a BP of 80/30 mm Hg, HR of 120/min, bilateral crackles, and a gallop. No murmurs are heard.

ANSWER: The diagnosis is acute AR. Select echocardiography, IV sodium nitroprusside, and dobutamine as a bridge to urgent surgery.

Mitral Stenosis

Diagnosis

Mitral stenosis usually presents 20 to 40 years after an episode of RF. The most common symptoms are orthopnea and paroxysmal nocturnal dyspnea. Patients may have a history of AF or systemic thromboembolism. Physical examination findings include:

- a prominent a wave in the jugular pulse
- a prominent tapping apical impulse
- signs of right-sided HF
- accentuation of the P_2 and an opening snap
- a low-pitched, rumbling diastolic murmur with presystolic accentuation

A chest x-ray shows an enlarged pulmonary artery, left atrium, right ventricle, and right atrium. The ECG shows RV hypertrophy and a notched P-wave duration >0.12 s in lead II (P mitrale).

TTE is used to assess disease severity of mitral stenosis by measuring valve area and transvalvular gradient. TEE provides better visualization for the presence of left atrial appendage thrombus.

Therapy

Percutaneous mitral balloon valvotomy is indicated for symptomatic patients (NYHA functional class II, III, or IV) with moderate or severe mitral stenosis and for asymptomatic patients with PH.

Valvular characteristics that favor a successful percutaneous valvulotomy include the presence of pliable leaflets, minimal commissural fusion, and minimal valvular or subvalvular calcification. Concurrent MR is a contraindication to valvulotomy.

Mitral valve surgery (repair if possible) is indicated in patients with symptomatic (NYHA functional class III–IV) moderate or severe mitral stenosis when balloon valvotomy is unavailable or contraindicated or the valve morphology is unfavorable.

Medical therapy for mitral stenosis consists of diuretics or long-acting nitrates, which may help improve symptoms such as dyspnea. In addition, β-blockers or nondihydropyridine calcium channel blockers can lower HR and improve LV diastolic filling time.

❖ **Test Yourself**

A 28-year-old woman who is 29 weeks pregnant has progressive dyspnea. Physical examination shows tachycardia, jugular venous distention, a parasternal impulse, an opening snap, and a grade 2/6 diastolic rumble with presystolic accentuation.

ANSWER: This is the classic presentation for mitral stenosis with associated increased intravascular volume in a pregnant patient. Select metoprolol to allow greater time for LV diastolic filling and relief of PH.

◆ **DON'T BE TRICKED**

- Treat all patients with mitral stenosis and AF, regardless of CHADS$_2$ score, with warfarin.

Mitral Regurgitation

Diagnosis

MR may be either acute or chronic. Acute MR most often occurs in patients with chordae tendineae rupture due to myxomatous valve disease or endocarditis. In the setting of an MI, consider papillary muscle dysfunction or rupture. Characteristic findings in acute MR include the abrupt onset of dyspnea, pulmonary edema, or cardiogenic shock. Physical examination shows left-sided HF associated with a holosystolic murmur at the apex that radiates to the axilla and occasionally to the base. The murmur may be short or absent in patients with acute MR.

Causes of chronic MR include:

- MVP
- IE
- HCM
- ischemic heart disease
- ventricular dilatation
- Marfan syndrome
- prolonged use of ergotamine, pergolide, or cabergoline

Characteristic findings include orthopnea, paroxysmal nocturnal dyspnea, and edema. Physical examination shows a holosystolic murmur that radiates to the left axilla or to the base if the posterior leaflet is involved; a displaced, hyperdynamic apical impulse; and decreased intensity of S_1, a widely split S_2, an S_3, and an increased P_2.

TTE serves as the main imaging modality in the evaluation and management of MR.

Therapy

Surgery is first-line therapy for:

- acute MR
- chronic symptomatic MR
- asymptomatic MR with LVEF <60% or LV end-systolic diameter >40 mm
- PH due to MR
- new onset AF

Options are mitral valve repair (preferred) or mitral valve replacement. MR resulting from ischemia-induced dysfunction of the papillary muscle should improve after appropriate revascularization.

Medical therapy is used to stabilize decompensated HF in patients with acute or chronic MR. Nitrates (nitroprusside) and diuretics reduce filling pressures in acute severe MR. Inotropic agents, an intra-aortic balloon pump, or other means of circulatory support may be added in the setting of hypotension.

◆ DON'T BE TRICKED

- ACE inhibitors and ARBs have not been shown effective in preventing progression of LV dysfunction in patients with chronic MR.

◈ Test Yourself

A 63-year-old man who is asymptomatic and active is found to have MR during a physical examination. LV systolic dimension is 51 mm and the EF is 52%.

ANSWER: Select mitral valve repair or replacement.

Mitral Valve Prolapse

Diagnosis

MVP is the most common cause of significant MR, but most patients with prolapse have either minimal or no MR. MVP syndrome is usually asymptomatic but can cause chest pain, palpitations, syncope, dyspnea, and embolic phenomena. On physical examination, a high-pitched midsystolic click is heard followed by a late systolic murmur that is loudest at the apex. Standing from a sitting position and performing the Valsalva maneuver causes the click and murmur to occur earlier (closer to S_1). Squatting from a standing position delays the click (moves closer to S_2) and murmur and decreases the intensity. The initial diagnostic study is echocardiography. Patients with symptoms of arrhythmia require ambulatory ECG monitoring.

Therapy

Treat patients with palpitations, chest pain, anxiety, or fatigue with β-blockers. Aspirin is appropriate for patients with unexplained TIA who have sinus rhythm and no atrial thrombi. Warfarin is indicated for patients with recurrent ischemic neurologic events despite aspirin. Surgery is required for significant MR, a flail leaflet caused by a ruptured chorda, or marked chordal elongation.

⬧ Test Yourself

A 28-year-old woman has palpitations. Cardiac examination is normal except for an isolated click. Echocardiography is also normal except for mild MR, and 24-hour ECG monitoring shows 728 isolated, unifocal PVCs.

ANSWER: Provide reassurance and counsel on lifestyle modification (reduction of caffeine and other stimulants).

Tricuspid Regurgitation

Diagnosis

Primary causes of TR include Marfan syndrome and congenital disorders such as Ebstein anomaly (abnormalities of the tricuspid valve and right ventricle) and AV canal malformations. Common secondary causes include IE, carcinoid syndrome, PH, and RF. Physical examination shows prominent v waves in the neck, increased CVP during inspiration, and hepatic pulsations. Patients with severe disease may have ascites and pedal edema. A holosystolic murmur is heard at the left lower sternal border, increasing in intensity during inspiration. Echocardiography is diagnostic.

Therapy

Consider tricuspid valve surgery only if other cardiac surgery is planned.

◆ **DON'T BE TRICKED**
- Mild or less severe TR is common, can be easily identified by echocardiography, is physiologically normal, and does not require treatment.

Prosthetic Heart Valves

Characteristics

Mechanical valves are more durable than bioprosthetic valves but require lifelong anticoagulation. Prosthetic valves in the aortic position are more durable and less prone to thromboembolism than valves in the mitral position.

Complications

Common complications include structural valve deterioration, valve thrombosis, embolism, bleeding, and endocarditis. In the immediate postoperative period, valve dehiscence or dysfunction should be suspected in patients who develop acute HF. Valve dysfunction is characterized by new cardiac symptoms, embolic phenomena, hemolytic anemia (with schistocytes on peripheral blood smear), or new murmurs. If valve dysfunction is suspected, TEE is the diagnostic procedure of choice.

◆ **DON'T BE TRICKED**
- Begin long-term anticoagulation only for patients with mechanical heart valves.

Anticoagulation

Lifelong oral anticoagulation with warfarin is recommended for all patients with a mechanical prosthesis. The target INR is based upon prosthesis location:

- 2.0 to 3.0 for an aortic prosthetic valve
- 2.5 to 3.5 for a mitral prosthetic valve

The addition of antiplatelet therapy (typically aspirin) should be considered in patients with a mechanical prosthesis and concomitant atherosclerotic disease, as well as those with a mechanical prosthesis after thromboembolism despite adequate INR.

Keep the following in mind:

- Interrupt anticoagulation in patients with a prosthetic heart valve before they undergo noncardiac or dental surgery (but not cataract surgery).
- For aortic valve prostheses, stop warfarin 4 to 5 days before the procedure and restart as soon as postprocedure control of bleeding allows.
- In patients at high risk for thrombosis (mitral prostheses, multiple prosthetic valves, AF, or previous thromboembolic events), stop warfarin 4 to 5 days before surgery and begin inpatient IV heparin and again within 24 hours after surgery. Warfarin is initiated after surgery, and heparin is discontinued when INR is therapeutic.

◆ **DON'T BE TRICKED**
- Select only warfarin for anticoagulation of mechanical heart valves. Do not select the new oral anticoagulants (e.g., dabigatran, rivaroxaban).

Atrial Septal Defect

Diagnosis

Findings of ASD include fixed splitting of the S_2, a pulmonary midsystolic murmur, and tricuspid diastolic flow murmur. The CVP may be normal, or equal a and v waves may be noted. An RV impulse is present.

The most common form of ASD is the ostium secundum defect, which usually occurs as an isolated abnormality. The ECG shows right axis deviation and partial RBBB. The ostium primum ASD is often associated with a cleft in the mitral or tricuspid valve with associated valve regurgitation. A VSD may also be present. The ECG characteristically shows first-degree AV block, left axis deviation, and RBBB. Chest x-ray may show right atrial, RV, and pulmonary artery enlargement and increased pulmonary vascularity.

Therapy

Closure is indicated for right atrial or ventricular enlargement, large left-to-right shunt, or symptoms (dyspnea, paradoxical embolism). Select percutaneous device closure for ostium secundum ASD and surgical closure for ostium primum ASD and associated mitral valve defects. Pregnancy in patients with ASD is generally well tolerated in the absence of PH.

◆ DON'T BE TRICKED

- Closure of an ASD is contraindicated if shunt reversal (right to left) is present.
- A small ASD with no associated symptoms or right heart enlargement can be followed clinically.

❖ Test Yourself

An asymptomatic 26-year-old woman who is 30 weeks pregnant has a recently discovered heart murmur. Physical examination shows a right parasternal lift, a normal S_1, fixed splitting of S_2, and a grade 2/6 early systolic murmur at the upper left sternal border.

ANSWER: The diagnosis is ASD. The murmur is often first discovered during pregnancy as a result of increased intravascular volume.

Ostium Secundum Atrial Septal Defect: The ECG shows right axis deviation, partial RBBB, and evidence of RV hypertrophy characteristic of ostium secundum ASD.

Coarctation of the Aorta

Diagnosis

Coarctation of the aorta is a congenital disorder that may not be discovered until young adulthood. Characteristic findings include hypertension, diminished femoral pulses, radial-to-femoral pulse delay, and a murmur of AS with a continuous murmur audible over the back.

A chest x-ray shows the classic "figure 3" sign (an indented aortic wall at the site of the coarctation with dilatation above and below the coarctation) and notching on the undersides of the posterior ribs. MRA confirms the diagnosis. In patients with aortic coarctation and a bicuspid aortic valve, an ejection click or a systolic murmur may be heard. An S_4 is often audible.

◆ DON'T BE TRICKED

- More than 50% of patients with aortic coarctation also have a bicuspid aortic valve.
- Obtain BP in the legs in young people presenting with unexplained hypertension.

Therapy

Schedule balloon dilation for patients with a discrete area of aortic narrowing, proximal hypertension, and a pressure gradient >20 mm Hg. Hypertension occurs in up to 75% of patients following coarctation repair.

✧ Test Yourself

A 35-year-old female immigrant reports cold feet and leg cramping when walking long distances. BP is 160/90 mm Hg. Cardiac examination shows a sustained apical impulse, an early systolic ejection sound, and an early systolic murmur at the upper right sternal border.

ANSWER: The diagnosis is coarctation of the aorta with an associated bicuspid aortic valve. Be alert for congenital heart disease in questions featuring an immigrant patient.

Aortic Coarctation: A chest x-ray shows inferior rib notching and the classic "figure 3" sign (an indented aortic wall at the site of the coarctation with dilatation above and below the coarctation).

Patent Ductus Arteriosus

Diagnosis

Patients with a moderate-sized PDA may present with symptoms of dyspnea and HF. A continuous "machinery" murmur is heard beneath the left clavicle. Bounding pulses and a wide pulse pressure may also be noted. A large PDA causes a large left-to-right shunt and, if unrepaired, may cause PH with eventual shunt reversal from right-to-left (Eisenmenger syndrome).

A characteristic feature of an Eisenmenger PDA is clubbing and oxygen desaturation that affects the feet but not the hands (differential cyanosis).

Therapy

Closure of a PDA is indicated for left-sided cardiac chamber enlargement in the absence of severe PH. A tiny PDA without other findings requires no intervention. A moderate-sized PDA is generally closed percutaneously. A large PDA with severe PH and shunt reversal should be observed as closure may be detrimental.

Patent Foramen Ovale

Diagnosis

The foramen ovale allows transfer of oxygenated placental blood to the fetal circulation and usually closes within the first few weeks of life. In 25% to 30% of the population, however, the foramen ovale remains patent. PFO is usually asymptomatic and identified incidentally and in these cases no treatment or follow-up is needed. PFO is diagnosed by visualizing the interatrial septum by echocardiography, and demonstrating shunting of blood across the defect by color flow Doppler imaging or by using agitated saline injected intravenously and observing subsequent transfer through the PFO from right to left atrium.

Therapy

Antiplatelet therapy is recommended as first-line therapy for patients with PFO and cryptogenic stroke.

◆ **DON'T BE TRICKED**

- Data are insufficient to recommend PFO closure for secondary stroke prevention after a first stroke.

Ventricular Septal Defect

Diagnosis

A small VSD causes a loud systolic murmur that obliterates the S_2. A displaced apical LV impulse and mitral diastolic flow rumble suggest a hemodynamically important VSD. TTE demonstrates the hemodynamic impact of a VSD.

Therapy

Consider closure in adults with progressive regurgitation of the aortic or tricuspid valve, progressive LV volume overload, and recurrent endocarditis. Device closure is possible in patients with muscular VSD. Without closure, large VSDs cause PH with eventual right-to-left shunt (Eisenmenger syndrome). At this stage, closure is contraindicated and pulmonary vasodilators may be used for progressive symptoms.

Infective Endocarditis

Prevention

Provide prophylaxis for IE only in patients with the highest risk, including those with:

- prosthetic cardiac valve
- history of IE
- unrepaired cyanotic congenital heart disease
- repaired congenital heart defect with prosthesis or shunt (≤6 months post-procedure) or residual defect
- valvulopathy following cardiac transplantation

Prophylaxis is only indicated for the highest-risk procedures:

- dental procedures that involve mucosal bleeding
- procedures that involve incision or biopsy of the respiratory mucosa
- procedures in patients with ongoing GI or GU tract infection

- procedures on infected skin, skin structures, or musculoskeletal tissue
- surgery to place prosthetic heart valves or prosthetic intravascular or intracardiac materials

Most patients requiring prophylaxis will be undergoing dental procedures, and the indicated antibiotic is oral amoxicillin 30 to 60 minutes before the procedure. If the patient is allergic to penicillin, use cephalexin, azithromycin, clarithromycin, or clindamycin.

Diagnosis

Fever, malaise, and fatigue are sensitive but nonspecific symptoms associated with IE. Suggestive physical examination findings include:

- new cardiac murmur
- new-onset HF
- conduction abnormalities on ECG (suggests perivalvular abscess)
- petechiae, splinter hemorrhages
- Osler nodes (violaceous, circumscribed, painful nodules found in the pulp of the fingers and toes)
- Janeway lesions (painless, erythematous, macular lesions found on the soles and palms)
- Roth spots (hemorrhagic lesions of the retina)
- leukocytosis, anemia, and hematuria
- focal neurologic signs (septic emboli)
- multiple bilateral small nodules on chest x-ray (septic emboli)

Osler Nodes: Osler nodes are red to purple painful papules, papulopustules, or nodules found in the pulp of fingers or occasionally hands and feet.

Septic Pulmonary Emboli: Septic pulmonary emboli are characterized by multifocal, patchy, and otherwise ill-defined infiltrates; cavitation may occur.

Janeway Lesions: Janeway lesions are macular, erythematous, nontender microabscesses in the dermis of the palms and soles caused by septic emboli that are considered pathognomonic for IE.

TTE is sufficient to rule out IE in low-probability patients but a TEE is indicated to rule in IE in patients with high probability of disease. Obtain a TEE particularly in the setting of *Staphylococcus aureus* bacteremia. TEE is the test of choice to identify a paravalvular abscess.

Diagnose endocarditis in patients with two major criteria or one major and three minor criteria.

STUDY TABLE: Diagnosing Endocarditis with Simplified Duke Criteria	
Major Duke Criteria	**Minor Duke Criteria**
Positive blood culture for endocarditis × 2	Predisposing heart condition or injection drug use
Positive echocardiogram	Fever
New valvular regurgitation	Embolic vascular phenomena
	Immunologic phenomena (GN or rheumatoid factor)
	Positive blood culture not meeting major criteria

◆ DON'T BE TRICKED

- Don't give antimicrobial prophylaxis to patients with MVP or other low-risk valvular abnormalities.
- The most common reason for negative or slow-growing cultures in endocarditis is antibiotic treatment before culture.
- Look for colon cancer in patients with *Streptococcus bovis* or *Clostridium septicum* endocarditis.

Therapy

Indications for surgery include:

- valvular dysfunction and acute HF
- infection with fungal or other highly resistant organisms
- heart block
- annular or aortic abscess
- systemic embolization on antibiotic therapy
- prosthetic valve endocarditis and HF or dehiscence
- *S. aureus* prosthetic valve endocarditis

Splinter Hemorrhages: Fingernails with splinter hemorrhages, which are non-blanching, linear, reddish-brown lesions found under the nail bed.

Patients with suspected IE and good cardiovascular function do not require empiric treatment before culture results. In decompensated patients, start empiric antibiotics immediately after blood cultures are obtained.

STUDY TABLE: Empiric Therapy for IE	
Condition	**Therapy**
Community-acquired native valve IE	Vancomycin or ampicillin-sulbactam plus gentamicin
Nosocomial-associated IE	Vancomycin, gentamicin, rifampin, and an antipseudomonal β-lactam
Prosthetic valve IE	Vancomycin, gentamicin, and rifampin

Narrow antibiotic selection after susceptibilities are known. Continue treatment for 4 to 6 weeks except in uncomplicated right-sided native valve endocarditis due to MSSA, which can be treated for 2 weeks with a combination of nafcillin and gentamicin.

◆ DON'T BE TRICKED

- Oral antibiotics are not recommended for treatment of IE.

Thoracic Aortic Aneurysm and Dissection

Perform screening echocardiography of first-degree relatives of patients with familial thoracic aneurysm syndromes such as familial thoracic aortic aneurysms and aortic dissections (TAAD), bicuspid aortic valve, Marfan syndrome, Turner syndrome, and Loeys-Dietz syndrome.

Diagnosis

Most thoracic aortic aneurysms are asymptomatic and are typically incidental findings on imaging studies. Patients present with symptoms attributable to compression or distortion of adjacent structures, such as hoarseness, dysphagia, recurrent pneumonia, and SVC syndrome. The more common risk factors in younger patients include Marfan syndrome, cocaine abuse, and a bicuspid aortic valve. Poorly controlled hypertension is a risk factor in older patients.

Signs and symptoms include chest and back pain. Physical examination findings may include new AR, HF, and a BP differential between the arms. A widened mediastinum is seen on chest x-ray. Patients may also have evidence of thromboembolism, dissection of branch arteries (stroke, MI), or cardiac tamponade. A low D-dimer level (<500 ng/mL) helps rule out an acute aortic syndrome. Dissections involving the ascending aorta are classified as type A, and all other dissections are classified as type B.

The diagnosis is established by TEE, a CT scan with contrast, or MRA. Bedside TEE is used for critically ill patients who cannot be moved.

Test Yourself

A 50-year-old man is evaluated for severe chest pain and left hemiparesis.

ANSWER: The diagnosis is aortic dissection with involvement of the right carotid artery.

Therapy

For thoracic aneurysms, β-blockers reduce the rate of thoracic aortic dilation in patients with Marfan syndrome. Prophylactic surgery is recommended for the following clinical situations:

- aortic diameter >55 mm (50 mm for Marfan syndrome)
- aortic diameter ≥45 mm for women with Marfan syndrome before pregnancy
- rapid growth >0.5 mm/year

For acute dissection, begin IV β-blocker therapy and nitroprusside, fenoldopam, or enalaprilat. Emergent surgery is required for type A dissection or intramural hematoma. Uncomplicated type B dissection is treated with continued medical therapy alone.

Follow-up

Annual echocardiography is recommended for all patients with thoracic aortic aneurysm that does not require immediate intervention.

Aortic atheroma is a coronary heart disease risk equivalent and should be aggressively treated to reduce the risk of future cardiovascular events with antiplatelet agents and statins.

DON'T BE TRICKED

- Do not use hydralazine for acute aortic dissection because it increases shear stress.
- Schedule surgery for type B dissection if major aortic vessels (renal arteries) are involved.

Test Yourself

A 73-year-old man has a 1-hour history of severe, tearing substernal chest pain. BP is 90/60 mm Hg in the right arm and 130/70 mm Hg in the left arm. A chest x-ray shows a widened mediastinum.

ANSWER: The diagnosis is dissection of the aortic arch. Choose β-blockers, sodium nitroprusside, and emergent imaging studies.

Abdominal Aortic Aneurysm

Screening

One-time ultrasonographic screening is indicated to detect an asymptomatic AAA in any man between the ages of 65 and 75 years who has ever smoked and in selected men ages 65 to 75 years who have never smoked (e.g., family history of AAA).

◆ DON'T BE TRICKED

- Do not screen women for AAA.

Diagnosis

Most chronic AAAs are asymptomatic and are detected by palpating a pulsatile mass in the mid abdomen. Signs and symptoms of a ruptured AAA include new abdominal, flank, or back pain; hypotension; syncope; and sudden collapse and shock. The diagnosis is confirmed by MRA or CT.

◆ DON'T BE TRICKED

- Ultrasonography is not accurate for diagnosing a ruptured AAA.

Therapy

Therapy includes treatment of cardiovascular risk factors. In the treatment of hypertension, no evidence supports the preferential use of β-blockers. Schedule surgical repair of symptomatic AAAs ≥5.5 cm in diameter, those growing ≥0.5 cm per year, or symptomatic AAAs. Ruptured AAA requires emergent surgery or endovascular repair.

Follow-up

Patients with an unrepaired AAA require ultrasonographic monitoring at 6-month intervals if the AAA measures 4.0 to 5.4 cm and every 2 to 3 years for smaller AAAs.

Aortic Atheroemboli

Diagnosis

Plaque in either the ascending or descending thoracic aorta is associated with an increased risk of clinical thromboembolism, including stroke. Characteristic findings include livedo reticularis, gangrene of the digits (blue toe syndrome), and transient vision loss (a golden or brightly refractile cholesterol body within a retinal artery [Hollenhorst plaque] is pathognomonic). Patients often present with stroke or AKI following recent cardiac or aortic surgery or other intravascular procedures (catheterization).

Thrombocytopenia and eosinophilia may be present. Biopsy of muscle, skin, kidney, or other organs confirms the diagnosis.

Therapy

Treatment is control of cardiovascular risk factors.

Livedo Reticularis: Livedo reticularis in the lower extremities due to cholesterol emboli following cardiac catheterization.

Hollenhorst Plaque: A highly refractile yellow body (cholesterol crystals) within a retinal artery.

❖ **Test Yourself**

A 67-year-old man has AKI following coronary angiography 10 days ago. BP is 168/100 mm Hg. Bruits are noted over the abdomen and femoral arteries. His legs have a lacy, purplish discoloration.

ANSWER: Look for cholesterol emboli to the skin and renal vasculature. Select skin biopsy and control all cardiovascular risk factors.

Peripheral Arterial Disease

Screening

The USPSTF has concluded that the current evidence is insufficient to assess the balance of benefits and harms of screening for PAD with the ABI in adults.

Diagnosis

PAD most commonly involves the lower extremities and is the result of atherosclerosis involving the aorta and branch vessels. Clinical risk factors include:

- age
- smoking
- diabetes mellitus
- hyperlipidemia

Intermittent claudication is the classic sign of PAD. Most patients with PAD have coexisting coronary artery and cerebrovascular disease. The absence of a femoral pulse suggests in-flow disease of the aorta or iliac arteries. Patients with a good femoral pulse and no femoral bruit but an absent popliteal pulse likely have disease confined to the arteries in the leg. Differentiate claudication due to PAD from claudication due to spinal stenosis. Spinal stenosis is associated with pain (often bilateral) that occurs when standing and resolves when sitting or lying down or flexing the spine (bending forward).

Interpret the ABI:

- ABI for each side is the ratio of the highest systolic arm BP (regardless of side) compared with the highest systolic ankle BP for that side.

- Normal ABI is >0.9 to ≤1.40.
- ABI ≤0.90 is compatible with PAD.
- ABI ≤0.40 is associated with ischemic rest pain.
- False-normal ABI occurs in patients with diabetes with calcified, noncompressible arteries (ABI >1.40).

Recall the "five Ps" to diagnose acute arterial ischemia:

- Pain
- Paresthesias
- Pallor
- Paralysis
- Pulselessness

Acute ischemia can be caused by in-situ thrombosis or remote embolization. Echocardiography is used to locate the embolic source of acute ischemia.

◆ DON'T BE TRICKED

- When the ABI is >1.40, select a toe-brachial index to provide a better assessment of lower extremity perfusion.

Therapy

PAD is a CAD risk equivalent. Therapy includes:

- BP goal <140/90 mm Hg
- aspirin (preferred over ticlopidine or clopidogrel)
- high-intensity statin therapy
- cilostazol for symptomatic PAD
- ramipril to reduce the risk of MI, stroke, or vascular death in PAD

Select angioplasty or surgery for patients who do not improve on medical therapy or have pain at rest or poorly healing ulcers.

Patients with acute arterial ischemia require antiplatelet agents and heparin anticoagulation as well as urgent surgical consultation.

◆ DON'T BE TRICKED

- Oral anticoagulation with warfarin has not been established to reduce cardiovascular events in patients with chronic PAD.
- Pentoxifylline is substantially less effective than either cilostazol or a supervised exercise program in relieving symptoms of PAD.
- Do not use cilostazol in patients with a low LVEF or history of HF.
- β-Blockers are not contraindicated in patients with PAD.

❖ Test Yourself

A 60-year-old man has a 6-month history of claudication in both thighs and calves. ABI is 0.66 on the right side and 0.55 on the left side. He is symptomatic despite an intensive lifestyle management program.

ANSWER: Begin cilostazol.

Myxoma

Diagnosis

The most common primary cardiac tumors in adults are myxomas. Myxomas may arise as part of the Carney complex:

- autosomal dominant disorder
- blue nevi
- cardiac and extracardiac myxomas
- schwannomas
- endocrine tumors

Patients with a myxoma may have constitutional symptoms, such as fever, anorexia, and weight loss. The auscultatory findings resemble mitral stenosis murmur with an accompanying sound of a "tumor plop." Embolization may cause neurologic symptoms.

Imaging (echocardiography, CT, or CMR imaging) is diagnostic for myxoma. Myxomas characteristically are pedunculated arising most commonly in the left atrium with the stalk adherent to the fossa ovalis.

◆ DON'T BE TRICKED

- Auscultatory findings of atrial myxoma may mimic those of mitral stenosis.

Therapy

Myxomas should be resected after diagnosis owing to the risk of embolization and cardiovascular complications, including the potential for sudden death.

Dermatology

Eczemas

Diagnosis

Eczematous dermatitis is a type of inflammation characterized by inflamed, dry, red, itchy skin.

- vesicles are typical of acute eczema
- lichenification defines chronic eczema

Lichenification is an exaggeration of skin markings, with skin thickening, scaling, and abnormal pigmentation.

There are several types of eczema. Common types include atopic, contact dermatitis, dyshidrotic, and asteatotic.

Atopic dermatitis is the development of eczema in patients with an inherited atopic diathesis. Look for:

- a waxing and waning course
- pruritic, erythematous papules and plaques that may be vesicular and weeping
- chronic lesions that may be lichenified and hyperkeratotic
- involvement of the periocular areas and flexural surfaces including posterior neck, antecubital and popliteal fossae, wrists, and ankles
- complicating staphylococcal infection evidenced by pustules, crusting, and erosions

There are two types of contact dermatitis: allergic contact dermatitis and irritant contact dermatitis.

Allergic contact dermatitis (type IV hypersensitivity reaction) is precipitated by local absorption of an allergen or irritant through the stratum corneum. With repeated exposure, an itchy eczematous dermatitis develops on the area that was exposed. A secondary "id" reaction may develop which is characterized by a generalized acute cutaneous reaction, in which pinpoint flesh-colored to red papules develop in areas not exposed to the allergen. Common allergens include:

- nickel
- topical anesthetics
- neomycin
- poison oak, poison ivy
- transdermal patches
- strong soaps or personal care products

Look for clues such as a neck rash caused by a necklace to identify the causative agent. For patients in whom treatment is refractory, consider patch testing for nickel, fragrance, and rubber.

Irritant contact dermatitis is a direct toxic effect from exposure to a chemical such as a cleaning agent or other caustic substance. For instance, over-washing will often lead to dry, irritated skin and is not immune mediated.

Dyshidrotic eczema (pompholyx) is an extremely itchy eruption of small vesicles on the sides of the fingers and palms that can occur from wetting and drying, sweating, or allergies; it also occurs as a reaction pattern to tinea pedis.

Xerotic eczema usually occurs on the anterior shins of older persons with dry skin. Affected skin is red, dry, and cracked with multiple fine fissures that resemble cracks in porcelain. The dermatitis is more common in winter or in dry conditions.

◆ **DON'T BE TRICKED**

- Food allergies are an uncommon cause of flares in atopic dermatitis.

Contact Dermatitis: Discretely grouped red vesicles and bullae in a linear distribution are characteristic of contact dermatitis due to poison ivy.

Atopic Dermatitis: The rash involves the antecubital fossae, with lichenification and surrounding excoriations.

Therapy

For irritant hand dermatitis, treat by washing less, moisturizing more, and wearing cotton gloves inside of rubber gloves when around chemicals or during activities such as dishwashing.

Contact dermatitis, atopic dermatitis, and dyshidrotic eczema may benefit from a short course of topical glucocorticoids for symptom relief.

- 1% topical hydrocortisone for the face and intertriginous areas (low-potency glucocorticoid)
- 0.1% triamcinolone for other body sites (medium-potency glucocorticoid)
- nighttime sedating antihistamines to reduce scratching
- topical tacrolimus for recalcitrant atopic eczema
- potent glucocorticoids for the palms, soles, and extremely thick eruptions (atopic eczema)

Xerotic Dermatitis: Asteatotic dermatitis is characterized by the location on the anterior shin of red, dry, and cracked skin with multiple fine fissures.

Treatment of xerotic eczema consists of regular emollient use. Mid- to low-potency topical glucocorticoids may minimize itching and facilitate healing.

Always select emollients as part of eczema treatment. Emollients work through various mechanisms, including trapping water in the skin (petrolatum), introducing water into the skin (aqueous cream), or increasing the water-holding capacity of the skin (urea).

◆ **DON'T BE TRICKED**

- Do not select potent glucocorticoids for the face because of the risk of steroid-induced acne and cutaneous atrophy.

❖ **Test Yourself**

A healthy 40-year-old female nurse has a 1-month history of vesicular eruptions on the dorsum and distal areas of her hands.

ANSWER: The diagnosis is acute eczema. Select a topical glucocorticoid.

Psoriasis

Diagnosis

Typical findings of chronic plaque psoriasis are erythema, scaling, and induration on the extensor surfaces, scalp, ears, intertriginous folds, and genitalia. The nails may be pitted, thickened, loose, or yellow and may be the only manifestation of psoriasis. Psoriatic arthritis and spondylitis may coexist in 25% of patients.

Psoriasis is exacerbated by systemic glucocorticoids, lithium, antimalarial drugs, tetracyclines, β-blockers, NSAIDs, and ACE inhibitors.

STUDY TABLE: Clinical Appearance of Common Psoriasis Subtypes	
Subtype	**Description**
Chronic plaque psoriasis	Thick, erythematous lesions with silvery, adherent scale anywhere on the body
Guttate psoriasis	Many small drop-like papules and plaques on the trunk often developing after infection with β-hemolytic *Streptococcus*
Erythrodermic psoriasis	Generalized erythema and scaling involving most of the body, often occurring after abrupt discontinuation of systemic glucocorticoids; potentially life-threatening
Inverse psoriasis	Red, thin plaques with variable amount of scale in the axillae, under the breasts or pannus, intergluteal cleft, and perineum
Nail psoriasis	Indentations, pits, and oil spots often involving multiple nails

Therapy

Select topical glucocorticoids for limited, localized plaques. Next, rotate therapy with topical vitamin D analogues (calcipotriene, tacalcitol), retinoids, anthralin, or tar preparations.

Patients with >10% body surface area or those with psoriatic arthritis, recalcitrant palmoplantar psoriasis, pustular psoriasis, or psoriasis in challenging anatomic areas (groin, scalp) are considered for systemic therapy including:

- phototherapy
- systemic agents (retinoids, methotrexate, cyclosporine)
- TNF inhibitors and interleukin-inhibitors

Patients receiving systemic glucocorticoids or cyclosporine are at risk for acute erythrodermic or pustular flares with sudden cessation of medication. Erythrodermic psoriasis is a dermatologic emergency, because patients are at high risk for infection and electrolyte abnormalities secondary to fluid loss.

Guttate Psoriasis: Guttate psoriasis is characterized by small, drop-like, scaly papules and plaques.

Nail Findings in Psoriasis: Psoriatic nails with characteristic discoloration, crumbling, subungual debris, and separation of the nail plate from the nail bed.

Chronic Plaque Psoriasis: Typical plaque psoriasis consists of a polymorphic red plaque covered with a thick, silvery scale.

◆ DON'T BE TRICKED

- Never select systemic glucocorticoids for the treatment of psoriasis.

✛ Test Yourself

A 28-year-old woman has a chronic extensive skin rash consisting of multiple small and large plaques with an adherent, thick, silvery scale covering 25% of her body surface area.

ANSWER: The diagnosis is psoriasis.

STUDY TABLE: Other Papulosquamous Disorders		
Condition	**Presentation**	**Therapy**
Lichen planus	Acute eruption of purple, pruritic, polygonal papules that most commonly presents on the wrists and ankles. Lichen planus can also present in the mouth, vaginal vault, penis, and in the nails (leading to thickening and distortion of the nail plate).	Topical glucocorticoids
Pityriasis rosea	Presents with one scaling patch that is a few centimeters wide (herald patch), followed by many 0.5- to 2.0-cm red scaling pruritic patches along the skin cleavage lines in a "Christmas tree" distribution on the back, and lasting 1 to 3 months.	Topical glucocorticoids and antihistamines for pruritus
Seborrheic dermatitis	An inflammatory scaling, itchy dermatosis that most commonly affects the scalp but can also affect the eyebrows, nasolabial folds, chin, central chest, and perineum. Explosive onset with wide distribution may be a sign of HIV infection.	Selenium sulfide or zinc pyrithione shampoos, ketoconazole shampoo

◆ DON'T BE TRICKED

- Pityriasis rosea can resemble secondary syphilis but does not involve the palms and soles; obtain rapid plasma reagin (RPR) in high-risk individuals.
- Extensive seborrheic dermatitis may be a clue to underlying HIV infection.

✛ Test Yourself

A 28-year-old man is evaluated for severe seborrheic dermatitis of acute onset.

ANSWER: Test for HIV infection.

Seborrheic Dermatitis: Seborrheic dermatitis, with fine, oily scale around the medial eyebrows.

Pityriasis Rosea

Diagnosis

Pityriasis rosea is an inflammatory, mildly pruritic eruption, possibly related to herpes-virus 6 or 7, which occurs in the spring and fall. It begins with a herald patch: a single, raised, bright-red, oval plaque that is 2 to 5 cm in diameter with a fine scale and is followed by smaller pink papules and plaques with the distinctive ring of scale at the periphery. The lesions follow the skin cleavage lines on the trunk and chest, producing a "Christmas tree" pattern.

Therapy

The rash spontaneously resolves in 1 to 3 months. Oral antihistamines or topical gluco-corticoids can be used for itching.

◆ **DON'T BE TRICKED**

- Secondary syphilis can mimic pityriasis rosea; check RPR if in doubt or if the patient has risk factors for STI.

Pityriasis Rosea: Pink plaques with a fine collar-ette of scale, characteristic of pityriasis rosea.

Acneiform Lesions

Diagnosis

Acne is a chronic inflammatory skin condition characterized by open and closed comedones (blackheads and whiteheads, respectively) and inflammatory lesions, including papules, pustules, or nodules. Consider hyperandrogenism in women whose acne is severe, cyclical, or unresponsive to conventional therapy and is associated with menstrual irregularities, virilization, hirsutism, or rapid onset of severe disease.

Rosacea is a chronic inflammatory skin disorder that affects the cheeks and nose and usually occurs after the age of 30 years. Rosacea is commonly associated with facial flushing in response to certain stimuli such as spicy foods. Erythema with telangiectasias, pustules, and papules without comedones is typically seen. In early stages, rosacea can resemble the malar rash of SLE. However, the rash of SLE spares the nasolabial folds. The development of papules, pustules, and flushing is inconsistent with SLE and supports the diagnosis of rosacea.

Hidradenitis suppurativa is a chronic inflammatory disease that predominantly affects the axillae, breasts and inframammary creases, inguinal folds, and gluteal cleft. It is characterized by comedones, inflammatory papules, nodules, cysts, and scarring.

Rosacea: Papules, pustules, and dilated blood vessels involving the central face are typical of rosacea.

STUDY TABLE: Differential Diagnosis of Acne	
Disease	**Characteristics**
Acne (acne vulgaris)	The microcomedone is the precursor to acne lesions. It is very common in adolescents, but also common in preadolescents and adults. Women may have premenstrual flare-ups. Physical examination: coexisting open and closed comedones, papules, pustules, and nodular lesions located primarily on the face, neck, and upper trunk.
Rosacea	Not true acne; primary lesion is not a comedone but an inflammatory papule; rhinophyma (bulbous, red nose) is a variant. Physical examination: central facial erythema, telangiectasias, papules, and pustules.
Medication-induced acneiform eruption	Onset weeks to months after start of the medication. Comedones are absent; inflammatory papules and pustules commonly appear on the upper trunk and arms when the cause is systemic. Common triggers include glucocorticoids, anabolic steroids, bromides, iodides, lithium, and EGFR inhibitors.
Bacterial folliculitis	Common in athletes. Physical examination: follicular papules; pustules; occasional furuncles on any hair-bearing area, especially scalp, buttocks, and thighs. Most common cause is *Staphylococcus aureus*.
Gram-negative folliculitis	Caused by overgrowth of bacteria during prolonged systemic antibiotic treatment for acne and presents as exacerbation of preexisting acne. Physical examination: many inflamed pustules, most often on the face. Positive culture for gram-negative bacteria, often *Escherichia coli*.
Periorificial dermatitis, idiopathic	More common in women. Physical examination: small (<2 mm) papules and pustules around mouth or eyelids. Similar to acne but without comedones.
Periorificial dermatitis, iatrogenic	Frequent causes are prolonged topical glucocorticoid therapy for atopic dermatitis and inappropriate use of these agents to treat acne. Similar in appearance to idiopathic type. Differentiation is by history.

◆ DON'T BE TRICKED

- The prominent papules and pustules seen in rosacea are not typical of the malar rash seen in SLE.

Perioral Dermatitis: Discrete papules and pustules on an erythematous base that are around the mouth is characteristic of perioral dermatitis.

Hidradenitis Suppurativa: Hidradenitis suppurativa is a chronic skin condition characterized by painful, recurrent, chronic, sterile abscesses; sinus tract formation; and scarring.

Therapy

STUDY TABLE: Drug Therapy for Acne	
Indication	**Drug**
Mild noninflammatory acne (comedones)	Comedolytic agent (topical retinoid)
Mild inflammatory acne (papules and pustules)	Topical retinoid and topical antibiotic (erythromycin or clindamycin)
Moderate noninflammatory acne	Topical retinoid and benzoyl peroxide or azelaic acid
Moderate to severe inflammatory acne	Topical retinoid, topical antibiotic, and an oral antibiotic (tetracycline or others)
Acne in women with hyperandrogenism	Oral contraceptive
Severe recalcitrant nodular acne	Oral isotretinoin (women require two forms of birth control when taking this drug because it is teratogenic)
Iatrogenic perioral acne	Stop topical glucocorticoid

Rosacea with inflammatory pustules and papules will respond to metronidazole gel and low-dose oral tetracycline.

Hidradenitis suppurativa is difficult to treat but clindamycin-rifampin combination antibiotics, infliximab, and surgical excision have the greatest evidence of effectiveness.

◆ DON'T BE TRICKED
- Topical tazarotene and oral isotretinoin are pregnancy category X drugs (teratogenic) and the tetracyclines are pregnancy category D drugs.
- Do not treat perioral dermatitis with topical glucocorticoids. Treat with topical or oral antibiotics.

❖ Test Yourself
An 18-year-old man has had nodular and cystic acne. Pustules and nodules with scarring are present on the chin, face, back, and chest.

ANSWER: The diagnosis is severe inflammatory acne. Select isotretinoin.

Dermatophyte and Yeast Infections

Diagnosis

Dermatophyte fungi invade epidermal stratum corneum, hair, and nails, causing tinea infections.

- Tinea pedis presents as chronic fissuring and scaling between the toes, but some patients have a chronic "moccasin-type" form of infection with a fine, silvery scale extending from the sole to heel and sides of the feet.
- Tinea corporis most typically presents as an annular lesion with an active erythematous border of small vesicles and scales, often with central clearing.
- Tinea cruris (jock itch) is dermatophyte infection of the inguinal folds presenting as erythematous patches with a rim of scale that does not involve the scrotum.
- Tinea versicolor is characterized by hypo- or hyperpigmented scaly macules on the trunk and proximal extremities.
- Onychomycosis is usually characterized by a thickened, yellow or white nail with scaling under the elevated distal free edge of the nail plate. Sometimes, however, the infecting organism invades the surface of the toenail.

Cutaneous candidiasis is characterized by red, itchy, inflamed skin. At sites of skin-to-skin contact, lesions have glazed, shiny, and at times eroded surfaces and may be characterized by burning more than pruritus. Satellite pustules (yellow, fluid-filled lesions at the edge of the confluent red eruption) are another key physical finding.

Diagnosis of dermatophyte infection can be performed by examination of the scale, nail plate, or hair follicle with KOH demonstrating the presence of branching hyphae. Tinea versicolor is associated with yeast spores characterized by "spaghetti and meatballs" microscopic appearance. Candida is associated with pseudohyphae and spores.

◆ DON'T BE TRICKED
- Candidal intertrigo, in contrast to tinea cruris, can involve the scrotum.
- Two feet–one hand tinea is a common presentation of concomitant tinea pedis and tinea manuum.
- Nail dystrophy may also be caused by psoriasis, other dermatologic conditions, aging, or peripheral vascular disease.

Tinea Pedis: Extension of tinea pedis onto the sole and sides of the foot ("moccasin" appearance) presents as chronic scaling.

Tinea Infection: Tinea most commonly presents as a round or oval erythematous scaling patch that spreads centrifugally with central clearing. It has an active border that is raised, consisting of tiny papules or vesicles and scale.

***Candida* Infection:** Bright red papules, vesicles, pustules, and patches with satellite papules and pustules are characteristic of candidiasis.

Onychomycosis: Distal subungual thickening and nail separation involving most of the nails are associated with onychomycosis.

Therapy

Select:

- topical antifungal creams (clotrimazole, terbinafine) for most dermatophyte infections except tinea capitis and onychomycosis
- oral terbinafine or itraconazole for confirmed onychomycosis, tinea capitis, extensive tinea corporis, or treatment-resistant dermatophytosis
- ketoconazole or fluconazole in a single dose to treat recurrent tinea versicolor
- topical nystatin, miconazole, clotrimazole, ketoconazole, and econazole for *Candida* infections

Treatment of onychomycosis is typically not necessary but is recommended for patients with peripheral vascular disease or diabetes mellitus to prevent development of cellulitis.

◆ DON'T BE TRICKED

- Do not select antifungal treatment for thick, yellow, and crumbling toenails without KOH scraping or positive culture for dermatophytes.
- Never select a combination of a topical antifungal agent and a glucocorticoid for treatment of an unknown skin rash or dermatophyte infection.
- PPIs and H_2-blockers impair the absorption of ketoconazole and itraconazole.

✣ Test Yourself

A 35-year-old man has a nonpruritic rash on his chest. He previously had a similar rash that became hypopigmented when he became suntanned. What is the diagnosis?

ANSWER: Choose tinea versicolor and KOH preparation of the scale to demonstrate a "spaghetti and meatballs" hyphae pattern.

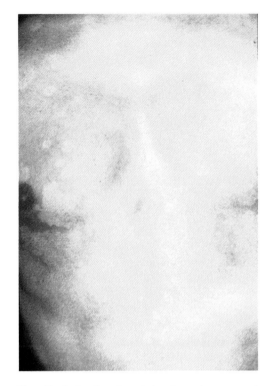

Tinea Versicolor: Hypopigmented, scaly macules are present on the chest.

Molluscum Contagiosum

Diagnosis

Molluscum contagiosum is a self-limited viral infection characterized by skin-colored, umbilicated papules that are typically found in children and sexually active adults. Associated HIV infection may cause multiple, large, disfiguring lesions.

Therapy

Treatment may include destructive techniques including cryotherapy, salicylic acid, cantharidin, or physical removal with curettage; topical imiquimod may be considered second-line therapy.

Molluscum Contagiosum: Molluscum contagiosum presents as small, flesh-colored, umbilicated papules in sexually active adults.

Leishmaniasis

Diagnosis

Leishmaniasis is a parasitic infection caused by several species of *Leishmania* and is transmitted by the sandfly. Military personnel returning from Afghanistan and Iraq and travelers to Saudi Arabia, Brazil, and Peru are at risk. The cutaneous form of the disease begins as a small, red, painless papule on the limb or face, usually 2 to 4 weeks after the sandfly bite. The papule enlarges to approximately 2 cm over the next 2 to 4 weeks, becomes dusky red to violaceous in color, and may ulcerate. Diagnosis is based on finding parasites on biopsy of the skin.

Leishmaniasis: The characteristic shallow ulcer of leishmaniasis is shown on an arm.

Herpes Zoster

Prevention

Administer varicella zoster virus vaccine to adults aged 60 years and older–regardless of previous history of varicella infection–who do not have contraindications for live vaccine (immunosuppression) to prevent or attenuate illness due to herpes zoster infection and reduce the risk of postherpetic neuralgia.

Diagnosis

Localized pain and a vesicular rash in a dermatomal distribution are characteristic features. Dermatomal neuropathic pain may develop before skin lesions occur. Be alert for two special syndromes:

- Lesions along the first division of the trigeminal nerve (zoster ophthalmicus), including the tip of the nose, may require referral to an ophthalmologist.
- Vesicles in the ears, diminished taste on the anterior two thirds of the tongue, and ipsilateral facial paralysis (Ramsay Hunt syndrome) require referral to an ENT specialist.

In patients with HIV or who are otherwise immunosuppressed, the lesions may be bullous and erosive; occur in multiple, widely separated dermatomes; be disseminated on the skin and internally; or produce recurrent disease. Severe, complicated, or recurrent herpes zoster should trigger testing for possible associated HIV infection.

Obtain rapid tests such as direct-fluorescent antibody and PCR studies on scrapings from active vesicular skin lesions that have not yet crusted, or viral culture from a vesicle when the diagnosis is not clear.

Therapy

Give valacyclovir, famciclovir, or acyclovir (7-day course) within 72 hours of lesion onset. Antiviral agents are used to treat zoster ophthalmicus even if more than 72 hours have elapsed. Treat postherpetic neuralgia with gabapentin, pregabalin, tricyclic antidepressants, or topical lidocaine or capsaicin.

Herpes Zoster: Herpes zoster is characterized by the dermatomal distribution of painful grouped vesicles on an erythematous base.

◆ DON'T BE TRICKED

- Do not select topical acyclovir or penciclovir for the treatment of herpes zoster.
- Serologic testing is not recommended for diagnosis of zoster because seroprevalence rates are high and do not correspond with active infection.
- Oral glucocorticoids provide symptomatic relief but do not reduce the risk of postherpetic neuralgia.

❖ Test Yourself

A 72-year-old man has a 4-day history of a painful vesicular rash in the distribution of the first division of the trigeminal nerve and conjunctival inflammation.

ANSWER: The diagnosis is zoster ophthalmicus. Select urgent referral to an ophthalmologist.

Scabies

Diagnosis

Look for itching (particularly at night) and burrows appearing as wavy, thread-like, grayish-white skin elevations capped with small vesicles at the terminal ends. Scabies is the correct answer when an "itchy rash" is described between the fingers and on the penis, scrotum, areolae, and nipples. Patients with AIDS and those in institutions may develop widespread scabies with extensive scaling that may not itch.

Microscopic identification of the mite, feces, or eggs using KOH or simple mineral oil is important. A skin biopsy may also establish the diagnosis.

Therapy

Treat all family members and close contacts of the patient simultaneously. Clothing, linens, and towels must be washed in hot water and dried at high heat. Topical permethrin is the preferred agent. Oral ivermectin is indicated for relapsed scabies, except when treating children and pregnant or lactating women.

◆ DON'T BE TRICKED

- Do not re-treat scabies because of persistent itching, which can continue for 2 weeks after successful treatment.
- Avoid topical lindane due to its associated neurotoxicity.

❖ Test Yourself

A 67-year-old woman and her 3-year-old granddaughter have a 3-week history of generalized pruritus. Both patients have widespread excoriations and a linear burrow between the thumb and index finger.

ANSWER: The diagnosis is scabies. Select topical permethrin for both patients and for other close contacts.

Scabies: Multiple pink papules, erosions, and excoriations with diffuse scaling are shown, predominantly in the finger webs.

Bedbugs

Diagnosis

Classic presentation is grouped, itchy papules in close configuration ("breakfast, lunch, and dinner") on exposed body areas. Bites are typically noticed in the morning, as bedbugs feed at night.

Therapy

Treatment is topical glucocorticoids and oral antihistamines as bedbugs do not actively live on humans. Eradication of bedbugs is necessary for "cure."

Bedbugs: Classic grouped pruritic papules ("breakfast, lunch, and dinner") presentation of bites from bedbugs.

Seborrheic Keratosis

Diagnosis

Seborrheic keratosis is a painless, nonmalignant growth that appears as a "stuck-on" waxy, brownish patch or plaque. It is more common in older adult patients and does not require treatment except for cosmetic reasons. Rapid onset of multiple pruritic seborrheic keratoses can be a sign of GI adenocarcinoma.

Therapy

Therapy is not required. A shave excision or liquid nitrogen destruction can be performed for lesions that are irritated (e.g., rubbed by clothing or jewelry).

Seborrheic Keratoses: Brown to tan, sharply demarcated, waxy-like papules, plaques, and nodules are characteristic of seborrheic keratoses.

Warts

Diagnosis

Look for flesh-colored, exophytic, hyperkeratotic papules or nodules.

- Verruca vulgaris is often present on hands but may be found anywhere.
- Verruca plantaris is a hyperkeratotic lesion on the plantar surface.
- Flat warts (verruca plana) are flat-topped papules that often are spread easily, especially from shaving.
- Anogenital warts (condyloma acuminata) present as single or multiple papules on the penis, vulva, or perianal area and may be flat-topped or cauliflower-like papules.

Therapy

Treat common warts with salicylic acid (a keratolytic agent). Alternatives to drug therapy include cryotherapy. "No therapy" is an acceptable answer, because spontaneous resolution is possible. Podophyllin is often used as the initial therapy for anogenital warts.

Actinic Keratosis

Diagnosis

Actinic keratosis is a precursor to SCC. Lesions are located on sun-exposed sites and appear as 2- to 3-mm, elevated, flesh-colored or red papules with adherent, whitish scale or "rough spots" that may be easier to palpate than to visualize. Biopsy is indicated for larger lesions (>5 mm); thick, indurated papules; lesions that have grown rapidly; and lesions that bleed, itch, or are painful.

Therapy

Destruction by liquid nitrogen or curettage is the preferred treatment for most single lesions. Select topical 5-FU or imiquimod cream for treatment of numerous lesions. Lesions suspicious for SCC require standard excision.

Actinic Keratoses: Multiple white, scaly patches measuring 1 to 3 mm on the hands, characteristic of actinic keratoses.

Squamous Cell Carcinoma

Diagnosis

SCC is the most common type of skin cancer seen in patients who are immunosuppressed from solid organ transplant. Cutaneous SCC presents as a slowly evolving, isolated, keratotic, or eroded macule, papule, or nodule that commonly appears on the scalp, neck, pinna, or lip. Bowen disease is a form of anaplastic in situ SCC that presents as circumscribed erythematous or pigmented patches that typically have a keratotic surface. Shave or punch biopsy confirms the diagnosis of SCC, and referral for definitive treatment is recommended.

Keratoacanthoma is a form of SCC generally appearing as a rapidly growing red nodule with a prominent central plug of scale and crust; its appearance is "volcaniform," resembling the cinder cone of a volcano.

Cutaneous Squamous Cell Carcinoma: Typically presents as a slowly evolving, isolated, keratotic, or eroded macule, papule, or nodule that commonly appears on the scalp, neck, pinna, or lip.

Therapy

Although small lesions can be treated with electrodesiccation and curettage, most lesions require excision.

Basal Cell Carcinoma

Diagnosis

The most characteristic lesion is a pink, pearly, translucent papule or nodule with telangiectasias, rolled borders, and central depression with ulceration. Superficial BCCs are well demarcated, irregularly bordered, red patches; they tend to enlarge radially rather than invading into deeper structures. Patients may have a history of radiation therapy, immunosuppression, arsenic exposure, or (most commonly) excessive sun exposure. Choose biopsy for clinically suspicious lesions.

Therapy

Most BCCs are treated with simple excision. Ill-defined lesions, high-risk histologic types, and tumors on the face and hands are often best treated with Mohs micrographic surgery, which is a staged tumor excision with mapping of specimens and preparation and interpretation of the frozen sections.

Dysplastic Nevi

Diagnosis

Dysplastic nevi are markers for melanoma diathesis. A low percentage transform into melanoma. Dysplastic nevi have some features of melanoma, including:

- diameter ≥5 mm
- asymmetric shape with indistinct borders
- a "fried egg" appearance with a darker, elevated, central portion and tan, flat shoulders blending into surrounding skin
- pigmentation ranging from light tan to dark brown and occasionally black

Autosomal-dominant familial melanoma/dysplastic nevus syndrome is defined by the presence of melanoma in at least two relatives and dysplastic nevi in other family members.

Therapy

Dysplastic nevi that develop increased characteristics associated with melanoma (fuzzy or ill-defined borders, multiple colors, diameter ≥5 mm), have otherwise changed, or stand out from other nevi must be removed and sent for pathology.

Melanoma

Prevention

Select sun avoidance and sun-protective clothing as first-line prevention. Use of sun screening agents is adjunctive therapy.

Diagnosis

Basal Cell Carcinoma: This pink, pearly, translucent, dome-shaped papule with telangiectasias is characteristic of BCC.

Dysplastic Nevi: Dysplastic nevi share similar characteristics with melanoma including asymmetry, indistinct and irregular borders, and variation in pigmentation.

STUDY TABLE: "ABCDE" Rule to Diagnose Melanoma	
Characteristic	**Description**
Asymmetry	Not regularly round or oval
Border irregularity	Notching, scalloping, or poorly defined margins
Color variegation	Shades of brown, tan, red, white, blue-black, or combinations
Diameter	Size >6 mm (early melanomas may be diagnosed at a smaller size)
Evolution	Lateral expansion or vertical growth

There are several subtypes of melanoma.

- Lentigo maligna begins as a uniformly pigmented, light brown patch on the face or upper trunk that is confined to the epidermis and resembles a solar lentigo. Over time, the lesion expands and becomes more variegated in color.
- Superficial spreading melanoma presents as a well-defined asymmetric patch or plaque with an irregular border, variation in color, and an expanding diameter. This type tends to occur on the back in men and the legs in women (areas that receive intermittent sun and are prone to sunburn).
- Nodular melanomas are the most aggressive form (invading deeper structures); they are responsible for the majority of deaths from melanoma.
- Acral lentiginous melanomas are the most common type of melanoma seen in patients with dark skin and usually occur on the hands and feet.

Lentigo Maligna: This carcinoma in situ appears as a brown patch on sun-exposed skin.

Melanoma: This asymmetric pigmented skin lesion has irregular, scalloped, notched, and indistinct borders with variegated coloration.

Therapy

Complete excision is the preferred biopsy technique for most varieties of melanoma, and sentinel lymph node biopsy is indicated for melanomas >1 mm thick. The extent of the surgical excision depends on the thickness of the primary melanoma.

Melanomas >4 mm thick or with lymph node involvement are associated with an increased risk of dying. In these patients adjuvant immunotherapy with interferon alfa improves relapse-free survival, but its impact on overall survival is not clear.

Surgical resection for metastatic disease limited to one or a few sites can result in prolonged survival. In these patients, immunotherapy (interleukin-2 and ipilimumab) or targeted therapy is preferred over chemotherapy.

For patients with the V600E *BRAF* mutation, targeted therapy with vemurafenib is recommended over immunotherapy for patients with poor performance status and/or more advanced disease.

Follow-up routine blood tests are not recommended, and the value of screening test radiography, CT scanning, or PET/CT scanning is questionable.

Acral Melanoma: Acral melanoma on the toe.

◆ **DON'T BE TRICKED**

- Lentigo maligna melanoma is treated with a broad, shallow shave biopsy, not excision as other melanomas are treated.

Urticaria

Diagnosis

The hallmark of urticaria (hives) is the wheal, a superficial itchy swelling of the skin. Wheals involving the skin around the mouth are considered an emergency, requiring careful observation and investigation for airway obstruction.

Individual lesions of acute urticaria last only a few hours but may recur. β-Lactams, sulfonamides, NSAIDs, opioids, insect stings, contrast dyes, latex (including condoms), nuts, fish, and eggs are common causes. Urticaria can also be initiated by pressure, cold, heat, vibration, water, or sunlight.

Lesions persisting >24 hours with purpura/ecchymoses upon resolution are likely due to urticarial vasculitis. In this situation, definitive diagnosis is made by skin biopsy.

◆ **DON'T BE TRICKED**

- Do not select ANA testing for acute or chronic urticaria.

STUDY TABLE: Differential Diagnosis of Urticaria

If you see this...	Select this...
↑ESR, ↑CRP, lesions persisting >24 hours	Vasculitic urticaria; perform skin biopsy and obtain serum complement levels, hepatitis B and C serology, cryoglobulins, and SPEP
Fever, adenopathy, arthralgia, and antigen or drug exposure	Serum sickness; measure IgE level (elevated)
Features of anaphylaxis, obvious allergen exposure	Immediate hypersensitivity reaction; treat emergently with epinephrine
Marked eosinophilia	Parasitic infection, possibly strongyloidiasis, filariasis, or trichinosis (especially with periorbital edema)

Therapy

Avoid aspirin and other NSAIDs. Select nonsedating antihistamines as first-line therapy. If no response is seen, add an H_2-blocker (cimetidine, ranitidine), although evidence for effectiveness is mixed. Doxepin blocks H_1, H_2, and serotonin receptors, and is often effective. Short-term oral glucocorticoids are indicated in very symptomatic patients with acute urticaria.

◆ **DON'T BE TRICKED**

- Systemic and topical glucocorticoids are not beneficial for patients with chronic urticaria.
- Measurement of C1 inhibitor levels is not indicated in patients with urticaria, because deficiency of C1 inhibitor is associated with angioedema, not with hives.

Urticaria: Urticaria is characterized by small white, pink, or flesh-colored pruritic papules.

✣ **Test Yourself**

A 31-year-old man has a 2-week history of hives. Individual lesions persist for less than 24 hours and are not worsened by cold, sunlight, or pressure. He has been taking diphenhydramine without relief.

ANSWER: The diagnosis is acute urticaria. Additional diagnostic studies are not indicated. Add an H_2-blocker.

Drug Allergy

Diagnosis

Immediate drug reactions (type I reactions) are usually IgE-mediated hypersensitivity reactions and cause symptoms of anaphylaxis within minutes to hours. Commonly implicated drugs are β-lactams, neuromuscular blocking agents, and platinum-containing chemotherapies.

Delayed drug reactions (type II-IV) typically present several days to months after treatment. Typical presentations include cytopenias (type II); vasculitis or serum sickness (type III); or rash, fever, and multiorgan involvement (type IV). Common causes include β-lactams, sulfa drugs, anticonvulsants, allopurinol, and abacavir. Radiocontrast agents, opiates, and NSAIDs cause a non–IgE-mediated degranulation of mast cells.

Penicillin is the most common self-reported medication allergy. Penicillin or one of its analogues should be avoided if the patient has a history of anaphylactic symptoms. If penicillin or one of its analogues must be used (treatment of neurosyphilis) in a patient with a penicillin allergy, choose skin testing, which identifies 95% of patients at risk for immediate reaction; do not select RAST or ELISA.

IgE-mediated cephalosporin reaction occurs in 2% of patients who are allergic to penicillin. Cephalosporins and carbapenems should be avoided in those with positive skin test for penicillin or convincing history of anaphylactic penicillin allergy.

Antibiotic therapy for syphilis or Lyme disease may precipitate the Jarisch-Herxheimer reaction, characterized by fever, headache, myalgia, rash, and hypotension. This reaction, related to dying spirochetes releasing endotoxin, begins within 2 hours of treatment, and resolves by 48 hours. Management is supportive. Continue antibiotic therapy.

STUDY TABLE: Common Drug-Mediated Skin Eruptions	
Type	**Description**
AGEP	Acute onset of widespread pustules, fever, leukocytosis, and possibly eosinophilia
	AGEP is usually self-limiting and clears without residual skin changes approximately 2 weeks after drug cessation
DRESS (also known as hypersensitivity syndrome)	Acute onset of generalized papular eruption, facial edema, fever, arthralgia, generalized lymphadenopathy, elevated serum aminotransferase levels, eosinophilia, and lymphocytosis
EM, SJS, TEN	Spectrum ranges from classic target lesions (EM), to involvement of mucous membranes with systemic symptoms (SJS), to a life-threatening loss of epidermis (TEN)
	SJS involves <10%, SJS/TEN overlap involves 10% to 30%, and TEN involves >30% detachment
Erythema nodosum	Tender subcutaneous nodules on lower leg; the eruption is often preceded by a prodrome of fever, malaise, and/or arthralgia
	Causes of EN fall into three broad categories: infections, drugs, and systemic diseases (usually inflammatory disorders)
Exfoliative and erythrodermic	Widespread generalized redness and scaling reaction
Fixed drug eruption	Discrete, often round or oval lesions that recur in exactly the same spot when rechallenged with the drug
Maculopapular and morbilliform (small discrete papules)	Most common type of drug reaction. Symmetric distribution, usually truncal, hardly ever on palms or soles; associated with fever and pruritus
Photosensitive skin reaction	Phototoxic reaction consists of severe sunburn after drug exposure (tetracycline)
	Photoallergic reaction presents as a rash after days or months of use (sulfonamides)
Red man syndrome	Body flushing, hypotension, and muscle pain associated with vancomycin and ciprofloxacin
	Not an allergic reaction
Urticarial	Second most common drug reaction type, with or without angioedema
AGEP = acute generalized exanthematous pustulosis.	

The most common drugs causing skin eruptions are antibiotics (penicillins and sulfa drugs) and anticonvulsants (phenytoin and carbamazepine).

The appearance of a maculopapular rash is associated with the use of ampicillin in EBV and CMV infections or underlying ALL. Duration of the rash is independent of whether the drug is continued. Subsequent reactions on re-exposure to the drug do not occur after resolution of the underlying medical condition.

Hypersensitivity is the most common cause of drug fever, and fever may be the only manifestation. Fever appears several days to 3 weeks after the drug has been started and resolves 1 to 3 days after drug withdrawal. Patients with HIV infection are more susceptible to drug reactions of all types, including fever.

◆ **DON'T BE TRICKED**

- The absence of eosinophilia does not rule out drug reaction or DRESS.

Therapy

Discontinue the offending medication. Treat anaphylaxis, if present, with epinephrine. AGEP is typically self-limited. Treat DRESS with glucocorticoids or IV immune globulin. SJS/TEN treatment is supportive (fluid and electrolyte management, wound care); IV immune globulin may decrease mortality, but the effect of glucocorticoids is uncertain.

Fixed Drug Eruption: Discrete round to oval lesions characteristic of a fixed drug eruption.

Drug Reaction with Eosinophilia and Systemic Symptoms: Acute facial edema in a patient with anticonvulsant-induced DRESS.

Morbilliform Drug Eruption: Morbilliform drug eruption consisting of symmetrically arranged erythematous macules and papules, some discrete and others confluent.

❖ **Test Yourself**

A 37-year-old man is prescribed ceftriaxone and a macrolide for CAP. Five days later, he is feeling better, coughs less, and produces less sputum, but he continues to have daily temperatures of up to 38.3 °C (100.9 °F).

ANSWER: Suspect drug fever for cause of persistent fever despite improvement in all other clinical parameters.

Pemphigus Vulgaris and Pemphigoid

Diagnosis

Pemphigus vulgaris often presents initially as painful, nonhealing oral erosions. Also look for flaccid, hemorrhagic, or seropurulent bullae and denuded areas that ooze serous fluid, bleed, or are covered with crusts. The esophagus and vulva may also be involved.

Look for a positive Nikolsky sign (erosion of normal-appearing skin by application of sliding pressure) or a positive Asboe-Hansen sign (ability to laterally extend bullae by applying gentle pressure).

STUDY TABLE: Differential Diagnosis of Blisters	
Condition	**Key Features**
Pemphigus vulgaris	Flaccid blisters that rapidly transform to large, weeping, denuded areas and appear most commonly on the oral mucosa, trunk, and proximal extremities. Nikolsky sign is positive. Only erosions may be clinically apparent. Direct immunofluorescence shows intercellular IgG deposition.
Paraneoplastic pemphigus	Polymorphous skin eruption marked by confluent erythema, bullae, erosions, and intractable stomatitis; patients also have painful oral, conjunctival, esophageal, and laryngeal erosions. Direct immunofluorescence shows IgG binding in intercellular pattern. Associated with lymphoma, CLL, and Castleman disease.
Bullous pemphigoid	Tense blisters most commonly seen in older adults on the trunk, limbs, and flexures. Oral lesions are uncommon. Nikolsky sign is negative. Direct immunofluorescence shows linear IgG deposition at the basement membrane.
Dermatitis herpetiformis	Severely pruritic vesicles on elbows, knees, back, and buttocks associated with celiac disease. Lesions occur in crops and are symmetrically distributed. Direct immunofluorescence shows granular IgA deposition.
Toxic epidermal necrolysis	A potentially lethal disease characterized by peeling of large areas of erythematous epidermis. Almost always due to a drug/medication. Immunopathologic findings are negative.
Porphyria cutanea tarda	Vesicles and bullae form in sun-exposed areas following minor trauma (typically back of the hands). Urine fluoresces dark orange with Wood lamp illumination. Direct immunofluorescence shows deposition of immune globulins and complement around the dermal capillaries and linear at the basement. Look for hepatitis C infection.

Pemphigus: This patient has multiple erosions and crusting with only an occasional intact blister; mucosal surfaces are typically involved.

Bullous Pemphigoid: An autoimmune blistering disease characterized by multiple tense bullae and occasional erosions; mucosal surfaces are typically not involved.

Dermatitis Herpetiformis: Dermatitis herpetiformis is characterized by pruritic papulovesicles over the external surface of the extremities and on the trunk; test for celiac disease.

Toxic Epidermal Necrolysis: Shedding of entire sheets of skin is characteristic of TEN.

◆ DON'T BE TRICKED

- The blisters of pemphigus vulgaris are so fragile that they are rarely seen; look instead for erosions, crusting, and sores in the mouth.

Therapy

Oral glucocorticoids are first-line therapy for pemphigus vulgaris and pemphigoid. Azathioprine and mycophenolate are often added as steroid-sparing agents. Patients who do not respond to conventional drug treatment may require plasmapheresis.

Dermatitis herpetiformis is always treated with gluten-free diet even in the absence of GI symptoms. Dapsone may be added initially to hasten resolution of symptoms.

❖ Test Yourself

A 72-year-old man has a 1-week history of a rash on his trunk and upper arms. He has lost 5 kg (11 lb). Oral erosions and numerous 1.5-cm bullae are present on his trunk. Pressure applied to the edge of one of the blisters causes it to extend laterally without eruption.

ANSWER: Choose either pemphigus vulgaris or paraneoplastic pemphigus. Biopsy is required for diagnosis.

Porphyria Cutanea Tarda: Bullae and erosions on the dorsal hands may be found in a patient with hepatitis C.

Erythema Multiforme

Diagnosis

Look for target-like erythematous macules or papules, each with an outer ring and a violaceous or dark center. Mucosal erosions may also be found. Recurrent HSV infection is the most common inciting factor. Drug allergy (most often to sulfonamides, penicillin, and phenytoin) is another common cause. Widespread blisters and mucosal lesions with systemic symptoms are seen in SJS, a severe form of EM.

Therapy

Treat EM by removing the offending agent, and provide supportive care. Depending on severity, antihistamines and topical or systemic glucocorticoids may be helpful. If EM is due to an active mycoplasma infection, antibacterial drugs may be helpful. Recurrent episodes of EM may be managed by antiviral suppressive therapy for HSV.

Erythema Multiforme: This flat, dull, red macule expands into a concentric ring, with the darkest part of the lesion in the center.

◆ **DON'T BE TRICKED**

- Don't confuse EM with erythema migrans, the rash of Lyme disease (red macule with central clearing as the macule expands).

❖ **Test Yourself**

A 24-year-old man is evaluated for target lesions on his hands and arms, which he says he has had twice before in recent years.

ANSWER: Diagnose recurrent EM due to HSV.

Stevens-Johnson Syndrome/ Toxic Epidermal Necrolysis

Diagnosis

SJS and TEN are severe mucocutaneous reactions, most commonly to a drug. These conditions are differentiated by the amount of epidermal detachment or necrosis.

- SJS: <10%
- TEN: >30%
- SJS-TEM overlap: 10% to 30%.

When due to drugs, SJS and TEN often occur between 4 and 28 days. Flu-like symptoms precede the skin eruption by 1 to 3 days. Initially, red-purple macules or papules develop on the trunk and extremities, which enlarge and coalesce. Skin pain is prominent. Vesicles, bullae, and Nikolsky sign are present. Two or more mucosal surfaces (eyes, nasopharynx, mouth, and genitals) are involved in >80% of patients.

Patients of Asian and South Asian ancestry positive for HLA-B*1502 have up to a 10% risk for SJS/TEN when exposed to aromatic anticonvulsants like carbamazepine, phenytoin, and phenobarbital. These patients should be tested for the presence of HLA-B*1502 antigen before these drugs are initiated.

Therapy

Stop the offending drug. Provide aggressive supportive care in a burn center or ICU. The role of glucocorticoids or IV immune globulin is controversial.

Dermatologic Signs of Systemic Disease

Diagnosis

Pruritus in the absence of primary skin lesions suggests an occult internal disease or medication effect. Causes of generalized pruritus without rash include liver disease (cholestatic and noncholestatic), CKD, Hodgkin disease, lymphoma, leukemia, and PV.

Specific dermatologic disorders may be associated with systemic diseases.

STUDY TABLE: Commonly Described Skin Lesions	
Description	**Diagnosis**
Violaceous papules around the nose including the ala, or periorbitally and periorificially (lupus pernio)	Sarcoidosis
Painful subcutaneous nodules or plaques with overlying red-brown discoloration, superimposed angulated purpuric patches with central necrosis	Calciphylaxis (end-stage kidney disease)
Tightening and thickening of the skin following gadolinium administration in patients with kidney disease (becoming rare now due to increased awareness by radiologists)	Nephrogenic systemic fibrosis
Painful, exudative ulcer with a purulent base and ragged, edematous, violaceous, "overhanging" border	Pyoderma gangrenosum
Pruritic eruption of papules and transient, almost immediately excoriated blisters on the elbows, knees, and buttocks	Dermatitis herpetiformis
Skin fragility and small, transient, easily-ruptured vesicles in sun-exposed areas, mainly on the hands, and hypertrichosis	Porphyria cutanea tarda
"Juicy" indurated edematous red-purple plaques and nodules, sharply demarcated from the adjacent skin	Sweet syndrome (acute febrile neutrophilic dermatosis)

STUDY TABLE: Important Associations	
If you see this...	**Consider diagnosis of...**
Porphyria cutanea tarda, palpable purpura	Hepatitis C
Severe or recalcitrant seborrheic dermatitis or abrupt onset of severe psoriasis	Initial manifestation of HIV infection
Erythema nodosum	IBD, TB, sarcoidosis, coccidioidomycosis, streptococcal infection; look particularly for Löfgren syndrome (bilateral hilar lymphadenopathy, erythema nodosum, and lower extremity arthralgia)
Dermatitis herpetiformis	Celiac disease
Livedo reticularis	Atheroemboli (previous vascular catheterization), thrombophilia, hyperviscosity syndrome, vasculitis
Pyoderma gangrenosum	IBD, inflammatory arthritis, lymphoproliferative disorders
Acanthosis nigricans (hyperpigmentation and velvety hyperkeratosis on flexural surfaces)	Diabetes
Xanthomas	Familial hypercholesterolemia

STUDY TABLE: Skin Conditions and Associated Malignancies

Skin Condition	Malignancy
Acanthosis nigricans	Gastric cancer, GU cancer
Acute febrile neutrophilic dermatosis (Sweet syndrome): acute onset of erythematous papules or plaques	Leukemia
Amyloidosis (primary systemic): pinch purpura, macroglossia, raccoon's eyes, and waxy skin	Multiple myeloma
Dermatomyositis: heliotrope-violaceous periorbital eruption; scaly red papules and plaques over bony prominences	Various cell types, but ovarian cancer is overrepresented
Paraneoplastic pemphigus: polymorphous erythematous plaques, blisters, and mucosal erosions	Lymphoma, Castleman disease, and CLL
Paget disease of the breast: nipple "eczema"	Breast cancer
Necrolytic migratory erythema: eczematous or psoriasiform eruption located around orifices and flexural and acral areas	Glucagonoma
Keratoderma of the palms and soles: bilateral thickening of the epidermis	SCC of the esophagus
Explosive onset of multiple pruritic seborrheic keratoses (Leser-Trélat sign)	GI adenocarcinomas
Rugal folds on palms and soles (tripe palms)	GI adenocarcinoma, SCC, head, neck, and lung.
Erythematous scaly plaque or patch on the perineal skin, scrotum, or perianal area (extramammary Paget disease)	GI or GU cancer
	Dermatosis is also a malignancy and requires removal

❖ **Test Yourself**

A 36-year-old woman has a rash around the left nipple that she attributes to jogging. No discharge, mass, or other abnormality of either breast is noted.

ANSWER: Select Paget disease of the breast, biopsy of the rash, and mammography.

A 25-year-old man presents with a painful leg ulcer and new-onset diarrhea.

ANSWER: The diagnosis is pyoderma gangrenosum. Select colonoscopy to diagnose IBD.

Acanthosis Nigricans: Acanthosis nigricans presents as a hyperpigmented hyperkeratosis on flexural surfaces and is most commonly associated with conditions such as diabetes mellitus and obesity.

Palpable Purpura: The hallmark of leukocytoclastic vasculitis is palpable purpura consisting of bright red macules and papules and occasionally hemorrhagic bullae confined to the lower leg and foot.

Erythema Nodosum: Tender, pink to dusky red, deep, subcutaneous nodules located on the anterior leg are characteristic of erythema nodosum.

Livedo Reticularis: Livedo reticularis is a net-like red or blue rash.

Pinch Purpura: "Raccoon's eyes" are characterized by purpura in the periorbital region; this sign is associated with amyloidosis.

Endocrinology and Metabolism

Diabetes Mellitus

Screening for Diabetes

The USPSTF recommends screening of all adults with risk factors for the development of diabetes.

Screen using the following tests: fasting plasma glucose, 2-hour postprandial glucose during an oral glucose tolerance test (OGTT), or hemoglobin A_{1c}. If 2 different tests are done simultaneously and both are abnormal, diagnose diabetes. If only 1 of the 2 tests is abnormal, repeat the abnormal test.

◆ **DON'T BE TRICKED**
- A random plasma glucose level ≥200 mg/dL with hyperglycemic symptoms is diagnostic of diabetes and does not warrant repeat measurement.

STUDY TABLE: Diagnosis and Classification of Type 2 Diabetes Mellitus				
Diagnosis	**Fasting Glucose**	**Random Glucose**	**2-Hour Glucose During OGTT**	**Hemoglobin A_{1c}**
Increased Risk for Diabetes (Prediabetes)	100-125 mg/dL	140-199 mg/dL	140-199 mg/dL	5.7%-6.4%
Diabetes	≥126 mg/dL	≥200 mg/dL with symptoms	≥200 mg/dL	≥6.5%

Type 1 Diabetes Mellitus

Type 1 diabetes is characterized by a beta cell destructive process that may eventually lead to absolute insulin deficiency. The onset of type 1 diabetes is typically abrupt and severe, with marked hyperglycemia developing over several days to weeks, and may be associated with a precipitating event, such as infection, pregnancy, or MI. Look for fatigue, polyuria, polydipsia, blurring of vision, weight loss, and dehydration.

More than 90% of cases of type 1 diabetes are autoimmune (type 1A). Several autoantibodies are directed against beta cells or their products. Measuring antibodies to GAD65 and IA-2 are recommended for initial confirmation. Approximately 20% of patients with type 1 diabetes develop other organ-specific autoimmune diseases, such as celiac disease, Graves disease, hypothyroidism, Addison disease, pernicious anemia, and vitiligo.

Type 1B diabetes is idiopathic, has no autoimmune markers, and occurs more commonly in patients of Asian or African ancestry. Some older patients with diabetes have autoimmune beta-cell destruction, albeit of a more gradually progressive nature, termed latent autoimmune diabetes of adulthood (LADA).

◆ **DON'T BE TRICKED**
- Look for other autoimmune diseases in patients with type 1 diabetes, including hypothyroidism and adrenal insufficiency.

Type 2 Diabetes Mellitus

Type 2 diabetes is characterized by a combination of insulin resistance and a beta-cell secretory defect. With time, progressive beta-cell dysfunction can develop, leading to absolute insulin deficiency.

In general, patients with type 2 diabetes present to medical attention less dramatically than those with type 1 diabetes. DKA is rare because patients maintain some degree of insulin secretion allowing for suppression of lipolysis. Because symptoms may be subtle, the time to diagnosis may be delayed. Consequently, approximately 20% of patients with type 2 diabetes have microvascular complications of the disease at presentation; an even higher percentage may have CAD or peripheral vascular disease. Most patients with type 2 diabetes are obese or at least have abdominal obesity. Characteristic findings of long-standing diabetes include:

- polyuria, polyphagia, and polydipsia
- retinal microaneurysms, dot-and-blot hemorrhages, macular edema
- symmetric sensory "stocking-glove" peripheral neuropathy
- cardiovascular and kidney disease

Nonproliferative Diabetic Retinopathy: Dot-and-blot hemorrhages and clusters of hard, yellowish exudates characteristic of nonproliferative diabetic retinopathy.

Five percent of patients with diabetes in the United States have an autosomal dominant form of the disease known as maturity-onset diabetes of youth (MODY). Presentation is generally before age 25 years.

Therapy

Intensive lifestyle modification (exercise, weight loss) is appropriate for all patients with prediabetes or type 2 diabetes. Metformin reduces the risk of diabetes in patients with prediabetes, although not as effectively as lifestyle interventions. Bariatric procedures can be considered in obese patients with type 2 diabetes.

Blood glucose monitoring includes self-monitoring of blood glucose (SMBG), hemoglobin A_{1c}, or continuous glucose monitoring.

- Obtain SMBG for patients on multiple daily injection insulin therapy or continuous subcutaneous insulin infusion therapy.
- Obtain postprandial blood glucose levels in patients with at-goal preprandial readings but with hemoglobin A_{1c} not at goal.
- Obtain overnight blood glucose monitoring to detect hypoglycemia or dawn phenomenon.

A reasonable goal for most patients is a hemoglobin A_{1c} <7.0% (guidelines vary).

Patients with type 1 diabetes are treated with intensive insulin therapy. Intensive insulin therapy includes intermediate or long-acting insulin for basal coverage and preprandial injections throughout the day with analog or regular insulin. Intensive insulin therapy can also include continuous subcutaneous insulin infusion therapy with meal-time boluses with an insulin pump.

Basal insulin dose accounts for half of the total daily dose of insulin, while the remaining insulin is divided to cover the preprandial doses. Examples of basal insulin options:

- Insulin glargine or insulin detemir: A single 10 PM dose controls nocturnal plasma glucose levels and glucose levels between meals. It also counters the early morning rise in glucose level ("dawn phenomenon") caused by hepatic gluconeogenesis.
- Isophane (NPH) intermediate-acting insulin: This insulin can be used in the morning and evening to provide basal plasma insulin levels and to suppress hepatic gluconeogenesis.

Examples of short-acting preprandial insulin options:

- Insulin aspart, insulin glulisine, and insulin lispro: Rapid-acting insulin given 5 to 15 minutes before meals to modulate the postprandial rise in glucose level.
- Regular insulin: Given 30 minutes before meals to prevent postprandial excursions in blood glucose.

Insulin pumps: Subcutaneous infusion of rapid-acting insulin is delivered continuously for basal insulin requirements and given in intermittent boluses for prandial needs.

◆ **DON'T BE TRICKED**

- If a patient is nonadherent with multiple insulin injections, adherence is unlikely to increase because a pump is prescribed.
- Hemoglobin A_{1c} will be falsely low in patients with hemolytic anemia, patients taking erythropoietin, or with renal failure.

Correctional insulin is the use of additional analog or regular insulin above usual dose to treat preprandial glucose that is not at target. A typical correction for type 1 diabetes is an additional 1 U of insulin for every 50 mg/dL above the preprandial target.

STUDY TABLE: Adjusting Insulin Dose in Diabetes Mellitus	
Condition	**Cause**
Fasting hyperglycemia	Not enough bedtime basal insulin
Prelunch hyperglycemia	Not enough rapid-acting insulin at breakfast or not enough morning NPH insulin
Predinner hyperglycemia	Not enough rapid-acting insulin at lunch or not enough morning NPH insulin
Bedtime hyperglycemia	Not enough rapid-acting insulin at dinner
Fasting or nocturnal hypoglycemia	Too much basal insulin at bedtime
Prelunch hypoglycemia	Too much rapid-acting insulin at breakfast or too much morning NPH insulin
Predinner or bedtime hypoglycemia	Too much rapid-acting insulin at lunch or dinner or too much morning NPH

Hypoglycemia unawareness describes the presence of severely low plasma glucose levels that occur without warning symptoms followed by sudden loss of consciousness. Treat immediately with rapid-acting carbohydrates or a glucagon injection followed by food. Lowering the insulin dose and allowing the average plasma glucose level to increase for several weeks restores sensitivity to hypoglycemia.

STUDY TABLE: Therapy for Type 2 Diabetes Mellitus	
First-Tier Validated Therapy (in suggested order)	**Notes**
1. Life style changes plus metformin	Avoid metformin in patients with a creatinine level >1.5 mg/dL, heart and liver failure, or alcoholism, and stop before procedures that require radiocontrast administration
2. Add basal insulin (± preprandial insulin) or add sulfonylurea	Insulin and sulfonylureas can cause hypoglycemia

STUDY TABLE: Adverse Effects Associated with Common Noninsulin Diabetes Medications		
Class	**Adverse Effect**	**Caution/Avoid**
Sulfonylureas (glipizide, glimepiride, others)	Weight gain, hypoglycemia, skin rashes	Reduced drug clearance in kidney failure for some sulfonylureas
Biguanides (metformin)	Diarrhea, abdominal discomfort, lactic acidosis	Contraindicated in progressive heart, liver, or kidney failure
		Avoid in the setting of IV iodinated contrast
α-Glucosidase inhibitors (acarbose, miglitol, voglibose)	Abdominal discomfort	Avoid in renal failure
Thiazolidinediones (rosiglitazone, pioglitazone)	Weight gain, edema, HF, macular edema, osteoporosis	Cardiovascular events and mortality increased with rosiglitazone
Meglitinides (repaglinide, nateglinide)	Weight gain, hypoglycemia	Reduced drug clearance in kidney failure
Amylinomimetics (pramlintide)	Nausea, vomiting	Increases hypoglycemia associated with insulin
GLP-1 mimetics (exenatide, liraglutide)	Nausea, vomiting	Possible increased risk of pancreatitis and kidney failure
DPP-4 inhibitors (sitagliptin, saxagliptin, vildagliptin, linagliptin, alogliptin)	Nausea, skin rashes, increased risk of infections	Possible increased risk of pancreatitis, HF exacerbation
SGLT2 inhibitors (dapagliflozin and canagliflozin)	Increased genital candidal infections and UTIs	Hypoglycemia with insulin secretagogues and insulin
DPP-4 = dipeptidyl peptidase-4; GLP-1 = glucagon-like peptide-1; SGLT2 = sodium-glucose transporter-2.		

If weight loss is a desired effect, GLP-1 mimetics, pramlintide, and SGLT2 inhibitors are the best choices.

STUDY TABLE: Screening Recommendations for Chronic Complications of Diabetes

Complication	Clinical Situation	Start	Frequency	Screening Test
Retinopathy	Type 1 diabetes	At 5 years after diagnosis	Annually	Comprehensive eye examination
	Type 2 diabetes	At diagnosis	Annually	Comprehensive eye examination
	Pregnancy	First trimester	Every trimester	Comprehensive eye examination
Nephropathy	Type 1 diabetes	At 5 years after diagnosis	Annually	Albumin-to-creatinine ratio
	Type 2 diabetes	At diagnosis	Annually	Albumin-to-creatinine ratio
Neuropathy (distal symmetric polyneuropathy)	Type 1 diabetes	At 5 years after diagnosis	Annually	10 g monofilament, 128-Hz tuning fork, ankle reflex
	Type 2 diabetes	At diagnosis	Annually	10 g monofilament, tuning fork, ankle reflex
Cardiovascular disease	Hypertension	At diagnosis	Every visit	BP measurement
	Dyslipidemia	At diagnosis	Annually	Fasting lipid profile

STUDY TABLE: Treatment of Diabetes Complications

Condition	Goal or Indication	Treatment
Hypertension	BP goal <140/90 mm Hg (JNC 8); <140/80 mm Hg (ADA); consider <130/80 mm Hg for nephropathy or some young patients (ADA)	Any first-line drug (JNC 8) ACE inhibitor or ARB (ADA)
Diabetes and average cardiovascular risk	Age >40 years, diabetes, and a 10-year ASCVD risk <7.5%	Moderate-intensity statin
Diabetes and increased cardiovascular risk	CAD, peripheral vascular disease, or ASCVD risk ≥7.5%	High-intensity statin
Nephropathy	Urine albumin excretion ≥30 mg/g of creatinine	ACE inhibitor or ARB BP <130/80 (ADA)
Diabetic retinopathy	Proliferative and nonproliferative retinopathy	Excellent blood glucose and BP control and smoking cessation Panretinal laser photocoagulation for PDR and severe NPDR Intraocular injections of bevacizumab or ranibizumab for severe NPDR and PDR or macular edema
Diabetic peripheral neuropathy	Numbness, tingling, burning, heaviness, pain, or sensitivity in stocking-glove distribution	Amitriptyline, venlafaxine, duloxetine, paroxetine, pregabalin, gabapentin, valproate, or capsaicin cream
Sexual dysfunction	Erectile dysfunction	Oral phosphodiesterase inhibitor (sildenafil, vardenafil, tadalafil)
Gastroparesis	Early satiety, nausea and vomiting	Small feedings; metoclopramide or erythromycin
Diabetic foot	Ulcer or osteomyelitis	See Infectious Disease, Diabetic Foot Infections

ADA = American Diabetes Association; NPDR = nonproliferative diabetic retinopathy; PDR = proliferative diabetic retinopathy.

◆ DON'T BE TRICKED

- Do not treat diabetic mononeuropathy (e.g., third nerve palsy); symptoms resolve spontaneously.

✣ Test Yourself

A 29-year-old woman with a 10-year history of type 1 diabetes has nocturnal hypoglycemia. Her insulin schedule includes 24 units NPH insulin/10 units regular insulin before breakfast and 14 units NPH insulin/10 units regular insulin before dinner. Her hemoglobin A$_{1c}$ is 7.2%. What change should be made to her insulin regimen?

ANSWER: Two answers are possible: delay the NPH insulin until bedtime or (an even better choice) stop the NPH insulin and substitute insulin glargine at bedtime.

A 58-year-old man with type 2 diabetes has a hemoglobin A$_{1c}$ value >9%. He takes metformin 1000 mg/d and glyburide 10 mg/d. His fasting and preprandial plasma glucose levels are >130 mg/dL.

ANSWER: Add evening basal insulin to control his hyperglycemia.

Proliferative Diabetic Retinopathy: A network of new vessels (neovascularization) is shown protruding from the optic nerve.

Hyperglycemic Hyperosmolar Syndrome

Diagnosis

Hyperglycemic hyperosmolar syndrome is defined as a plasma osmolality >320 mOsm/kg H$_2$O, a plasma glucose level 600 mg/dL, either no or low serum levels of ketones, and a relatively normal arterial pH and bicarbonate level. The diagnosis is considered in any older adult patient with altered mental status and dehydration.

Therapy

Manage hyperglycemic hyperosmolar syndrome mainly by identifying the underlying precipitating illness and restoring the contracted plasma volume. Choose normal saline first to replenish the extracellular space. When BP is restored and urine output is established, administer hypotonic solutions. Administer IV insulin only after expansion of the intravascular space has begun. After the plasma glucose level decreases to <200 mg/dL and the patient is eating, begin subcutaneous insulin injections.

Diabetic Ketoacidosis

Diagnosis

DKA is the most life-threatening acute complication of diabetes and is often the presenting manifestation of type 1 diabetes. The major manifestations of DKA (hyperglycemia, ketosis, and dehydration) are directly or indirectly related to insulin deficiency.

Laboratory findings include a plasma glucose level ≥250 mg/dL, arterial blood pH ≤7.30, bicarbonate level ≤15 mEq/L, widened anion gap, and positive serum ketone levels. Evaluate patients for underlying precipitants of DKA, such as medication nonadherence, infection, and MI.

Therapy

Give normal saline solution for immediate volume replacement. Switch to 0.45% sodium chloride after the initial bolus if the serum sodium level is high or normal. Then give:

- insulin infusion (delay if serum potassium level is <3.3 mEq/L)
- potassium replacement when the serum potassium level is <5.5 mEq/L
- glucose infusion (5% dextrose with 0.45% normal saline) when the plasma glucose level is <250 mg/dL
- continuation of insulin infusion and glucose infusion until the serum anion gap is normal

Treatment of severe acidosis with bicarbonate is controversial and evidence of benefit is lacking.

◆ **DON'T BE TRICKED**

- DKA can present with abdominal pain.
- Reducing the insulin infusion before complete clearing of ketones will cause a relapse of DKA.

Diabetes Care for Hospitalized Patients

Therapy

Insulin is the preferred therapy for achieving inpatient glycemic control. Critically ill patients with type 2 diabetes are treated with IV insulin infusion when plasma glucose levels exceed 180 to 200 mg/dL. Glucose goals are 140 to 200 mg/dL.

For non–critically ill patients, the insulin regimen should incorporate both basal and prandial coverage. Prandial coverage can be supplemented with additional insulin (correction factor insulin) for preprandial hyperglycemia.

◆ **DON'T BE TRICKED**

- Do not select sliding scale insulin alone to treat in-hospital hyperglycemia.

Oral agents and noninsulin injectable agents do not have safety or efficacy data in the hospital setting. In particular, hold metformin in patients who are hemodynamically unstable or at risk for AKI. Continuation of oral agents can be considered in a stable patient with glycemic control at goal and no anticipated changes in nutrition or hemodynamic status.

Pregnancy and Diabetes

Screening

Screen women for gestational diabetes at 24 to 28 weeks of gestation with the 75-gram 2-hour OGTT.

◆ **DON'T BE TRICKED**

- Women with a history of gestational diabetes are at very high risk for developing type 2 diabetes and require annual screening following delivery.

Therapy

Untreated gestational diabetes is associated with congenital malformations and increased fetal loss. Lowering the hemoglobin A_{1c} value to within 1% of normal decreases the risk of congenital malformations and fetal loss. Try lifestyle interventions as initial therapy, with the addition of insulin if glycemic targets are not met. Glycemic targets in pregnancy include preprandial plasma glucose <95 mg/dL, 1-hour postprandial values <140 mg/dL, and 2-hour postprandial values <120 mg/dL.

Management strategies in pregnant women are different from those in other patients with diabetes:

- Insulin should replace oral hypoglycemic agents.
- ACE inhibitors, ARBs, and cholesterol-lowering drugs should be stopped before pregnancy.
- A comprehensive eye examination should be done once per trimester.

Employ aggressive control of BP to avoid worsening of nephropathy and retinopathy. Antihypertensive agents that can be safely used during pregnancy include methyldopa, β-blockers (except atenolol), calcium channel blockers, and hydralazine.

Hypoglycemia in Patients Without Diabetes

Diagnosis

In persons without diabetes, hypoglycemia is defined as a plasma glucose level <70 mg/dL. Look for the Whipple triad:

- symptoms of hypoglycemia
- low plasma glucose levels
- resolution of symptoms after glucose administration

Hypoglycemic disorders are classified as postprandial or fasting. A common cause of postprandial hypoglycemia is previous gastrectomy or gastric bypass surgery. Clinical manifestations include hypoglycemia approximately 30 to 60 minutes after meals due to rapid intestinal absorption of glucose triggering excessive secretion of insulin.

Fasting hypoglycemia is associated with several serious conditions.

STUDY TABLE: Diagnosis of Nondiabetic Fasting Hypoglycemia	
Condition	**Diagnosis**
Surreptitious use of oral hypoglycemic agents	Patient has access to hypoglycemic agents. Serum C-peptide levels are inappropriately elevated at time of hypoglycemia. Perform urine screen for sulfonylurea and meglitinide metabolites.
Surreptitious use of insulin	Patient has access to insulin. Serum C-peptide levels are low at time of hypoglycemia.
Insulinoma	Perform 72-hour fast and document fasting plasma glucose level <45 mg/dL and serum insulin >5-6 mU/L and elevated C-peptide levels. If positive, schedule abdominal CT.
Substrate deficiency	Starvation, hepatic failure, or sepsis; suppressed hepatic glucose production (alcoholism, cortisol or GH deficiencies)

Begin the evaluation of all patients with fasting hypoglycemia with screening for surreptitious use of a sulfonylurea or insulin.

MEN1 can present as hyperparathyroidism, pituitary neoplasms, or pancreatic NETs (gastrinomas that can cause PUD and insulinomas that can cause hypoglycemia).

◆ **DON'T BE TRICKED**

- Home glucose meters may be inaccurate in the hypoglycemic range.
- Asymptomatic hypoglycemia with a plasma glucose level <60 mg/dL is often found after fasting in patients without underlying disease and does not require evaluation.

Therapy

Treat acute hypoglycemia with oral carbohydrates, IV glucose, or IM glucagon.

For management of postprandial hypoglycemia associated with previous gastrectomy or gastric bypass surgery, choose small mixed meals containing protein, fat, and high-fiber complex carbohydrates.

❖ **Test Yourself**

A previously healthy 28-year-old woman is found unconscious on the ward where she works as a registered nurse. Her plasma glucose level is 28 mg/dL. She regains consciousness following IV glucose administration. Serum insulin level is 42 mU/L (normal, 2-20 mU/L), and serum C-peptide level is 7.2 ng/mL (normal, 0.9-4.0 ng/mL).

ANSWER: Select factitious hypoglycemia and screening for surreptitious ingestion of sulfonylureas. Demographically, women in the health professions are most likely to self-induce hypoglycemia.

Hypopituitarism

Diagnosis

Hypopituitarism may be partial or complete. Most commonly, hypopituitarism is the result of a pituitary tumor that causes progressive hypofunction by applying pressure to the normal gland. Pituitary surgery and cranial irradiation are other common causes. Pituitary apoplexy causes acute hypopituitarism, results from sudden pituitary hemorrhage or infarction, and is often associated with sudden headache, visual change, ophthalmoplegia, and altered mental status.

Postpartum pituitary necrosis (Sheehan syndrome) is due to silent pituitary infarction and is usually associated with obstetric hemorrhage and hypotension. Acutely, vascular collapse may occur, but more commonly the syndrome presents with amenorrhea, a postpartum inability to lactate, and fatigue.

Lymphocytic hypophysitis causes hypopituitarism and, possibly, symptoms of a mass lesion. Most cases of lymphocytic hypophysitis occur during or after pregnancy.

Symptoms of anterior hypopituitarism are identical to primary target–organ hypofunction. However, the presence of headache and loss of peripheral vision suggest a pituitary mass effect.

Look for:

- history of cranial radiation therapy or pituitary surgery
- difficult delivery with hemorrhage or hypotension
- amenorrhea, loss of libido, or erectile dysfunction
- fatigue, nausea, vomiting, weight loss, or abdominal pain (ACTH deficiency)
- cold intolerance, weight gain, or constipation (TSH deficiency)
- loss of muscle mass (GH deficiency)
- polydipsia, polyuria, and nocturia (DI secondary to ADH deficiency)
- visual field diagram showing bitemporal loss of vision (mass effect on the optic chiasm)

Diagnosis is confirmed by documenting target-organ hormone deficiency and a corresponding low or "normal" serum pituitary hormone level. Stimulation testing may be needed to document hypopituitarism.

STUDY TABLE: Key Hormone Tests for Hypopituitarism	
Hormone	**Findings**
GH	Depressed IGF-1
	Diminished response to insulin tolerance test (insulin-induced hypoglycemia)
FSH/LH	Depressed FSH, LH, and estradiol or testosterone levels
TSH	Depressed free T_4 and TSH
ACTH	Low cortisol level and depressed ACTH
	Depressed response of 11-deoxycortisol and cortisol to metyrapone
	Positive cortisol response to ACTH
Prolactin	Level may be elevated from loss of tonic inhibition

After documenting hypopituitarism or hyperprolactinemia, select MRI of the pituitary gland.

◆ DON'T BE TRICKED

- Measurement of serum FSH/LH levels is not needed in women who have normal menstrual cycles.
- Do not measure GH, because its release is pulsatile; measure the serum marker of GH instead (IGF-1).

Therapy

Hydrocortisone is indicated for patients with adrenal insufficiency. Androgen replacement therapy is appropriate for men with hypogonadism, and estrogen replacement therapy is used for premenopausal women with hypogonadism. Consider GH replacement for biochemically confirmed deficiency and consistent symptoms.

Pituitary apoplexy requires acute administration of glucocorticoids until acute adrenal insufficiency has been ruled out and may also require urgent neurosurgical decompression.

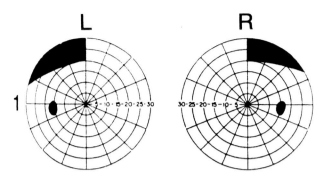

Visual Field Defects: Bitemporal quadrant visual field defects secondary to a pituitary mass.

◆ DON'T BE TRICKED

- Thyroxine dosing for central hypothyroidism is based on serum free T_4 rather than TSH levels.
- T_4 replacement is indicated only after hypoadrenalism has been ruled out or treated.

❖ Test Yourself

A 65-year-old man was diagnosed with SCLC 20 years ago and received chemotherapy and chest and cranial irradiation. Physical examination shows hypotension, tachycardia, and small testes. Serum sodium is 123 mEq/L.

ANSWER: The diagnosis is hypopituitarism. Select immediate replacement with stress doses of hydrocortisone followed by confirmatory testing.

Pituitary Tumors

Diagnosis

Pituitary tumors are benign adenomas that originate from one of the different anterior pituitary cell types. They are classified based on size as microadenomas (<10 mm) or macroadenomas (≥10 mm). Pituitary adenomas become symptomatic by two different mechanisms:

- mass effect causing hypopituitarism (anterior hormone deficiencies more common than posterior), headaches, visual disturbance/visual field defects, and cranial nerve dysfunction
- endocrine hyperfunction caused by excess secretion by the tumor

◆ DON'T BE TRICKED

- The pituitary gland is enlarged diffusely in untreated primary hypothyroidism and normally during pregnancy.

STUDY TABLE: Diagnosis of Pituitary Tumors		
If you see this...	**Think this...**	**Order this...**
Galactorrhea, amenorrhea	Prolactinoma	Serum prolactin level
Enlargement of hands, feet, nose, lips, or tongue; increased spacing of teeth	Acromegaly	Serum IGF-1
		OGTT (fails to suppress GH)
Proximal muscle weakness, facial rounding, centripetal obesity, purple striae, diabetes mellitus, and hypertension	Cushing disease	24-hour urine cortisol excretion or late night salivary cortisol level (elevated), serum ACTH level (elevated or inappropriately "normal")

Order MRI if testing indicates hormonal hypersecretion due to a pituitary source. If mass effect is the presenting symptom (headache, visual disturbances), obtain MRI first and endocrine testing later.

Screen patients with at least one component of MEN1 (usually hyperparathyroidism), and a family history of MEN1, for a pituitary adenoma.

Test all patients with an incidentally discovered pituitary adenoma for hormone hypersecretion.

Psychotropic agents, tricyclic antidepressants, antiseizure medications, metoclopramide and domperidone, calcium channel blockers, methyldopa, opiates, and protease inhibitors can cause hyperprolactinemia.

◆ DON'T BE TRICKED

- Hyperprolactinemia caused by drugs and other nonprolactinoma conditions is usually <150 ng/mL.
- Obtain a pregnancy test in all women with hyperprolactinemia.
- Obtain a serum TSH level in all patients with hyperprolactinemia (hypothyroidism can cause hyperprolactinemia).

Prolactinoma: Discrete area of hypolucency (*arrow*) in otherwise normal-sized pituitary gland of homogeneous density.

Therapy

Choose observation for women with microprolactinoma and normal menses. Otherwise, choose a dopamine agonist (cabergoline preferred to bromocriptine) for symptomatic prolactinoma. Consider withdrawal of dopamine agonist therapy for prolactinomas no longer visible on neuroimaging if the prolactin level has normalized. Close follow-up is required because of recurrence rates of up to 50%.

Choose surgery for adenomas secreting GH, ACTH, or TSH; for adenomas associated with mass effect, visual field defects, or hypopituitarism; and for prolactinomas unresponsive to dopamine agonists.

Radiation therapy may be indicated for the management of hormonal hypersecretion that persists after surgery or to treat residual tumor after resection. It may also be given as primary therapy for patients who are not surgical candidates. Radiation therapy frequently results in hypopituitarism.

❖ Test Yourself

A 32-year-old woman has a 4-mm hypointense area in the pituitary gland discovered incidentally on an MRI. Medical history, including menstrual function, and physical examination are normal. The serum prolactin level and thyroid function tests are normal.

ANSWER: The patient has an incidental nonfunctioning pituitary adenoma. Repeat the MRI and recheck the prolactin level in 6 months.

Diabetes Insipidus

Diagnosis

DI is characterized by an inability to concentrate urine because of insufficient arginine vasopressin (AVP, ADH) release (central DI) or activity (nephrogenic DI). Signs and symptoms of central DI are cravings for water or cold liquids, urinary frequency, nocturia, and depending on mass effect of a pituitary tumor, visual field deficits. Important clues are a history of head trauma, recent neurosurgery, pituitary mass lesion, evidence of anterior hypopituitarism (adrenal insufficiency, hypothyroidism), history of an infiltrative disorder (such as sarcoidosis), kidney disease (tubulointerstitial disease), or medications such as lithium.

Patients typically have large-volume polyuria with urine osmolality <200 mOsm/kg H_2O. Measure a plasma glucose level to rule out diabetes mellitus and a serum calcium level to rule out hypercalcemia. The inability to increase the concentration of the urine during a water deprivation test confirms the diagnosis. When DI has been confirmed, a desmopressin challenge test is done to differentiate between central and nephrogenic forms. If the desmopressin challenge test is positive (urine concentrates, indicating central DI), order an MRI of the pituitary gland. If the test is negative (urine does not concentrate, indicating nephrogenic DI), order kidney ultrasonography.

Therapy

Treatment of DI depends on the cause.

STUDY TABLE: Treating Diabetes Insipidus	
If you see...	**Choose...**
DI after neurosurgery or head trauma	If unable to drink, 5% dextrose in 0.45% sodium chloride IV
	Add desmopressin if urine output is high or hypernatremia develops
Chronic central DI	Intranasal or oral desmopressin
Lithium-induced nephrogenic DI	Stop lithium or add amiloride
Non-drug-induced nephrogenic DI	Thiazide diuretic and salt restriction

❖ **Test Yourself**

A previously healthy 27-year-old woman has a 1-month history of polydipsia and polyuria. She has had amenorrhea since giving birth 9 months ago. The plasma glucose level is 90 mg/dL, urine output is 4 L/d, and urine osmolality is 95 mOsm/kg H_2O.

ANSWER: The patient has probable central DI. Select a water deprivation test.

Empty Sella Syndrome

Diagnosis

Empty sella is diagnosed when the normal pituitary gland is not visualized or is excessively small on MRI. Causes include:

- increased CSF entering and enlarging the sella
- tumor
- previous pituitary surgery, radiation, or infarction

In asymptomatic persons, obtain measures of cortisol, TSH, and free (or total) T_4. A patient with symptoms of hormone deficiency requires testing of all pituitary hormones.

If examination reveals normal hormone functioning, repeated imaging is not necessary.

Hyperthyroidism

Diagnosis

The term *thyrotoxicosis* encompasses any cause of thyroid hormone excess, including primary and secondary hyperthyroidism, excessive thyroid hormone release due to thyroid destruction, and excessive exogenous thyroid hormone ingestion. The term *hyperthyroidism* refers specifically to disorders of increased thyroid hormone production and release, such as destructive thyroiditis, Graves disease, autonomous thyroid nodules, and toxic multinodular goiter.

Thyrotoxicosis occurs in destructive thyroiditis because thyroid damage results in release of preformed thyroid hormone into the circulation. Forms of destructive thyroiditis include subacute (de Quervain), silent (painless), and postpartum thyroiditis. Subacute thyroiditis is a nonautoimmune inflammation that generally presents with a firm and painful thyroid gland. Postpartum thyroiditis is a painless autoimmune thyroiditis occurring within a few months of delivery. Permanent hypothyroidism may follow all forms of destructive thyroiditis.

Look for symptoms of thyrotoxicosis:

- nervousness, emotional lability
- increased sweating, heat intolerance
- palpitations
- increased defecation
- weight loss
- menstrual irregularity

Look for signs of thyrotoxicosis:

- tachycardia
- lid lag
- fine tremor
- muscle wasting, proximal muscle weakness
- hyperreflexia

Ancillary laboratory testing may reveal:

- mild hypercalcemia
- elevated alkaline phosphatase level
- low total and HDL cholesterol levels

The most common causes of hyperthyroidism are Graves disease and toxic adenoma(s). Physical examination findings specific for Graves disease include goiter, ophthalmopathy (proptosis, chemosis, and extraocular muscle palsy), and pretibial myxedema.

Older adult patients with hyperthyroidism may present with depression, AF, and HF.

Order serum TSH and free T_4 levels to make the diagnosis of thyrotoxicosis. If TSH is suppressed but T_4 is normal, order free T_3 to diagnose T_3 toxicosis (rare).

STUDY TABLE: Interpreting Thyroid Function Tests in Hyperthyroidism	
If you see this...	**Choose this...**
↓ TSH, ↑ free T_4	Primary hyperthyroidism
↓ TSH, ↑ T_3, normal free T_4	Primary hyperthyroidism with T_3 toxicosis
↓ TSH, normal T_3 and free T_4, without symptoms	Subclinical hyperthyroidism
↑ TSH, ↑ T_3, ↑ free T_4	Secondary hyperthyroidism from a pituitary tumor (central hyperthyroidism)

A thyroid scan and radioactive iodine uptake test can differentiate thyrotoxicosis caused by increased production of thyroid hormone (high uptake) from thyroiditis or surreptitious ingestion of thyroid hormone (low uptake).

STUDY TABLE: Radioactive Iodine Uptake and Scan Interpretation	
Result	**Diagnosis**
Diffuse homogeneous increased uptake	Graves disease
Patchy areas of increased uptake	Toxic multinodular goiter

(Continued on next page)

STUDY TABLE: Radioactive Iodine Uptake and Scan Interpretation (*Continued*)	
Result	**Diagnosis**
Focal increased uptake with decreased uptake in the rest of the gland	Solitary adenoma
Decreased or no uptake	Iodine load (IV contrast or amiodarone)
	Thyroiditis (silent, subacute, postpartum, or amiodarone induced)
	Surreptitious ingestion of excessive thyroid hormone

Thyroglobulin levels can be elevated in both hyperthyroidism and thyroiditis. Intake of exogenous thyroid hormone suppresses thyroglobulin levels, which makes its measurement useful in patients with thyrotoxicosis due to surreptitious use of thyroid hormone.

An elevated serum ESR supports thyroiditis, whereas TSH-receptor antibodies are associated with Graves disease. However, antibodies need not be checked routinely in the evaluation of hyperthyroidism unless the diagnosis is unclear.

Thyroid storm is the development of life-threatening hyperthyroidism associated with cardiac decompensation, fever, delirium, and psychosis. It may occur following surgery, infection, or administration of an acute iodine load (contrast agents) and may also develop in patients with untreated Graves disease. Thyroid storm is a clinical diagnosis; no level of thyroid hormone elevation is diagnostic.

Therapy

Available strategies for managing hyperthyroidism include antithyroid drugs, radioactive iodine therapy (^{131}I), and thyroid surgery. Radioactive iodine therapy is associated with few adverse effects and preferred in most patients but may lead to painful radiation thyroiditis and sialadenitis; it is not used during pregnancy or when breastfeeding. Choose ^{131}I therapy or surgery to treat toxic multinodular goiter or toxic adenoma. With ^{131}I ablation, hyperactive nodules take up iodine preferentially, while suppressed normal tissue receives minimal radiation exposure. Treatment frequently restores euthyroidism.

Antithyroid drugs may lead to a drug-free remission of Graves disease in 30% to 50% of patients after treating for 1 year. Antithyroid drugs may also be used short term as a bridge to more definitive therapy (radioactive iodine or thyroidectomy).

STUDY TABLE: Comparison of Antithyroid Drugs		
Treatment	**Indicated for...**	**Watch for...**
Methimazole	First-line antithyroid medication for most patients	Agranulocytosis, drug rash, hepatotoxicity
Propylthiouracil	Treatment of choice in first trimester of pregnancy; preferred in thyroid storm (inhibits peripheral T_4 to T_3 conversion)	Same as methimazole, except more frequent hepatotoxicity

A thyroidectomy is preferred when definitive therapy for hyperthyroidism is required in a patient with severe Graves ophthalmopathy. Thyroidectomy may also be considered if radioactive iodine or antithyroid cannot be given or are not tolerated.

STUDY TABLE: Management of Thyrotoxicosis	
If you see this...	**Choose this...**
Sympathetic nervous system symptoms	Atenolol or propranolol
Preparation for thyroidectomy	Methimazole
Severe Graves ophthalmopathy	Methimazole or thyroidectomy
	Avoid radioactive iodine (may cause worsening of ophthalmopathy unless pretreated with glucocorticoids)
Pregnancy	Propylthiouracil in first trimester of pregnancy, methimazole thereafter
	Radioactive iodine is contraindicated
Subclinical hyperthyroidism	Methimazole if TSH <0.1 μU/mL
Subacute thyroiditis	NSAIDs or glucocorticoids
Suspicious nodule (malignancy)	FNAB followed by thyroidectomy (if malignant)
Thyroid storm	Propylthiouracil (preferred) or methimazole, iodine-potassium solutions, glucocorticoids, and β-blockers

◆ DON'T BE TRICKED

- A fever or sore throat in a patient taking methimazole or propylthiouracil should be presumed agranulocytosis until proven otherwise.

❖ Test Yourself

An asymptomatic 78-year-old woman has a serum TSH level of 0.2 μU/mL. Serum T_3 and T_4 levels are normal.

ANSWER: The diagnosis is subclinical hyperthyroidism. Repeat the thyroid tests in 4 to 6 months, because thyroid studies will normalize in 50% of patients without intervention.

Hypothyroidism

Diagnosis

The most common causes of hypothyroidism include:

- chronic lymphocytic (Hashimoto) thyroiditis
- thyroidectomy
- previous radioactive iodine ablation
- history of external beam radiation to the neck

Hashimoto thyroiditis increases in prevalence with age and is usually associated with a goiter.

Transient mild hypothyroidism typically occurs during the second phase of destructive thyroiditis (initial phase is hyperthyroidism). Permanent hypothyroidism may follow either postpartum thyroiditis (more common) or subacute thyroiditis (less common).

Certain medications may be associated with hypothyroidism, including lithium carbonate, interferon alfa, interleukin-2, and amiodarone.

Central hypothyroidism results from pituitary disease or previous surgery or radiation therapy to the sella. TSH and free T_4 are suppressed.

Look for symptoms suggesting hypothyroidism:

- weakness, lethargy, fatigue
- depression, impaired concentration
- myalgia
- cold intolerance
- constipation
- weight gain
- menstrual irregularity or menorrhagia
- carpal tunnel syndrome

Examination findings include bradycardia, hypothermia, diastolic hypertension, husky voice, goiter, cool dry skin, brittle hair, edema, and delayed relaxation phase of deep tendon reflexes.

Hypothyroidism may be associated with hyperprolactinemia, hyponatremia, and increased CK, AST, and cholesterol levels.

Order TSH and free T_4 to make the diagnosis. Measurement of T_3 levels is generally not necessary. An anti–thyroid peroxidase antibody assay is associated with Hashimoto thyroiditis but is not needed to make the diagnosis; high levels are associated with an increased risk of permanent hypothyroidism.

◆ DON'T BE TRICKED

- Thyroid scan and radioiodine uptake tests are not needed to make the diagnosis of hypothyroidism.

STUDY TABLE: Interpreting Thyroid Function Tests in Hypothyroidism	
If you see this...	**Choose this...**
↑TSH, ↓ free T$_4$	Primary hypothyroidism
↑TSH, normal T$_4$	Subclinical hypothyroidism
↓TSH, ↓ free T$_4$	Secondary (central) hypothyroidism; consider hypopituitarism
↓TSH, ↓ or normal free T$_4$ and critical illness	Euthyroid sick syndrome; no treatment required

Euthyroid sick syndrome occurs in patients acutely ill with a nonthyroidal illness. Testing reveals low or normal free T$_4$, and suppressed TSH (initially) followed by elevated TSH (recovery phase). Normalization of thyroid function tests occurs 4 to 8 weeks after recovery.

Myxedema coma is defined as severe hypothyroidism leading to decreased mental status, hypothermia, hypotension, bradycardia, hyponatremia, hypoglycemia, hypoxemia, and hypoventilation. It occurs in patients with severe, long-standing, untreated hypothyroidism and may be precipitated by an acute medical or surgical event or the administration of opiates.

Therapy

Levothyroxine is the only agent used to treat hypothyroidism. Therapy is indicated for subclinical hypothyroidism when the serum TSH is >10 μU/mL.

Treat women with subclinical hypothyroidism who are pregnant or want to become pregnant, because greater maternal and fetal risk is associated with this disorder.

Check thyroid function tests frequently during pregnancy in women with a known diagnosis of hypothyroidism taking thyroxine, because maternal thyroxine demand increases to 30% to 50%.

Recall that celiac disease, calcium and iron supplements, and PPIs can decrease levothyroxine absorption.

STUDY TABLE: Treatment of Hypothyroidism	
Condition	**Treatment**
Age <60 years	Begin full-dose levothyroxine (about 100 μg/d)
Age >60 years	Begin levothyroxine at 25-50 μg/d
	Increase by 25 μg every 6 weeks until TSH level is 1.0-2.5 μU/mL
Heart disease	Begin levothyroxine at 12.5-25 μg/d
	Increase by 12.5-25 μg every 6 weeks until TSH level is 1.0-2.5 μU/mL
Myxedema coma	Begin levothyroxine and hydrocortisone
	Hydrocortisone should be given until concomitant adrenal insufficiency has been ruled out

Thyroid Nodules

Diagnosis

Thyroid nodules are common and are often found incidentally on imaging tests. When a nodule is discovered, assess thyroid function with a serum TSH level.

A low TSH level suggests a benign, autonomously functioning thyroid adenoma. If TSH is suppressed, order a radioisotope scan to confirm the diagnosis and to rule out additional nonfunctioning nodules within a multinodular goiter. The serum TSH level is normal (and unhelpful) in most other patients with thyroid nodules.

Thyroid ultrasonography allows for accurate detection and sizing of all nodules on the thyroid gland, and ultrasound characteristics can be used to further delineate cancer risk.

Look for risk factors for thyroid cancer, including family history of thyroid malignancy, personal history of radiation therapy to the head and neck, or other radiation exposure in childhood.

FNAB is indicated for:

- all thyroid nodules >1 cm associated with a normal TSH level
- nodules <1 cm in patients with risk factors for thyroid cancer or suspicious ultrasound characteristics

The risk for malignancy is the same for multiple nodules in a multinodular goiter as it is for a solitary nodule; therefore, the evaluation and management is identical. Biopsy should be performed on the three or four nodules (>1 cm) with the most suspicious ultrasound features. In the absence of suspicious features, the largest nodules should be chosen for aspiration. Evaluate patients with multinodular goiter for compressive symptoms:

- dysphagia
- hoarseness
- dyspnea (tracheal compression from substernal goiter)

Consider evaluation with barium swallow, direct vocal cord visualization, spirometry with flow volume loops, and/or chest CT as needed.

◆ DON'T BE TRICKED

- Serum thyroglobulin measurement is not helpful in distinguishing benign and malignant thyroid nodules.
- Calcitonin measurement is only considered in patients with hypercalcemia or a family history of thyroid cancer or MEN2.

Therapy

Follow benign nodules with periodic ultrasonography. Although benign thyroid nodules usually remain stable or decrease in size, one third may increase in size. Malignancy must be ruled out when a nodule increases in size or if a nodule develops concerning ultrasound characteristics.

Treat hyperfunctioning solitary thyroid nodules with radioactive iodine ablation or hemithyroidectomy.

Surgery is indicated for patients with continued nodule growth despite normal initial FNAB results or nondiagnostic results on repeat FNAB and for patients with malignant cytology. Surgery is also indicated for large multinodular goiters associated with compressive symptoms.

◆ DON'T BE TRICKED

- Do not prescribe T_4-suppression therapy for benign thyroid nodules.

❖ Test Yourself

An 18-year-old man has a 2-cm right-sided thyroid nodule. The serum TSH level is 1.4 μU/mL.

ANSWER: Perform an FNAB.

Thyroid Nodule: A hyperfunctioning nodule is shown on the lateral aspect of the left thyroid lobe on thyroid scan.

Hypercortisolism (Cushing Syndrome)

Diagnosis

The most common cause of Cushing syndrome is the use of glucocorticoids (systemic, topical, intra-articular, or inhaled). Doses of prednisone (or equivalent) ≤5 mg/d are unlikely to cause clinically significant hypothalamic-pituitary-adrenal axis suppression, while those >10-20 mg/d can cause hypothalamic-pituitary-adrenal axis suppression after ≥3 weeks of consecutive use.

Endogenous causes of Cushing syndrome can be ACTH-dependent or ACTH-independent. ACTH-dependent causes of Cushing syndrome is defined by ACTH levels elevated or inappropriately "normal" for level of cortisol:

- ACTH-secreting pituitary adenomas (Cushing disease)
- ACTH-secreting carcinomas and carcinoid tumors

ACTH-independent causes of Cushing syndrome is defined by low or "normal" ACTH levels for level of cortisol:

- Adrenal adenomas
- Adrenal carcinomas

Clinical findings that are highly specific for Cushing syndrome include:

- centripetal obesity
- facial plethora
- supraclavicular or dorsocervical ("buffalo hump") fat pads
- wide (>1 cm) violaceous striae

First-line diagnostic studies include:

- low-dose dexamethasone suppression test (failure to suppress serum cortisol to <5 µg/dL)
- 24-hour urine cortisol level (elevated)
- late night salivary cortisol level (elevated)

If cortisol level is elevated (or not suppressible), order an ACTH level to differentiate ACTH-dependent from ACTH-independent hypercortisolism.

STUDY TABLE: Evaluation of Hypercortisolism	
If you see this...	**Do this...**
Morning ACTH elevated (>20 pg/mL)	Pituitary MRI or CT
Morning ACTH suppressed or normal (<5 pg/mL)	Adrenal CT

If ACTH is elevated but no pituitary tumor is visualized, perform high-dose (8-mg dexamethasone) suppression test to differentiate between pituitary and ectopic tumor ACTH production.

If high-dose dexamethasone does not suppress cortisol production, an ectopic tumor is releasing ACTH. The most common ACTH-secreting malignant tumors are SCLC, bronchial carcinoid, pheochromocytoma, and medullary thyroid carcinoma. Begin investigation with chest and abdomen CT.

If high-dose dexamethasone suppresses pituitary ACTH production and adrenal cortisol secretion, the source is the pituitary. In this case, obtain intrapetrosal sinus sampling for ACTH to confirm pituitary source.

◆ DON'T BE TRICKED

- False-positive results (failure to suppress cortisol) with the 1-mg dexamethasone suppression test are commonly due to alcohol use, obesity, and psychological disorders.

Therapy

Surgical resection of the adrenal gland, pituitary gland, or ectopic tumor is the optimal therapy for Cushing syndrome. Bisphosphonates are the treatment of choice for low bone density caused by hypercortisolism.

❖ Test Yourself

A 43-year-old woman has diabetes mellitus, hypertension, hirsutism, and central obesity. The serum cortisol level is 26 μg/dL after administration of 1 mg of dexamethasone and 8.2 μg/dL after 8 mg of dexamethasone. The serum ACTH level is 50 pg/mL.

ANSWER: The diagnosis is a pituitary tumor. Select pituitary gland MRI.

Cushing Syndrome: Wide purple striae characteristic of Cushing syndrome.

Adrenal Incidentaloma

Diagnosis

An adrenal incidentaloma is a mass >1 cm that is discovered incidentally. The two goals of evaluation are to determine if an adenoma is functioning and if it is malignant. All asymptomatic patients with adrenal incidentaloma should have a 1-mg overnight dexamethasone suppression test and a measurement of 24-hour urine levels of metanephrines and catecholamines. Patients with hypertension or spontaneous hypokalemia also require measurement of the plasma aldosterone–plasma renin ratio.

Adrenal metastases are common in patients with a known nonadrenal malignancy. Adenomas >6 cm are more likely to be malignant.

Therapy

Choose surgery for adrenal masses >6 cm in diameter or functioning tumors. Controversy exists regarding the optimal management for adrenal masses 4 to 6 cm in diameter, whereas masses <4 cm in size are monitored radiographically.

Follow-up

Repeat imaging in 6 to 12 months for all patients with nonfunctioning tumors that fail to meet surgical criteria. Also repeat screening for hormonal hypersecretion.

Hypoadrenalism (Addison Disease)

Diagnosis

Adrenal insufficiency may be due to disease of the adrenal glands (primary) or disorders of the pituitary gland (secondary).

- Autoimmune adrenalitis is the most common cause of primary insufficiency (also look for type 1 diabetes, hypothyroidism, and vitiligo).
- Glucocorticoid use is the most common cause of secondary insufficiency (hypothalamic-pituitary suppression).

Primary disease results in loss of cortisol, aldosterone, and adrenal androgens; secondary insufficiency causes only cortisol and adrenal androgen deficiencies (aldosterone synthesis is not ACTH dependent).

Characteristic findings include:

- weight loss
- fatigue, anorexia, nausea, vomiting, abdominal pain
- orthostatic hypotension
- hypoglycemia
- eosinophilia
- hyperpigmentation (primary adrenal insufficiency only)
- hyponatremia and hyperkalemia (primary adrenal insufficiency only)
- hypercalcemia

Look for patients who recently discontinued glucocorticoid therapy or did not increase their glucocorticoid dose in times of stress.

An 8:00 AM serum cortisol <3 µg/dL diagnoses cortisol deficiency and values >18 µg/dL exclude the diagnosis.

For patients with unequivocally low cortisol levels, a morning ACTH level can help distinguish between primary and secondary adrenal insufficiency.

STUDY TABLE: Evaluation of Hypocortisolism	
If you see this...	**Do this...**
Morning ACTH elevated (>20 pg/mL)	Adrenal CT
Morning ACTH suppressed or "normal" (<5 pg/mL)	Pituitary MRI

For nondiagnostic cortisol values, select stimulation testing with synthetic ACTH (cosyntropin). A stimulated serum cortisol >20 µg/dL excludes adrenal insufficiency.

◆ DON'T BE TRICKED

- Approximately 50% of patients with autoimmune adrenal insufficiency have other autoimmune endocrine disorders (thyroid disease, type 1 diabetes) and testing for these disorders is indicated.

Therapy

If acute adrenal insufficiency is suspected, treat empirically with high-dose (4 mg) dexamethasone and IV saline before obtaining cortisol and ACTH levels and without waiting for the ACTH and cortisol level results to return from the laboratory. Dexamethasone does not interfere with the serum cortisol assay.

After a diagnosis is made, hydrocortisone 10 to 30 mg/d is the standard therapy. Increase the hydrocortisone dose 2 to 10 times the standard replacement dose during periods of physiological stress, including surgery. Oral fludrocortisone is only appropriate for treatment of primary adrenal insufficiency.

◆ DON'T BE TRICKED

- Do not prescribe dexamethasone for chronic replacement therapy.

❖ Test Yourself

A 32-year-old man with hypothyroidism has a 3-month history of fatigue, weakness, nausea, and a 13.9-kg (30-lb) weight loss. He has orthostatic hypotension and increased pigment in the palmar creases. The serum sodium level is 132 mEq/L, and the serum potassium level is 5 mEq/L.

ANSWER: Diagnose autoimmune adrenalitis.

Pheochromocytoma

Diagnosis

Pheochromocytomas are rare tumors arising in the chromaffin cells of the adrenal medulla that secrete biogenic amines (nor-epinephrine, epinephrine, or dopamine) or their metabolites.

Characteristic findings may be remembered by the 7 H's:

- hypertension
- headache
- hypermetabolism
- hyperhidrosis
- hyperglycemia
- hypokalemia
- hypotension (during anesthesia induction)

Orthostatic hypotension (due to vasoconstriction-related volume depletion) is also a helpful physical examination clue.

Pheochromocytoma is associated with MEN2, von Hippel-Lindau disease, and neurofibromatosis type 2. Suspect a familial form in patients with a family history of pheochromocytoma, those with bilateral disease or an extra-adrenal location, and younger patients with a history of MEN2 or neurofibromatosis.

24-hour urine measurements of metanephrines and catecholamines are recommended when the pretest probability of disease is relatively low (adrenal mass without typical radiographic appearance or symptoms), while measurement of plasma metanephrines is preferred when clinical suspicion is higher (known hereditary syndrome or compatible symptoms).

Positive biochemical tests are followed by MRI or CT of the abdomen and pelvis. A ^{131}I or ^{123}I-MIBG scan may aid in localization when CT or MRI scans are negative.

Therapy

Surgery is the treatment of choice. Use phenoxybenzamine to control BP preoperatively. Give IV normal saline to maintain intravascular volume; nitroprusside or phentolamine is indicated for treating intraoperative hypertensive crisis.

◆ DON'T BE TRICKED

- Select β-adrenergic blockade only after adequate α-adrenergic blockade is achieved.

Primary Hyperaldosteronism

Diagnosis

Primary hyperaldosteronism is diagnosed in up to 14% of unselected patients with hypertension. Primary hyperaldosteronism is caused by aldosterone-producing adrenal adenomas (40%) and the remainder is due to bilateral adrenal hyperplasia. Characteristic findings are:

- difficult-to-treat or resistant hypertension
- hypokalemia

Screen patients with hypertension with unprovoked hypokalemia, a family history of primary hyperaldosteronism, or resistant hypertension with simultaneous measurements of plasma aldosterone and plasma renin activity.

A plasma aldosterone–plasma renin ratio >20, with a plasma aldosterone level >15 ng/dL, strongly suggests primary hyperaldosteronism.

Testing can be done in patients receiving treatment with any antihypertensive agent except spironolactone and eplerenone, both of which antagonize the aldosterone receptor. The diagnosis is confirmed by demonstrating nonsuppressibility of elevated plasma aldosterone in response to a high salt load given intravenously or orally. In patients without an adenoma, the plasma aldosterone level is suppressed to <5 ng/dL.

After autonomous hyperaldosteronism is diagnosed, select either CT or MRI of the adrenal glands. Adrenal vein sampling is needed in most patients to determine the source of aldosterone secretion when imaging is unrevealing and to confirm lateralization when imaging demonstrates an adrenal adenoma.

◆ DON'T BE TRICKED

- Almost 50% of patients with hyperaldosteronism do NOT have hypokalemia.
- Nonfunctioning adrenal adenomas are common and the source of aldosterone secretion must be confirmed before surgery with adrenal vein sampling.

Therapy

Spironolactone or eplerenone is the treatment of choice for adrenal hyperplasia, and laparoscopic adrenalectomy is indicated for an aldosterone-producing adenoma. If additional antihypertensive medications are required to control BP, select a thiazide diuretic agent.

Primary Amenorrhea

Diagnosis

Primary amenorrhea is the failure of menstruation (never occurred). Approximately 50% of primary amenorrhea is caused by chromosomal disorders, commonly Turner syndrome. Approximately 15% of patients have an anatomic abnormality of the uterus, cervix, or vagina, such as müllerian agenesis, transverse vaginal septum, or imperforate hymen.

Most important studies:

- pregnancy test
- karyotype
- FSH, LH, TSH, prolactin level
- pelvic ultrasound

STUDY TABLE: Most Common Causes of Primary Amenorrhea	
Diagnosis	**Characteristics**
Turner syndrome	45 XO karyotype
	Lack of secondary sexual characteristics, growth retardation, webbed neck, and frequent skeletal abnormalities
Hypothalamic/pituitary disorders	Functional (stress, excessive exercise, weight loss), developmental defects of cranial midline structures, tumors, or infiltrative disorders (sarcoidosis)
Androgen-resistance syndromes	XY karyotype
	Absence of or minimal pubic and axillary hair, a shallow vagina, and often a labial mass (testes)
PCOS	Most commonly associated with secondary amenorrhea but can cause primary amenorrhea. See Polycystic Ovary Syndrome

Secondary Amenorrhea

Diagnosis

Look for absence of menstruation for three cycle intervals or 6 consecutive months in women with previous menstrual flow. Test all women with secondary amenorrhea for pregnancy, the most common etiology.

Look for structural causes of secondary amenorrhea. Asherman syndrome is a complication of dilatation and curettage and intrauterine device placement; it is caused by a lack of basal endometrium proliferation and formation of adhesions (synechia).

Next assess the hormonal status with estradiol, FSH, LH, TSH, and prolactin level.

Low estradiol and inappropriately normal FSH and LH indicate hypogonadotrophic hypogonadism. Causes include:

- hypothyroidism
- hyperprolactinemia
- hypothalamic (stress, weight loss, exercise)
- pituitary (tumor, Sheehan syndrome)

Low estradiol and elevated FSH and LH levels indicates hypergonadotrophic hypogonadism. Consider:

- premature ovarian insufficiency (autoimmune)
- chemotherapy
- pelvic radiation

A progesterone challenge is sometimes used to determine cause of secondary amenorrhea, especially if estrogen level is difficult to interpret.

- Withdrawal bleeding within 1 week of completing a course of progesterone confirms ovarian estrogen production.
- If no withdrawal bleeding occurs, the patient has a low-estrogen state (no ovarian function).

STUDY TABLE: Common Causes of Secondary Amenorrhea

Diagnosis	Characteristics	Evaluation
PCOS	Ovulatory dysfunction, evidence of hyperandrogenism, and polycystic ovaries on ultrasonography	Mild elevation in testosterone and DHEAS (not needed for diagnosis)
	See Polycystic Ovary Syndrome	
Hyperprolactinemia	May be associated with galactorrhea	First rule out hypothyroidism
	Related to medications (tricyclic antidepressants, phenothiazines, and metoclopramide), tumors that secrete prolactin or compress the pituitary stalk, history of cranial radiotherapy	If TSH is normal and serum prolactin level >100 ng/mL, obtain brain MRI to diagnose tumor
Hypothalamic amenorrhea	Most commonly functional (related to stress, weight loss, excessive exercise)	Low or normal LH level, and low estradiol level
Hypothyroidism	Causes secondary increase in serum prolactin levels	High TSH, high prolactin
Adrenal tumor	Signs of hyperandrogenism and virilization, usually acute onset and severe	Decreased LH and FSH, increased or normal estradiol, and increased testosterone and DHEAS levels
Sheehan syndrome (postpartum pituitary necrosis)	History of difficult delivery (blood loss, hypotension) and inability to breastfeed	Varying levels of panhypopituitarism
Asherman syndrome (uterine synechiae)	History of previous dilatation and curettage amenorrhea due to fibrous uterine scarring	Normal LH and estradiol levels; no response to estrogen and progesterone challenge
		Abnormal pelvic ultrasound or hysterogram

Therapy

Treat the underlying disorder. Prevent osteoporosis by choosing estrogen and progesterone replacement until menstruation returns to normal or age 50 years. For hypothalamic amenorrhea, choose reduced exercise, improved nutrition, and attention to emotional needs.

Polycystic Ovary Syndrome

Diagnosis

PCOS is the most common etiology of hirsutism with oligomenorrhea. Symptoms normally start at puberty or several years later and are slowly progressive. Diagnosis requires two of the following:

- ovulatory dysfunction (amenorrhea, oligomenorrhea, infertility)
- laboratory or clinical evidence of hyperandrogenism (hirsutism, acne)
- ultrasonographic evidence of polycystic ovaries

Insulin resistance is an important feature of the disorder, as is being overweight or obese. A mild elevation in testosterone and DHEAS levels and an LH/FSH ratio greater than 2:1 are typical.

◆ DON'T BE TRICKED

- Do not routinely order testosterone or DHEAS testing, because PCOS is a clinical diagnosis and laboratory evaluation is only necessary when androgen-producing neoplasms must be ruled out.
- An androgen-secreting ovarian or adrenal tumor should be suspected in a woman with acute onset of rapidly progressive hirsutism or virilization.

Therapy

Instruct patients in intensive lifestyle modification to reduce weight, control abdominal obesity, and restore insulin sensitivity. Treatment follows two models:

- If fertility is not desired, first-line treatment of hirsutism and regulation of menses is an oral contraceptive; spironolactone can be added if hirsutism remains a problem.
- If fertility is desired, ovulation induction can be brought about with clomiphene citrate or letrozole.

✧ Test Yourself

A 27-year-old woman has had oligomenorrhea since age 14 years. She also has acanthosis nigricans and hirsutism but no galactorrhea; she is obese. She does not desire pregnancy.

ANSWER: The diagnosis is PCOS. Begin intensive lifestyle modification and an oral contraceptive.

Infertility

Diagnosis

Infertility is defined as the inability to conceive after 1 year of intercourse without contraception. Regular menses is correlated with regular ovulation. If oligomenorrhea is present, evaluate like secondary amenorrhea. Consider structural abnormalities and evaluate with pelvic ultrasound or hysterography.

Semen analysis can be performed at any time.

Male Hypogonadism

Diagnosis

Characteristic findings are fatigue, decreased strength, poor libido, hot flushes, erectile dysfunction, and gynecomastia.

Testosterone deficiency is diagnosed with two 8:00 AM total testosterone levels below the reference range.

- If the testosterone measurement is equivocal, measure free testosterone level by equilibrium dialysis or mass spectrometry.
- If the testosterone level is low, measure LH, FSH, and prolactin levels.

Elevated LH and FSH values indicate primary testicular failure. Some common causes include:

- Klinefelter syndrome (check karyotype)
- atrophy secondary to mumps orchitis
- autoimmune destruction
- previous chemotherapy or pelvic irradiation
- hemochromatosis

Low or normal LH and FSH levels indicate secondary hypogonadism. Important causes include:

- sleep apnea
- hyperprolactinemia
- hypothalamic or pituitary disorders (hemochromatosis, pituitary/hypothalamic tumor)
- use of opiates, anabolic steroids or glucocorticoids

If secondary hypogonadism is confirmed, in addition to measuring prolactin, check iron studies to rule out hemochromatosis and obtain an MRI to evaluate for hypothalamic or pituitary lesions.

Men who self-administer anabolic steroids can come to medical attention because of infertility. Physical examination typically reveals acne, muscular hypertrophy, testicular atrophy, and gynecomastia (if the patient is using testosterone). Aromatase inhibitors are frequently used concurrently with testosterone preparations to prevent adipose conversion of androgens to estrogens and development of gynecomastia. Laboratory data show suppressed LH and FSH levels, variable testosterone levels, and otherwise normal pituitary function.

◆ DON'T BE TRICKED

- Do not measure serum testosterone if a patient is having regular morning erections, has no gynecomastia on examination, and the genital examination is normal.

Therapy

Testosterone can be administered as a transdermal (preferred by patients but expensive), buccal, implantable pellets, or IM preparation. Before initiation of testosterone replacement and during therapy, routinely monitor hematocrit and PSA to screen for the development of erythrocytosis and prostate cancer, respectively.

◆ DON'T BE TRICKED

- Don't provide testosterone replacement therapy for nonspecific symptoms, such as fatigue and weakness, in the absence of unequivocal testosterone deficiency.
- Testosterone replacement therapy (and anabolic steroid abuse) results in small testicles and male infertility.

Hyperparathyroidism and Hypercalcemia

Diagnosis

Primary hyperparathyroidism is the most common cause of hypercalcemia in outpatients. Primary hyperparathyroidism commonly presents as asymptomatic hypercalcemia. Less common presentations are kidney stones, osteoporosis, pancreatitis, and fractures (osteoporosis). Malignancy is the most common cause of hypercalcemia in hospitalized patients. Hypercalcemia may also occur with the use of lithium (PTH-mediated) or thiazide diuretics (non–PTH-mediated) and in the setting of excessive ingestion of vitamin D and calcium. Sarcoidosis may be associated with hypercalcemia (10% of patients) and hypercalciuria (50% of patients).

Measure the ionized calcium to exclude pseudohypercalcemia caused by an increase in plasma proteins capable of binding calcium; total calcium will be increased and ionized calcium will be normal.

If hypercalcemia is confirmed, check calcium, PTH, phosphate, creatinine, and 25-hydroxyvitamin D levels. If PTH is elevated or inappropriately "normal" in the setting of elevated serum calcium, the most likely cause is primary hyperparathyroidism.

◆ **DON'T BE TRICKED**

- **In patients with hypercalcemia and normal PTH levels, measure urinary calcium excretion to exclude familial hypocalciuric hypercalcemia.**

If hyperparathyroidism is confirmed and surgery is indicated, do a sestamibi parathyroid scan to look for an adenoma.

STUDY TABLE: Causes of Hypercalcemia	
Diagnosis	**Key features include hypercalcemia and …**
Primary hyperparathyroidism	PTH elevated (80%) or inappropriately normal (20%); phosphorus low
	X-rays may show chondrocalcinosis or osteitis fibrosa cystica (rare)
Humoral hypercalcemia of malignancy	PTH suppressed; phosphorus normal or low
	PTH-related protein may be elevated but is not needed for diagnosis
Local osteolytic lesions	PTH suppressed; phosphorus normal or low
	Lytic bone metastases result in increased mobilization of calcium from the bone
Multiple myeloma	PTH suppressed; phosphorus elevated
	Look for patients presenting with new kidney injury and anemia
	Diagnose with serum and urine protein immunoelectrophoresis
Granulomatous disease (sarcoidosis and TB) and B-cell lymphoma	PTH suppressed; phosphorus elevated; calcitriol elevated (particularly in sarcoidosis)
Milk-alkali syndrome	PTH suppressed; phosphorus, creatinine, carbon dioxide elevated
	Consider in healthy persons in whom primary hyperparathyroidism has been excluded
	Excessive ingestion of calcium-containing antacids is a cause (rare)
Hyperthyroidism	Hypercalcemia is a frequent incidental finding in hyperthyroidism due to direct stimulation of osteoclasts by thyroid hormone

Primary hyperparathyroidism is the most common manifestation of MEN1.

STUDY TABLE: Multiple Endocrine Neoplasia Types 1 and 2	
MEN1	**MEN2**
Multigland hyperparathyroidism is the most common manifestation	Multigland hyperparathyroidism is the least common manifestation
Pituitary neoplasms associated with prolactinoma (amenorrhea and erectile dysfunction), acromegaly (enlargement of hands, feet, tongue, frontal bossing), Cushing disease (bruising, hypertension, central obesity, hirsutism)	Medullary thyroid cancer is the most common manifestation and may be associated with a palpable neck mass
Pancreatic NETs associated with gastrinoma (diarrhea, ulcers), insulinoma (fasting hypoglycemia), vasoactive intestinal polypeptide-secreting tumor (watery diarrhea, hypokalemia), carcinoid syndrome (diarrhea, flushing, right heart valvular lesion)	Pheochromocytoma (hypertension and palpitations)

◆ DON'T BE TRICKED

- About 50% of patients with primary hyperparathyroidism have coexisting vitamin D deficiency, and serum and urine calcium levels may be decreased. Select measurement of serum vitamin D levels in all patients with hyperparathyroidism.

Therapy

Parathyroidectomy is indicated for patients with primary hyperparathyroidism and hypercalcemic complications, such as kidney stones, bone disease, or previous episodes of hypercalcemic crisis. Asymptomatic patients are surgical candidates if they have any of the following:

- serum calcium level >1 mg/dL above upper limit of normal
- estimated GFR <60 mL/min/1.73 m^2
- reduction in bone mineral density (T-score <−2.5)
- age <50 years

Watch for a precipitous fall in the serum calcium level caused by relative hypoparathyroidism after parathyroidectomy ("hungry bone" syndrome). Monitor serum calcium after surgery, and give oral calcium if mild hypocalcemia develops.

Treat patients who are not candidates for parathyroidectomy with cinacalcet or bisphosphonates.

Hypercalcemia requiring acute intervention is most common in the setting of malignancy. Select:

- volume resuscitation with normal saline
- furosemide if the calcium level has not normalized following volume repletion
- IV bisphosphonates
- oral glucocorticoid therapy if hypercalcemia is due to multiple myeloma or sarcoidosis

❖ Test Yourself

A 44-year-old man has a 1-year history of fatigue and poor concentration. His serum calcium level is 10.9 mg/dL, serum phosphorus level is 2.8 mg/dL, and PTH level is 75 pg/mL.

ANSWER: Diagnose primary hyperparathyroidism, measure serum vitamin D levels, and select parathyroidectomy.

Hypocalcemia

Diagnosis

Most cases of hypocalcemia are due to low serum albumin levels; the ionized calcium concentration is normal. Total calcium declines by 0.8 mg/dL for each 1 g/dL decrement in serum albumin concentration.

The most common cause of acquired hypocalcemia is surgical excision of or vascular injury to the parathyroid glands. Other causes include:

- neck irradiation
- congenital hypoparathyroidism (DiGeorge syndrome)
- autoimmune destruction
- infiltrative diseases
- complication of plasmapheresis

Autoimmune hypoparathyroidism occurs as an isolated defect or as part of polyglandular autoimmune syndrome type 1 in association with mucocutaneous candidiasis, adrenal insufficiency, hypogonadism, and malabsorption.

In addition to hypoparathyroidism, hypocalcemia may result from pseudohypoparathyroidism, vitamin D deficiency, hypomagnesemia, or pancreatitis, or may occur in the setting of rhabdomyolysis, kidney failure, and tumor lysis syndrome.

Look for:

- circumoral and acral paresthesias
- carpal-pedal spasm
- positive Trousseau sign
- positive Chvostek sign

Order calcium, phosphate, magnesium, creatinine, PTH, 25-hydroxyvitamin D, albumin, and/or ionized calcium tests. Order an ECG to evaluate for QTc interval prolongation.

STUDY TABLE: Differential Diagnosis of Hypocalcemia	
Diagnosis	**Key features include hypocalcemia and...**
Hypoparathyroidism	Hyperphosphatemia; low PTH and variable vitamin D levels
Pseudohypoparathyroidism (resistance to PTH)	Hyperphosphatemia; elevated PTH and normal vitamin D levels
CKD	Hyperphosphatemia; elevated PTH and low 1,25-dihydroxyvitamin D levels
Vitamin D deficiency	Hypophosphatemia; bone tenderness or fibromyalgia-like syndrome, weakness, gait difficulty, osteomalacia
Impaired PTH secretion and PTH resistance	Magnesium deficiency (small bowel bypass, diarrhea, alcoholism, diuretic therapy)
"Hungry bone" syndrome	Recent parathyroidectomy

Therapy

Treat acute symptomatic hypocalcemia with IV calcium gluconate and vitamin D. Chronic hypocalcemia is treated with oral calcium supplements and vitamin D. Choose the type of vitamin D based on the presence of underlying disease:

- kidney disease: calcitriol (1,25-dihydroxyvitamin D)
- liver disease: 25-hydroxycholecalciferol
- any other cause of hypocalcemia: cholecalciferol (D_3) or ergocalciferol (D_2)

The main side effect of therapy is hypercalciuria and nephrolithiasis. Remember to correct hypomagnesemia with magnesium supplements.

❖ Test Yourself

A 46-year-old woman has cramps in her hands and feet. She has pernicious anemia and Hashimoto thyroiditis. Her serum calcium level is 7.9 mg/dL and her serum phosphorus level is 4.1 mg/dL.

ANSWER: Diagnose autoimmune hypoparathyroidism and select a serum PTH level.

Osteoporosis

Screening

DEXA is indicated for all women >65 years of age and in women <65 years with risk factors for osteoporosis:

- glucocorticoid therapy
- low body weight
- current cigarette smoking
- alcohol use
- family history of hip fracture

Screen men and women with risk factors for secondary osteoporosis (glucocorticoid use, hyperparathyroidism, ADT [men], malabsorption).

◆ DON'T BE TRICKED

- Do not repeat annual DEXA in women with normal DEXA results without risk factors. Although the optimal screening interval is unknown, most experts recommend 10 to 15 years for women with normal or slightly low bone mineral density and no risk factors.

Diagnosis

Osteoporosis is a silent skeletal disorder characterized by compromised bone strength and an increased predisposition to fractures.

- DEXA T-score of -1.0 to -2.4 defines osteopenia
- DEXA T-score of ≤-2.5 defines osteoporosis
- Osteoporosis is also diagnosed by a history of fragility fracture (fracture from a fall at standing height or lower).

The most common cause of osteoporosis in women is estrogen deficiency and in men, testosterone deficiency. Secondary causes include:

- hyperthyroidism, hyperparathyroidism, Cushing syndrome
- malabsorption (Crohn disease, intestinal resection, celiac disease)
- rheumatoid arthritis
- medications (excessive thyroid hormone, glucocorticoids, phenobarbital, phenytoin, thiazolidinediones)
- multiple myeloma
- CKD, chronic liver disease
- vitamin D deficiency

Reasonable tests include: CBC; TSH; calcium, phosphorus, and creatinine levels; liver chemistry tests; ESR; serum 25-hydroxy-vitamin D level (if vitamin D deficiency is suspected); and tTG antibodies (if celiac disease is suspected). In the absence of fractures, primary osteoporosis is associated with no abnormalities on laboratory testing.

Therapy

Encourage all patients to stop smoking, reduce alcohol intake, and begin resistance exercises. Exposure to sunlight is especially important for home-bound persons or nursing-home residents. Supplement calcium and vitamin D intake.

Indications for antiresorptive therapy:

- osteoporosis
- osteopenia (if additional high-risk factors are present)
- previous fragility fracture
- vertebral or hip fracture

The Fracture Risk Assessment Tool (FRAX) estimates the 10-year probability of hip fracture and major osteoporotic fracture. Antiresorptive treatment is cost effective when the risk of major osteoporotic fracture is ≥20% or the risk of hip fracture is ≥3%.

Treatment options:

- alendronate, ibandronate, or risedronate as first-line therapy
- raloxifene for patients who cannot tolerate bisphosphonates
- teriparatide (synthetic recombinant human PTH 1-34) for severe osteoporosis with fractures
- calcitonin for pain from osteoporotic fractures

Oral bisphosphonates are taken on an empty stomach, and patients must remain upright for at least 30 minutes. These agents are contraindicated in patients with CKD or esophageal disease. IV zoledronate (once yearly) or IV ibandronate (once every 3 months) are alternative therapeutic options.

No recommended duration of therapy is available. Stopping therapy after 5 years is reasonable in women who have a stable BMI, no history of fracture, and are at low risk for fracture. The duration of the drug holiday is unknown but may be determined by changes in DEXA measurements.

Drugs for osteoporosis have various adverse effects:

- oral bisphosphonate therapy may lead to erosive esophagitis and atypical hip fracture
- IV bisphosphonate therapy can lead to osteonecrosis of the jaw
- raloxifene is associated with thromboembolic disease
- teriparatide is associated with osteosarcoma

Treatment with teriparatide should be limited to 2 years.

◆ DON'T BE TRICKED

- Do not use estrogen replacement therapy for osteoporosis in postmenopausal women.
- Do not combine teriparatide with a bisphosphonate.
- IV bisphosphonates are contraindicated in patients with severe hypocalcemia and CKD.
- Raloxifene has not been shown to reduce hip fracture risk.

Follow-up

Although no consensus exists, DEXA 24 months after beginning therapy for osteoporosis is reasonable.

❖ Test Yourself

An 82-year-old woman has been taking thyroid hormone since age 31 years. She has lost about 7.6 cm (3.0 in) in height. Serum TSH level is <0.01 µU/mL (normal 0.5 to 5.0 µU/mL).

ANSWER: The diagnosis is thyroid hormone–induced osteoporosis. Reduce the thyroid hormone dose and schedule DEXA.

Osteomalacia

Diagnosis

Osteomalacia is a metabolic bone disease resulting from failure of the organic matrix of bone to mineralize because of lack of available calcium or phosphorus. Many cases of osteomalacia are related to abnormalities in vitamin D but may also result from deficiencies of calcium or phosphate.

Look for:

- fatigability, malaise, and bone pain
- generalized bone tenderness
- proximal muscle weakness
- Looser zones (bands perpendicular to the bone surface visible on x-rays)
- hypocalcemia and hypophosphatemia
- elevated serum alkaline phosphatase level

Evaluate for underlying conditions that may lead to intestinal malabsorption of vitamin D, such as celiac disease, or abnormalities in vitamin D metabolism, such as liver and kidney disease. Diagnosis is confirmed with bone biopsy when necessary.

Therapy

If osteomalacia is secondary to vitamin D deficiency, treat with oral ergocalciferol 1000 to 2000 U/d and elemental calcium 1 g/d.

◆ DON'T BE TRICKED

- Not all fractures in older adult patients are due to osteoporosis. Look for osteomalacia, particularly in nursing-home residents.

Vitamin D Deficiency

Diagnosis

Most patients are asymptomatic. Prolonged and severe vitamin D deficiency will cause secondary hyperparathyroidism; osteomalacia in adults; and symptoms of bone pain, muscle weakness (including difficulty walking), and fracture. In assessing serum levels of vitamin D, concentrations of 25-hydroxyvitamin D are the best indicator of vitamin D status.

There is disagreement as the desired level of vitamin D. Most expert panels define a sufficient level ≥30 ng/mL. The Institute of Medicine has determined that ≥20 ng/mL is sufficient.

Special populations will have lower levels of vitamin D owing to medical conditions or medication side effects:

- obesity
- glucocorticoids
- orlistat
- malabsorption disorders (including bariatric surgery)

Therapy

Maintenance dose for adults 19-70 years of age is at least 600 U/d of vitamin D to maximize bone health; for adults >70 years of age, 800 U/d is recommended.

In treating the deficient patient, 50,000 U of either ergocalciferol or cholecalciferol is recommended, followed by maintenance therapy of 1500 to 2000 U/d.

Paget Disease

Diagnosis

Paget disease is a focal disorder of bone remodeling that leads to greatly accelerated rates of bone turnover, disruption of the normal architecture of bone, and sometimes gross deformities of bone (enlargement of the skull, bowing of the femur or tibia). Most patients are asymptomatic, and the disease is suspected when an isolated elevation of alkaline phosphatase is detected in the absence of liver disease.

Characteristic findings of symptomatic Paget disease include:

- bone pain, fractures
- cranial nerve compression syndromes, spinal stenosis, nerve root syndromes
- high-output cardiac failure
- angioid retinal streaks

If the serum alkaline phosphatase (bone) level is elevated in an asymptomatic patient, order a bone scan and follow-up x-rays of areas that localize radionuclide. In symptomatic patients, obtain x-rays of the painful area. X-rays will reveal these pathognomonic pagetic lesions: focal osteolysis with coarsening of the trabecular pattern, cotton wool skull, and cortical thickening.

Therapy

Indications to treat Paget disease include bone pain, radiculopathy, or involvement of a weight-bearing bone or a joint, regardless of symptoms. Bisphosphonates are the first-line agents.

Paget Disease: X-ray showing "cotton wool" appearance of the skull typical of Paget disease.

Gastroenterology and Hepatology

Dysphagia

Diagnosis

Dysphagia is defined as difficulty swallowing and is classified as oropharyngeal or esophageal.

Patients with oropharyngeal dysphagia have difficulty initiating swallowing and present with:

- coughing
- choking
- nasal regurgitation of fluids

Oropharyngeal dysphagia frequently results from muscular or neurologic disorders, most commonly stroke, Parkinson disease, ALS, MG, and muscular dystrophy. Patients with pharyngoesophageal (Zenker) diverticulum often present with regurgitation of undigested food and severe halitosis. Select videofluoroscopy to evaluate suspected oropharyngeal dysphagia.

Patients with esophageal dysphagia report food "sticking" or discomfort in the retrosternal region. Solid-food dysphagia is most often due to a structural esophageal abnormality. Dysphagia for solids and liquids or for liquids alone suggests an esophageal motility abnormality such as achalasia. Solid-food dysphagia that occurs episodically for months to years suggests an esophageal web or a distal esophageal ring (Schatzki ring). Progressively increasing solid-food dysphagia suggests a peptic stricture or carcinoma.

Therapy

Oropharyngeal dysphagia is managed with dietary adjustment and incorporation of swallowing exercises with the assistance of a speech pathologist. Therapy for esophageal dysphagia is dictated by the underlying cause.

✧ Test Yourself

A 75-year-old man with Parkinson disease has difficulty initiating a swallow.

ANSWER: The diagnosis is probably neuromuscular pharyngeal dysphagia; order oropharyngeal videofluoroscopy.

Achalasia

Diagnosis

Achalasia is caused by degeneration of the myenteric plexus with the loss of inhibitory neurons, failure of the lower esophageal sphincter (LES) to relax in response to swallowing, and absent peristalsis. This leads to the retention of food and liquids in the body of the esophagus, the characteristic findings of dysphagia with solids and liquids,

Barium Esophagogram: The "bird's beak" finding reflects narrowing of the distal esophagus and is characteristic of achalasia.

and "bird's beak" narrowing of the GE junction on barium swallow. If the patient has a history of travel to South America, suspect Chagas disease as the cause of achalasia.

Diagnostic evaluation should be done in the following order:

- barium swallow: the preferred screening test when diagnosis is suspected clinically
- esophageal manometry: documents the absence of peristalsis and incomplete relaxation of the LES with swallows
- upper endoscopy: to rule out adenocarcinoma (pseudoachalasia) at the GE junction

Therapy

Laparoscopic surgical myotomy of the LES and endoscopic pneumatic dilatation of the esophagus are first-line therapies for achalasia. Second-line therapy is botulinum injection which will relieve symptoms for about 6 months. Third-line therapy is calcium channel blockers, or nitrates if the patient cannot tolerate dilation, surgery, or injection therapy.

Gastroesophageal Reflux Disease

Diagnosis

GERD is caused by reflux of gastric contents into the esophagus. Characteristic findings of GERD are heartburn and/or regurgitation. Extraesophageal symptoms may include wheezing, cough, hoarseness, and chest pain. In a patient without alarm features (dysphagia, weight loss, anemia, vomiting) symptom relief with PPI therapy confirms the diagnosis.

STUDY TABLE: GERD Diagnostic Studies	
Indication	**Test**
GERD symptoms refractory to empiric therapy with PPIs	Upper endoscopy; if normal, then choose ambulatory esophageal pH monitoring or impedance pH testing while taking a PPI for symptom-reflux correlation
Dysphagia, odynophagia, and weight loss	Upper endoscopy to rule out cancer
Confirmed Barrett esophagus	Periodic upper endoscopy to monitor for dysplasia and cancer

◆ DON'T BE TRICKED

- If symptoms fail to respond to once daily PPI, administer twice daily PPI for 4 to 8 weeks before performing upper endoscopy.
- Do not order barium x-rays to diagnose GERD.

Therapy

PPIs are first-line therapy for GERD and GERD with extraesophageal manifestations (asthma, chronic laryngitis, chronic cough). PPI therapy is associated with an increased risk for *Clostridium difficile* infection, pneumonia, osteoporosis, and hip fractures.

Select antireflux surgery for patients who are refractory to medical management or those who have an excellent response to a PPI but do not want long-term medical therapy. Patients should undergo pH monitoring to demonstrate true reflux with symptom correlation and manometry to rule out a motility disorder prior to surgery. Antireflux surgery does not prevent BE or adenocarcinoma.

❖ Test Yourself

A 34-year-old woman has frequent heartburn. She has tried a PPI, once before breakfast and once before dinner, without improvement.

ANSWER: The probable diagnosis is GERD. Order upper endoscopy and, if normal, 24-hour esophageal pH monitoring while the patient is taking a PPI to confirm acid reflux is the cause of her symptoms.

Barrett Esophagus

Screening

Screen men age >50 years with chronic GERD symptoms (symptoms for more than 5 years) and additional risk factors (nocturnal reflux symptoms, hiatal hernia, elevated BMI, tobacco use, and intra-abdominal distribution of fat) to detect esophageal adenocarcinoma and BE.

Diagnosis

The diagnosis of BE is based on the endoscopic finding of columnar epithelium above the normally located GE junction. The pathway of progression of BE is from intestinal metaplasia to low-grade dysplasia to high-grade dysplasia to invasive adenocarcinoma.

Therapy

Treatment to remove BE is recommended for patients with confirmed high-grade dysplasia and can be done with endoscopic therapies that include radiofrequency ablation, photodynamic therapy, or endoscopic mucosal resection. Endoscopic therapies have had similar outcomes to esophagectomy.

Follow-up

In patients with BE and no dysplasia, surveillance examinations should occur at intervals no more frequently than 3 to 5 years. More frequent intervals of every 6 to 12 months are indicated in patients with BE and low-grade dysplasia.

Esophagitis

Diagnosis

Odynophagia is the most common presenting symptom of esophagitis. *Candida albicans* is the most common infectious cause, followed by CMV and HSV. Two-thirds of patients with candidal esophagitis have oral thrush. Patients with viral esophagitis rarely have associated ulcerative oropharyngeal lesions. Upper endoscopy and biopsy/brushings establish the diagnosis.

In patients with odynophagia who are immunosuppressed, begin empiric therapy for esophageal candidiasis. In patients with AIDS and odynophagia, the presence of oral candidiasis is 100% predictive of esophageal candidiasis. Perform upper endoscopy if empiric therapy for candidiasis is unsuccessful.

Pill-induced esophagitis may be caused by tetracycline, NSAIDs, potassium chloride, iron, and alendronate. Symptoms of severe substernal chest pain with swallowing occur several hours to days after taking the medication.

Young adults with eosinophilic esophagitis (EE) present with extreme dysphagia and food impaction. Macroscopic findings at upper endoscopy are nonspecific but may show mucosal furrowing, stacked circular rings, white specks, and mucosal friability. Endoscopic biopsies show marked infiltration with eosinophils. GERD has been associated with esophageal eosinophilia and can mimic EE. Evaluation includes an 8-week trial of a PPI; clinical response to the PPI trial indicates GERD-associated eosinophilia rather than EE. Persistent esophageal eosinophilia following PPI therapy confirms a diagnosis of EE.

❖ **Test Yourself**

A 30-year-old man has frequent heartburn and recurrent episodes of food impaction.

ANSWER: Diagnose eosinophilic esophagitis.

◆ **DON'T BE TRICKED**
- Do not select barium esophagography to evaluate suspected esophagitis.
- The absence of oral *Candida* lesions does not rule out esophageal candidiasis.

Therapy

Address the underlying cause of esophagitis:

- fluconazole or itraconazole for esophageal candidiasis
- acyclovir, famciclovir, or valacyclovir for HSV esophagitis
- ganciclovir and/or foscarnet for CMV esophagitis
- swallowed fluticasone or budesonide for EE
- supportive care for pill esophagitis (spontaneously resolves)

❖ **Test Yourself**

A 28-year-old man with HIV infection has a 2-month history of odynophagia. On physical examination, oral thrush is present.

ANSWER: Choose empiric treatment with fluconazole.

Peptic Ulcer Disease

Diagnosis

Most PUD is caused by *Helicobacter pylori* infection or NSAID use. Upper endoscopy is the gold standard to diagnose PUD. Gastric ulcers should be biopsied to rule out malignancy. Duodenal ulcers carry little risk of malignancy and do not require biopsy unless they are refractory to therapy. All patients with PUD should be tested for *H. pylori* infection regardless of NSAID use. In patients undergoing upper endoscopy, select biopsy and histologic assessment for *H. pylori* or rapid urease testing for *H. pylori*.

In patients aged <50 years with dyspepsia without alarm symptoms, use the "test-and-treat" approach for *H. pylori* without performing upper endoscopy. Noninvasive strategies for diagnosing *H. pylori* include urea breath tests, and stool test for *H. pylori* antigens. False-negative rapid urease tests, urea breath tests, and stool antigen results for *H. pylori* may occur in patients who recently took antibiotics, bismuth-containing compounds, or PPIs; these drugs should be stopped before testing (28 days for antibiotics, 2 weeks for PPIs) or histologic assessment of *H. pylori* should be performed.

For older patients and those with persistent symptoms or alarm features at any age, obtain upper endoscopy and *H. pylori* testing.

Look for complications of PUD:

- penetration characterized by a gradual increase in the severity and frequency of abdominal pain, with pancreatitis as a common presentation
- perforation characterized by severe, sudden abdominal pain that is often associated with shock and peritoneal signs
- outlet obstruction characterized by nausea, vomiting, and/or early satiety and a succussion splash
- bleeding characterized by hematemesis, melena, or hematochezia (see Upper GI Bleeding)

◆ **DON'T BE TRICKED**
- Do not order serum antibody testing for *H. pylori* (<20%); it will not differentiate between past and current infection.
- Do not routinely order any tests other than *H. pylori* testing and upper endoscopy as indicated for the evaluation of PUD.

Therapy

STUDY TABLE: Treating NSAID-Induced Peptic Ulcer Disease	
If you see this...	**Do this...**
Aspirin, NSAID-induced PUD	Stop NSAIDs, treat with H_2-blocker or PPI
Aspirin, NSAID-induced PUD, unable to stop aspirin or NSAID	Treat with long-term PPI
High risk for developing NSAID-induced PUD but needs NSAID treatment*	Initiate prophylaxis with PPI or misoprostol

*High risk is associated with a history of PUD; a history of UGI bleeding; receiving dual antiplatelet therapy or anticoagulation; and age 60 years or older plus glucocorticoid use, dyspepsia, or GERD.

◆ DON'T BE TRICKED

- A selective COX-2 inhibitor provides no better gastric protection compared to a nonselective NSAID plus a PPI.
- The beneficial gastric effect of COX-2 inhibitors is lost when taken concomitantly with low-dose aspirin.

Initial *H. pylori* therapy includes a PPI and two antibiotics (typically clarithromycin and either amoxicillin or metronidazole) for 2 weeks. If unsuccessful, give a second course of antibiotics that the patient has not already received. The initial treatment of gastric outlet obstruction is nasogastric suction and an IV PPI.

Surgery is reserved for complications of PUD because of the risk of postoperative complications.

Follow-up

Documentation of *H. pylori* eradication with noninvasive testing (fecal antigen test or urea breath test) is indicated only for patients with persistent symptoms and *H. pylori*–associated ulcer. Follow-up upper endoscopy for gastric ulcers is indicated only if the patient remains symptomatic after treatment, the cause is uncertain, or biopsies were not performed during initial upper endoscopy.

◆ DON'T BE TRICKED

- Duodenal PUD without complications does not require follow-up upper endoscopy.
- Do not order an *H. pylori* antibody assay for eradication testing because antibody titers remain elevated after treatment.

❖ Test Yourself

A 42-year-old man was treated with a PPI, amoxicillin, and clarithromycin for an *H. pylori*–positive duodenal ulcer. He returns 9 weeks after treatment because of recurrent symptoms.

ANSWER: Order a urea breath test. If positive, re-treat with different antibiotics than those prescribed initially.

Nonulcer Dyspepsia

Diagnosis

Nonulcer dyspepsia is defined as nonspecific upper abdominal discomfort or nausea not attributable to PUD or GERD. Various drugs may cause dyspepsia, including NSAIDs, antibiotics, bisphosphonates, and potassium supplements. Diagnosis is based on satisfying one or more of the following criteria:

- bothersome postprandial fullness
- early satiety
- epigastric pain
- epigastric burning

Patients aged >55 years or patients with alarm features require investigation with upper endoscopy. Alarm features include unexplained iron deficiency anemia, heme-positive stools, progressive dysphagia, weight loss, new-onset dyspepsia, vomiting, and family history of GI malignancy.

Therapy

For patients aged ≤55 years without alarm features, a test-and-treat approach for *Helicobacter pylori* is reasonable. For those who test negative for *H. pylori*, an empiric trial of acid suppression using a PPI for 4 to 6 weeks is recommended.

◆ DON'T BE TRICKED

- Patients with refractory symptoms despite empiric therapy should undergo upper endoscopy.

Gastroparesis

Diagnosis

Consider delayed gastric emptying (gastroparesis) in patients with recurrent nausea, early satiety, bloating, and weight loss. Look for SSc, diabetes mellitus, hypothyroidism, and administration of anticholinergic agents and narcotics. A viral cause is suggested by rapid onset of gastroparesis after a presumed viral infection.

In patients with acute symptoms, upper endoscopy is the initial study to rule out pyloric channel obstruction due to PUD. Patients with chronic symptoms or negative findings on upper endoscopy should have a nuclear medicine solid-phase gastric emptying study.

◆ DON'T BE TRICKED

- Patients with diabetes mellitus should have a blood glucose level <275 mg/dL during testing, because marked hyperglycemia can acutely impair gastric emptying.

Therapy

Provide nutritional support with liquid supplements or pureed meals. Specific diet recommendations include small low-fat meals consumed four to five times per day. Use IV erythromycin for acute gastroparesis and metoclopramide for chronic gastroparesis. Dystonia, parkinsonism-type movements, and tardive dyskinesia are serious complications of metoclopramide therapy and the drug must be stopped at the first sign of these disorders.

❖ Test Yourself

A 64-year-old woman with a 20-year history of type 2 diabetes mellitus has a 3-year history of postprandial nausea.

ANSWER: The probable diagnosis is diabetic gastroparesis. Order a gastric emptying study.

Complications of Bariatric and Gastric Surgery

Diagnosis

Major complications following Roux-en-Y gastric bypass include cholelithiasis, nephrolithiasis (due to increased urinary oxalate excretion), dumping syndrome, anastomotic stricture or ulceration, small-bowel obstruction, and gastrogastric fistula. Small intestinal bacterial overgrowth occurs most often with Roux-en-Y gastric bypass.

Micronutrient deficiencies can develop following bariatric surgery.

STUDY TABLE: Possible Micronutrient Deficiency Following Bariatric Surgery	
Nutrient	**Features of Deficiency**
Calcium	Short term: muscle contractions, pain, spasms, paresthesia
	Long term: drop in bone density, osteopenia/osteoporosis
Cobalamin (Vitamin B$_{12}$)	Macrocytic anemia, neurocognitive impairment, peripheral neuropathy, proprioceptive loss, spasticity, weakness, glossitis, cheilosis, angular stomatitis
Copper	Microcytic anemia, leukopenia, myelopathy (weakness, numbness, spasticity, hyperreflexia, painful paresthesia), poor wound healing
Folate	Macrocytic anemia, glossitis, cheilosis, palpitations, fatigue
Iron	Microcytic anemia, fatigue, white fingernail beds
Magnesium	Muscle contractions, muscle pain, muscle spasms
Selenium	Dilated cardiomyopathy, myopathy, myositis, connective tissue abnormalities (hair, nails, skin)
Thiamine (Vitamin B$_1$)	Cerebellar ataxia, nystagmus, ophthalmoplegia, confusion, confabulation (Wernicke-Korsakoff), HF, edema, ascites, peripheral neuropathy, weakness
Vitamin A	Night vision impairment, Bitot spots, corneal ulceration, blindness, itching, dry hair, loss of immunity
Vitamin D	Osteomalacia, osteoporosis, myalgia, arthralgia, depression, fasciculations
Zinc	Dermatitis, poor wound healing, blunting of taste sense, hair loss, glossitis

Data from: Stein J, Stier C, Raab H, Weiner R. Review article: the nutritional and pharmacological consequences of obesity surgery. Aliment Pharmacol Ther. 2014 Jul 30. [PMID: 25078533]

Complications following gastrectomy include:

- anastomotic leaks and strictures
- delayed gastric emptying
- dumping syndrome
- fat malabsorption

STUDY TABLE: Complications of Gastric Surgery	
If you see this...	**Do this...**
Abdominal cramps, nausea, and loose stools 15 minutes after eating followed within 90 minutes by lightheadedness, diaphoresis, and tachycardia following gastric resection or bypass surgery	Diagnose dumping syndrome
	Treat with small frequent feedings and low-carbohydrate meals
Loose stools and malabsorption following bypass surgery	Diagnose blind loop syndrome
	Treat with antibiotics and nutritional supplements
Abdominal pain, bloating, difficulty belching following fundoplication	Diagnose gas-bloat syndrome
	Treat with diet modification; most treatments are untested

Acute Pancreatitis

Diagnosis

Patients with acute pancreatitis usually have the sudden onset of epigastric pain, often radiating to the back, accompanied by nausea, vomiting, fever, and tachycardia. Causes of acute pancreatitis in the United States include:

- gallstone biliary obstruction and alcohol (most common)
- sulfonamides, estrogens, didanosine, valproic acid, thiazide diuretics, azathioprine/6-MP, pentamidine, and furosemide
- hypertriglyceridemia (>1000 mg/dL)

- endoscopic retrograde cholangiopancreatography (ERCP)
- CF (young people with pancreatitis)
- hypercalcemia

Diagnosis of acute pancreatitis requires at least two of the following criteria:

- acute onset of upper abdominal pain
- serum amylase or lipase increased ≥3 ULN (upper limit of normal)
- characteristic findings on cross-sectional imaging (ultrasound, CT, MRI)

Lipase is more specific and sensitive than amylase.

Mildly increased amylase values can be caused by kidney disease, intestinal ischemia, appendicitis, and parotitis. All patients require abdominal ultrasonography to evaluate the biliary tract for obstruction. A CT scan of the abdomen is also indicated if the pancreatitis is severe, lasts longer than 48 hours, or complications are suspected. Severe pancreatitis is associated with hemoconcentration as suggested by elevated (or rising) creatinine, and BUN. Pancreatic pseudocysts are the most common complication of acute pancreatitis. Repeated episodes of acute pancreatitis may result in chronic pancreatitis.

◆ DON'T BE TRICKED

- Do not routinely obtain abdominal CT for acute pancreatitis.
- Uncomplicated pancreatitis is not typically associated with rebound abdominal tenderness, absent bowel sounds, high fever, or melena. When these findings are present, consider abscess, pseudocyst, or necrotizing pancreatitis.

Therapy

In addition to supportive therapy with vigorous IV hydration and pain relief, look for indications for the following treatments:

- resume oral feeding when nausea, vomiting, and abdominal pain resolve
- enteral jejunal feedings (preferred) or total parenteral nutrition for moderate to severe pancreatitis
- antibiotics for cholangitis, infected pancreatic necrosis, and infected pseudocysts
- cholecystectomy prior to discharge for uncomplicated gallstone pancreatitis
- ERCP for ascending cholangitis within 24 hours of presentation
- ERCP for nonresolving biliary obstruction

Fluid collections arise from disruption of the pancreatic ductal system. They are known as acute peripancreatic fluid collections for the first 4 weeks after presentation and pancreatic pseudocysts after becoming encapsulated. Most resolve spontaneously. Symptomatic fluid collections are treated with transgastric or transduodenal drainage. Walled-off necrosis often resolves spontaneously but may require decompression or debridement if symptomatic.

◆ DON'T BE TRICKED

- Fluid resuscitation (250-500 mL/h) is most beneficial in the first 12-24 hours and may be detrimental after this therapeutic window.
- Do not withhold oral feeding on the basis of persistent elevations in pancreatic enzyme levels.
- Do not select antibiotics for interstitial (nonnecrotizing) pancreatitis without evidence of infection.

❖ Test Yourself

A 71-year-old woman is hospitalized with gallstone pancreatitis. On the sixth day, she has increased pain, fever, and leukocytosis. A CT scan of the abdomen with contrast shows hypodense, nonenhancing areas involving 50% of the pancreas.

ANSWER: The diagnosis is pancreatic necrosis. Arrange a surgical consultation.

Chronic Pancreatitis

Diagnosis

Common diagnostic criteria:

- history of pain, recurrent attacks of pancreatitis, weight loss
- pancreatic calcifications on imaging
- ductal dilation or inflammatory masses
- exocrine pancreatic insufficiency (steatorrhea)
- diabetes

Chronic alcohol abuse is the most common cause in industrialized countries. Abdominal CT is the most sensitive imaging test to document pancreatic calcifications. If calcifications are absent, a pancreas-protocol CT or magnetic resonance cholangiopancreatography (MRCP) should be done to detect abnormalities of the main and branch pancreatic ducts. Young adults with chronic pancreatitis require genetic testing for CF. Disease onset in older patients requires exclusion of AIP and pancreatic cancer.

◆ **DON'T BE TRICKED**

- Normal amylase and lipase levels do not rule out chronic pancreatitis.

Therapy

Treatment of chronic pancreatitis is directed at controlling pain and alleviating the manifestations of diabetes mellitus, malabsorption, and steatorrhea. Administer pancreatic enzymes as initial therapy for malabsorption. If enzyme supplements do not control diarrhea, begin antidiarrheal agents.

Persistent pain is treated in a stepwise approach:

- simple analgesics
- tramadol
- nonenteric coated pancreatic enzymes
- low-dose tricyclic antidepressants
- gabapentinoids (gabapentin and pregabalin)

In patients with persistent or refractory pain look for a dilated pancreatic duct and intraductal calcifications. These patients may benefit from endoscopic stenting, lithotripsy, or surgical drainage (pancreaticojejunostomy).

Autoimmune Pancreatitis

Diagnosis

Patients with AIP typically present with painless obstructive jaundice or acute pancreatitis (rare). Cross-sectional imaging reveals "sausage-shaped" pancreatic enlargement with an indistinct border. It is important to exclude pancreatic cancer; biopsy may be necessary.

Type I AIP

- pancreatitis, Sjögren syndrome, PSC, and IBD
- older men
- increased serum IgG4 level

Type II AIP

- chronic pancreatitis
- no systemic disease
- normal IgG4 levels

Therapy

Most patients with type I or II respond to glucocorticoids. Patients with relapse typically respond to glucocorticoid retreatment.

Acute Diarrhea

Diagnosis

The majority of acute diarrhea in developed countries is due to viral gastroenteritis or food poisoning and is self-limited. A careful review of medication history (including nonprescription medications and supplements) is indicated to look for drugs that cause diarrhea. If diarrhea does not resolve in 1 week, evaluation is recommended with stool testing for common bacterial pathogens, including *Clostridium difficile.*

STUDY TABLE: Foodborne Acute Diarrhea	
When Symptoms Develop...	**Make this Diagnosis...**
6 hours after ingestion	*Staphylococcus aureus* or *Bacillus cereus*
8-14 hours after ingestion	*Clostridium perfringens*
>14 hours after ingestion	Viral or enterotoxigenic or EHEC

Ten percent of patients with enterohemorrhagic *Escherichia coli* O157:H7 (EHEC) colitis develop HUS or TTP. *Yersinia enterocolitica* colitis can mimic appendicitis or Crohn disease. Cryptosporidiosis develops most often in patients with AIDS, but outbreaks also occur in immunocompetent patients and cause a self-limited secretory diarrhea.

Therapy

Supportive care with oral hydration and antidiarrheal medications is sufficient for most patients with acute diarrhea. Antibiotic treatment is reserved for patients with diarrhea lasting >7 days or with symptoms of fever, abdominal pain, or hematochezia. Diarrhea due to parasites (*Giardia lamblia* or *Entamoeba histolytica*) requires therapy with metronidazole.

◆ DON'T BE TRICKED

- Do not order stool cultures for acute diarrhea of <1 week duration.
- Do not choose antibiotics for EHEC colitis.
- Do not choose loperamide or diphenoxylate for acute diarrhea with fever or blood in the stool. Both agents are associated with HUS in EHEC colitis and toxic megacolon in *C. difficile* infection.

Chronic Diarrhea

Diagnosis

Chronic diarrhea is arbitrarily defined as lasting longer than 4 weeks and is often due to noninfectious causes, except for infection with *Giardia lamblia*. This diagnosis should be considered in patients with exposure to young children or potentially contaminated water (lakes and streams).

Medications are often overlooked as a cause of chronic diarrhea. Look for PPIs, magnesium-containing antacids, metformin, colchicine, antibiotics, and sorbitol (added as a sweetener to gum and candy).

Select colonoscopy for most patients with chronic diarrhea. Patients undergoing colonoscopy should have the terminal ileum viewed to assess for Crohn disease and undergo random biopsies of the colonic mucosa to assess for microscopic colitis.

If the colonoscopy is nondiagnostic, a 48- to 72-hour stool collection with analysis of fat content measures the amount of diarrhea and steatorrhea. Fat excretion above 14 g/d is diagnostic of steatorrhea. Patients with steatorrhea should undergo evaluation for small-bowel malabsorption disorders (e.g., celiac disease), bacterial overgrowth, and pancreatic insufficiency.

Stool electrolytes (sodium and potassium) can be measured in liquid stool to calculate the fecal osmotic gap, which helps to diagnose osmotic diarrhea. The gap is calculated as $290 - 2 \times [Na + K]$; an osmotic gap >100 mOsm/kg H_2O indicates an osmotic diarrhea. A gap <50 mOsm/kg H_2O indicates a secretory diarrhea. Measured stool osmolarity <250 mOsm/kg H_2O suggests factitious diarrhea associated with chronic laxative abuse or adding water to the stool.

Osmotic diarrhea is most commonly caused by lactase deficiency. Osmotic diarrhea is associated with eating, improves with fasting, and typically is not nocturnal. Secretory diarrhea is characterized by large-volume, watery, nocturnal bowel movements and is unchanged by fasting (see also Celiac Disease).

STUDY TABLE: Differential Diagnosis of Chronic Diarrhea	
If you see this...	**Diagnose or do this...**
Bloating, abdominal discomfort relieved by a bowel movement, no weight loss or alarm features	IBS; test for celiac disease
Diarrhea mainly in women aged 45-60 years, unrelated to food intake (nocturnal diarrhea), normal colonoscopy	Microscopic colitis; stop NSAIDs, PPIs; biopsy
Diarrhea with dairy products	Lactose intolerance; dietary exclusion or hydrogen breath test
Use of artificial sweeteners or fructose	Carbohydrate intolerance; attempt dietary exclusion or hydrogen breath test
Nocturnal diarrhea and diabetes mellitus or SSc	Small bowel bacterial overgrowth; hydrogen breath test or empiric antibiotic trial
Coexistent pulmonary diseases and/or recurrent *Giardia* infection	CVI and selective IgA deficiency; obtain measurement of immune globulins
Somatization or other psychiatric syndromes, history of laxative use	Self-induced diarrhea; obtain tests for stool pH, sodium, potassium, and magnesium
Severe secretory diarrhea and flushing	Carcinoid syndrome; obtain test for 24-hour urinary excretion of 5-HIAA

❖ Test Yourself

A 36-year-old woman has watery diarrhea that is not nocturnal. She has six to seven high-volume bowel movements daily, and her symptoms improve with fasting. Fecal leukocytes and stool culture are negative. Stool sodium is 70 mEq/L and stool potassium is 10 mEq/L.

ANSWER: The diagnosis is osmotic diarrhea.

A 55-year-old woman who takes daily NSAIDs for OA has watery diarrhea without weight loss. Colonoscopy is normal.

ANSWER: The diagnosis is likely microscopic colitis.

Malabsorption

Diagnosis

Patients with chronic diarrhea, especially those who report an oily residue in their stool, should be evaluated for possible fat malabsorption. The four most common disorders causing malabsorption with steatorrhea are celiac disease, small bowel bacterial overgrowth, short-bowel syndrome, and pancreatic insufficiency.

STUDY TABLE: Chronic Diarrhea and Malabsorption Syndromes	
If you see this...	**Do this...**
History of IBS and iron deficiency anemia	Diagnose celiac disease
	Obtain IgA anti-tTG or IgA anti-endomysial antibody assays and small bowel biopsy if positive
	Order a gluten-free diet
Chronic pancreatitis, hyperglycemia, history of pancreatic resection, CF	Diagnose pancreatic insufficiency
	Obtain tests for excess fecal fat, x-rays for pancreatic calcifications, and consider pancreatic function tests
	Treat with pancreatic enzyme replacement therapy
Previous surgery, small bowel diverticulosis, dysmotility (SSc or diabetes mellitus), combination of vitamin B_{12} deficiency and elevated folate level	Diagnose bacterial overgrowth
	Order empiric trial of antibiotics or hydrogen breath test
Resection of >200 cm of distal small bowel (or viable small bowel <180 cm)	Diagnose short-bowel syndrome
	Replace nutrient and electrolyte deficiencies
History of resection of <100 cm of distal ileum, now with voluminous diarrhea, weight loss, and evidence of malnutrition	Diagnose short-bowel syndrome with bile acid enteropathy
	Order empiric trial of cholestyramine
Arthralgia; fever; neurologic, ocular, or cardiac disease	Diagnose Whipple disease
	Select small bowel biopsy and PCR for *Tropheryma whippelii*
	Order antibiotics for 12 months
Travel to India or Puerto Rico, malabsorption, weight loss, malaise, folate or vitamin B_{12} deficiency, and steatorrhea	Diagnose tropical sprue
	Order a small bowel biopsy
	Treat with a sulfonamide or tetracycline and folic acid
Prolonged traveler's diarrhea, diarrhea after a camping trip, or outbreak in a day-care center	Diagnose giardiasis
	Identify *Giardia* parasites or *Giardia* antigen in the stool
	Treat with metronidazole

◆ DON'T BE TRICKED

- Do not use cholestyramine if ileal resection is >100 cm (will worsen bile salt deficiency and steatorrhea).
- Use cholestyramine if diarrhea begins after cholecystectomy.

❖ Test Yourself

A 54-year-old woman has a 4-month history of diarrhea and weight loss. Laboratory studies show hypocalcemia, microcytic anemia, and an increased PT.

ANSWER: The probable diagnosis is celiac disease. Order an IgA anti-tTG antibody assay and, if positive, follow with a small bowel biopsy.

Celiac Disease

Diagnosis

Celiac disease occurs secondary to ingestion of wheat gluten or related rye and barley proteins in genetically predisposed persons. Characteristic findings are:

- chronic diarrhea or steatorrhea
- bloating, weight loss, and abdominal pain
- pruritic papulovesicular rash on the extensor surfaces (dermatitis herpetiformis; see Dermatology, Pemphigus Vulgaris and Pemphigoid)

- isolated abnormalities of liver chemistry tests
- iron deficiency anemia
- fat-soluble vitamin deficiencies
- osteoporosis

Celiac disease is often misdiagnosed as IBS. Diagnostic tests include an IgA anti–tTG or IgA anti–endomysial antibody assay. An association between celiac disease and IgA deficiency can lead to false-negative IgA-based tests. In patients with IgA deficiency, assays for IgG anti–tTG or IgG anti–endomysial antibodies are necessary. Definitive diagnosis requires small bowel biopsy or presence of dermatitis herpetiformis.

Type 1 diabetes mellitus and autoimmune thyroid disease occur more commonly in patients with celiac disease. Patients with celiac disease and thyroiditis can have problems absorbing thyroid hormone. The first sign of celiac disease may be malabsorption of thyroid hormone (inability to increase total T_4 with increasing doses of thyroxine). Small bowel lymphoma is more common in patients with celiac disease. Measure the bone mineral density in all patients with newly diagnosed celiac disease.

◆ DON'T BE TRICKED

- Do not select empiric treatment with a gluten-free diet because it may result in false-negative serologic test results with subsequent testing.

Therapy

Select a gluten-free diet for treatment of celiac disease or dermatitis. All patients, regardless of symptoms, are treated to prevent intestinal lymphoma, including patients with isolated dermatitis herpetiformis. Patients with osteomalacia should also receive supplemental vitamin D and calcium. The effectiveness of diet therapy is determined by remeasuring IgA anti–tTG antibody titers or repeating small bowel biopsies. Nonadherence is the most common reason for failure of a gluten-free diet. Adherent patients with recurrent malabsorption should be evaluated for intestinal lymphoma. Other causes of continued symptoms include inadvertent exposure to gluten and microscopic colitis.

Inflammatory Bowel Disease

Diagnosis

IBD comprises a group of related conditions characterized by idiopathic inflammation of the GI tract. The two most common IBDs are Crohn disease and ulcerative colitis, both of which cause macroscopic inflammation. Microscopic colitis is the least common IBD and does not cause significant macroscopic abnormalities. Although several features may differentiate Crohn disease from ulcerative colitis, overlap is significant.

STUDY TABLE: Differentiating Ulcerative Colitis from Crohn Disease	
Ulcerative Colitis	**Crohn Disease**
Mucosal edema, erythema, loss of the vascular pattern, granularity, friability, ulceration, and bleeding	Linear, stellate, or serpiginous ulcerations with "skip" areas of inflammation involving entire GI tract
Altered crypt architecture with shortened, branched crypts, crypt abscesses	Granulomas are characteristic but are often not found; transmural involvement
Diarrhea (prominent), tenesmus, urgency hematochezia, weight loss, and fever	Abdominal pain (prominent), diarrhea, inflammatory masses, fever, weight loss, intestinal strictures and fistula (to skin, bladder, vagina, or enteric-enteric)
Smoking alleviates symptoms	Smoking is a risk factor for disease

The most common extraintestinal manifestations are oral aphthous ulcers, arthralgia, and back pain (indicating ankylosing spondylitis or sacroiliitis). Eye symptoms (redness, pain, swelling) may be due to uveitis or scleritis. Skin manifestations include pyoderma gangrenosum and erythema nodosum. Liver involvement most commonly includes PSC.

Colonoscopy and biopsy confirm the diagnosis. Stool studies are indicated for *Shigella, Salmonella, Campylobacter, Escherichia coli* O157:H7, ova and parasites, and *Clostridium difficile* toxin.

◆ **DON'T BE TRICKED**

- Some ulcerative colitis patients have inflammation extending into the ileum for a few centimeters (backwash ileitis) but this finding alone is not indicative of Crohn disease.
- Do not do a barium enema examination in patients with moderate to severe ulcerative colitis because this procedure may precipitate toxic megacolon.
- In patients with Crohn disease and cystitis, consider the possibility of enterovesical fistula.

Therapy

Treatment of Crohn disease and ulcerative colitis is divided into active and maintenance strategies. Specific treatment choices depend on the type, extent, and severity of the disease.

The 5-ASA drugs are first-line therapy for inducing and maintaining remission in ulcerative colitis. They deliver 5-ASA topically to the bowel lumen, primarily to the colon, with the exception of the time-release formulation of mesalamine, which is able to deliver the drug throughout the small bowel as well as the colon.

STUDY TABLE: Treatment of Ulcerative Colitis	
Indications	**Principal Therapy**
Mild disease: <4 bowel movements daily; occasional blood in stool; and normal vital signs, hemoglobin, and ESR	5-ASA agents: mesalamine or sulfasalazine (not effective for small bowel disease)
Moderate disease	Prednisone or budesonide for remission induction
	Maintenance therapy with either a 5-ASA agent or 6-MP or azathioprine
Severe disease: >6 bowel movements daily, bleeding, fever, pulse >90/min, ESR >30 mm/h, anemia	IV glucocorticoids followed by anti-TNF antibody
	Surgery for refractory disease

Anti-TNF antibodies are approved for inducing and maintaining remission in ulcerative colitis (e.g., infliximab, adalimumab, and golimumab). Patients whose symptoms do not respond to glucocorticoids are treated with an anti-TNF biologic agent, or colectomy.

STUDY TABLE: Treatment of Crohn Disease	
Indications	**Principal Therapy**
Mild to moderate disease: No fever or abdominal tenderness, <10% weight loss	5-ASA agent as initial therapy for small- or large-bowel disease (often not effective)
	Prednisone or budesonide for ileal or right colonic disease followed by 6-MP, azathioprine, or methotrexate for maintenance
Moderate to severe disease: Fever, >10% weight loss, anemia, abdominal pain, and nausea or vomiting	Prednisone for remission induction
	6-MP, azathioprine, or methotrexate for maintenance
	Anti-TNF antibodies for refractory disease
Severe to fulminant disease: Despite oral glucocorticoids, high fever, cachexia, vomiting, rebound tenderness, obstruction, or abscess	IV glucocorticoid for remission
	Anti-TNF antibodies in glucocorticoid-refractory disease
	Surgical intervention with colectomy if patient is extremely toxic or does not benefit from medications
Fistula	Azathioprine, 6-MP, anti-TNF antibodies

The level of thiopurine methyltransferase should be checked before starting azathioprine or 6-MP; 1 in 300 patients lack enzyme activity and are at high risk of drug toxicity, and azathioprine and 6-MP should not be used in these patients.

Anti-TNF agents (e.g, infliximab, adalimumab, and certolizumab) are effective for inducing and maintaining remission and closing fistulas. Natalizumab is a monoclonal antibody that is effective for induction and maintenance of remission in Crohn disease that has failed to respond to other medications.

Beginning 8 years after diagnosis, surveillance colonoscopy for colon cancer is needed every 1 to 2 years for patients with ulcerative colitis or Crohn disease involving most of the colon. If dysplasia is found, proctocolectomy is required.

◆ **DON'T BE TRICKED**

- Prior to initiating an anti-TNF agent, all patients should be screened for TB, HBV, and HCV.

❖ **Test Yourself**

An 18-year-old man has a 3-month history of five or more bowel movements daily, fever, and abdominal pain. Vital signs are stable. Colonoscopy shows ulcerative colitis.

ANSWER: Begin prednisone for remission and oral sulfasalazine for maintenance.

Microscopic Colitis

Diagnosis

Microscopic colitis is characterized by chronic diarrhea without abdominal pain or weight loss, most commonly in women between ages 45 and 60 years. In certain cases, NSAIDs and PPIs have been implicated as causative agents. Colonoscopy with biopsies is required for diagnosis. The colonic mucosa appears normal on gross examination. Microscopic colitis is further classified into collagenous colitis or lymphocytic colitis based on histology.

The association with celiac disease is of particular clinical importance because the symptoms of these conditions are similar. Therefore, in patients with celiac disease or microscopic colitis whose symptoms do not respond to appropriate therapy, the other condition must be considered and ruled out with appropriate testing.

Therapy

Microscopic colitis is best treated with supportive treatment with antidiarrheal agents such as loperamide or bismuth subsalicylate; diphenoxylate may be effective for mild cases. Otherwise, budesonide has the best documented efficacy. Stop NSAIDs, which may contribute to symptoms.

Chronic Constipation

Diagnosis

Diagnosis of chronic constipation requires presence of symptoms for ≥3 months. If secondary causes of constipation are excluded based on history, structural testing, and biochemical testing, constipation is classified as functional.

Classification of functional constipation:

- normal-transit constipation
- slow-transit constipation
- dyssynergic defecation

Dyssynergic defecation can be suspected if the following findings are present when the patient is asked to "bear down" as if performing a bowel movement:

- failure of or weak abdominal muscle contraction
- no relaxation of the external anal sphincter
- lack of perineal descent

Anorectal manometry can confirm the diagnosis of dyssynergic defecation.

Therapy

Chronic constipation can be approached in a stepped fashion:

- increase physical activity and dietary fiber
- soluble fibers such as psyllium or methylcellulose
- surfactants such as docusate sodium or docusate calcium (most appropriate for very mild, intermittent constipation)
- osmotic laxatives include magnesium hydroxide, lactulose, sorbitol, and PEG 3350 (PEG is superior)
- stimulant laxatives such as anthraquinone, senna, and the diphenylmethanes (fastest-acting agents)

If chronic constipation does not respond to initial stepped approach, prosecretory agents, including lubiprostone and linaclotide, are available by prescription.

Physical therapy with biofeedback is utilized for the treatment of dyssynergia and is effective.

◆ DON'T BE TRICKED

- Medications (particularly narcotic analgesics) are the most common cause of chronic constipation.
- Chronic senna use can lead to benign pigmentation of the colon, known as melanosis coli.

Irritable Bowel Syndrome

Diagnosis

IBS has been defined as abdominal pain associated with altered bowel habits (change in stool form or frequency) over a period of at least 3 months. Other symptoms include straining, urgency, a feeling of incomplete evacuation, passing mucus, and bloating. IBS is further subtyped based on the predominant stool pattern as IBS with constipation (IBS-C), IBS with diarrhea (IBS-D), or mixed IBS (IBS-M).

The clinical diagnosis of IBS can be made in the absence of alarm symptoms (anemia; weight loss; and family history of colorectal cancer, IBD, or celiac disease). Routine CBC, serum chemistry studies, TSH, stool studies for ova and parasites, and abdominal imaging are unnecessary. Screening for celiac disease with serum tTG should be considered in patients with IBS-D or IBS-M symptoms. Patients older than 50 years of age or with severe or refractory symptoms require colonoscopy.

◆ DON'T BE TRICKED

- Routine colonoscopy (every 10 years) should be pursued only in patients between the ages of 50-75 years who otherwise meet criteria for colon cancer screening.

Therapy

Management of IBS focuses on controlling symptoms rather than on cure.

- Modify sdiet to control symptoms.
- Hyoscyamine and dicyclomine are used for the short-term treatment of abdominal pain in IBS-D or IBS-C.
- Tricyclic antidepressants and SSRIs are effective for abdominal pain; tricyclic antidepressants are preferred in IBS-D and SSRIs are preferred in IBS-C.
- The osmotic laxative PEG is effective in IBS-C.
- Lubiprostone and linaclotide are indicated for IBS-C unresponsive to PEG; lubiprostone is FDA approved for women with IBS-C, and linaclotide is FDA approved for the treatment of IBS-C in adults.
- Loperamide is effective for IBS-D.

◆ DON'T BE TRICKED

- Alosetron should not be used to treat IBS because of the risk of ischemic colitis.

Diverticular Disease

Diagnosis

Diverticular disorders of the colon include diverticulosis, diverticular bleeding, and diverticulitis.

Diverticulosis refers to an asymptomatic herniation (diverticulum) of the intestinal wall.

Diverticulitis is an inflammatory response following microperforation of a diverticulum and is characterized by LLQ abdominal pain and fever. If clinical features are highly suggestive of diverticulitis, imaging studies are unnecessary. If the diagnosis is not clear or if an abscess is suspected (severe pain, high fever, palpable mass), CT imaging is indicated. Dysuria, urinary frequency, and urgency may reflect bladder irritation. Pneumaturia, fecaluria, or recurrent/polymicrobial UTI suggest a colovesical fistula. A colonoscopy is performed following recovery to rule out cancer.

Diverticular bleeding occurs following rupture of an artery that has penetrated a diverticulum, is typically painless, and usually stops without therapy.

◆ DON'T BE TRICKED

- Avoid colonoscopy in the setting of acute diverticulitis, because air insufflation may increase the risk for perforation.

Therapy

For stable patients with diverticulitis, select a clear-liquid diet and a 7- to 10-day course of antibiotics, such as ciprofloxacin and metronidazole. Hospitalize patients if they are unable to maintain oral intake for IV fluids and antibiotics. A small abscess may resolve with antimicrobial therapy alone. CT-guided drainage can facilitate nonsurgical management of larger abscesses. Emergent surgery is required when conservative treatment fails or for peritonitis, sepsis, or perforation. After recovering from acute diverticulitis, 30% of patients will have recurrent episodes. After a second episode, the risk of subsequent attacks increases to 50%, and surgical resection of the affected colon is indicated. After the patient has recovered, follow-up colonoscopy is needed to exclude colon cancer.

Mesenteric Ischemia and Ischemic Colitis

Diagnosis

The two most common GI ischemic disorders are acute mesenteric ischemia (AMI) and ischemic colitis. Embolism to the mesenteric arteries causes 50% of cases of AMI due to AF or left ventricle thrombus. Arterial thrombosis is usually due to atherosclerotic disease. Mesenteric vein thrombosis (rare) may result from malignancy, hypercoagulable states, abdominal or cardiac surgery, or pancreatitis. Nonocclusive mesenteric ischemia is caused by low-flow states such as HF, sepsis, profound hypotension, or hypovolemia, or use of vasoactive medications (vasopressors, ergots, triptans, cocaine, digitalis). Leukocytosis, hemoconcentration, ion gap metabolic acidosis, and elevations in LDH and/or amylase levels are seen.

STUDY TABLE: Differential Diagnosis of GI Ischemic Syndromes		
Problem	**Symptoms**	**Diagnosis**
AMI	Poorly localized severe abdominal pain, often out of proportion to physical findings; peritoneal signs signify infarction	CTA or selective mesenteric angiography
Chronic mesenteric ischemia	Postprandial abdominal pain, fear of eating, and weight loss	CTA, selective angiography, or MRA
Ischemic colitis	LLQ abdominal pain and self-limited bloody diarrhea	Colonoscopy: patchy segmental ulcerations

Ischemic Colitis: Thumbprinting (submucosal hemorrhage and edema) is shown in the transverse colon on this barium x-ray.

Therapy

Patients will require hospitalization, fluid resuscitation, correction of electrolyte and acid-base disorders, and broad-spectrum antibiotics.

STUDY TABLE: Therapy for Mesenteric Ischemia and Ischemic Colitis	
Condition	**Therapy**
AMI with peritoneal signs	Urgent laparotomy. Resection of necrotic bowel. Embolectomy or thrombectomy and surgical revascularization.
AMI without peritoneal signs	Angiography. Surgical embolectomy or intra-arterial thrombolysis. Intra-arterial papaverine for nonocclusive mesenteric ischemia.
Chronic mesenteric ischemia	Surgical reconstruction or angioplasty with stenting.
Ischemic colitis	Supportive care with IV fluids and bowel rest.

◆ DON'T BE TRICKED

- The diagnosis of colonic ischemia is based on clinical history; there is no role for angiography.

Differentiating Cholestatic and Hepatocellular Diseases

Key Considerations

Hepatocellular injury primarily results in elevated AST and ALT values, usually >500 U/L.

- Virus- or drug-induced acute hepatitis usually causes serum aminotransferase elevations >1000 U/L (ALT > AST) and serum total bilirubin levels >15 mg/dL.
- ALT values >5000 U/L are usually due to acetaminophen hepatotoxicity or hepatic ischemia.
- An AST/ALT ratio >2.0 is highly suggestive of AH.
- An AST/ALT ratio >1.0 may suggest cirrhosis in patients with chronic viral hepatitis.
- Abnormal PT and serum albumin values imply severe hepatocellular dysfunction.
- AST and ALT elevations in chronic hepatitis are less marked than elevations in acute hepatitis.
- Minimal ALT and AST elevations in a patient with obesity, hyperlipidemia, and hypertension suggest nonalcoholic liver disease.

Cholestatic liver diseases primarily cause elevated serum bilirubin and alkaline phosphatase values with proportionally lesser elevations of aminotransferase levels. Cholestatic diseases affect microscopic ducts, large bile ducts, or both.

Overproduction (hemolysis) or impaired uptake (Gilbert disease) of bilirubin is characterized by >80% indirect (unconjugated) bilirubin, whereas hepatocyte dysfunction or impaired bile flow (obstruction) is characterized by >20% direct (conjugated) bilirubin.

◆ **DON'T BE TRICKED**

- Extensive testing is not required to establish the diagnosis of Gilbert disease; verify normal aminotransferase levels and absence of hemolysis with normal hemoglobin and reticulocyte count.
- Early common bile duct obstruction with a biliary stone may be associated with a hepatocellular pattern or changes to a cholestatic pattern with the passage of time.

Hepatitis A

Prevention

Hepatitis A vaccine is indicated for travelers to endemic areas, injection drug users, men who have sex with men, and patients with chronic liver disease and clotting factor disorders. Immunization or immune globulin should be given within 2 weeks to household, sexual, and day-care contacts of patients with hepatitis A or persons who ate foods contaminated with HAV. Immune globulin should be administered to travelers leaving for endemic areas in <2 weeks who did not previously receive the hepatitis A vaccine. Hepatitis A immunization should also be provided.

Diagnosis

HAV is transmitted by the fecal-oral route and spreads primarily by close personal contact with a person infected with HAV. It is associated with abrupt onset of fatigue, anorexia, malaise, nausea, vomiting, and jaundice. Laboratory findings include marked elevations of serum aminotransferases (usually >1000 U/L). Approximately 50% of patients with HAV have no identifiable source for their infection. Patients with unexplained acute hepatitis or acute liver failure should be tested for IgM anti-HAV. The clinical course of relapsing HAV infection is characterized by clinical recovery with near normalization of the serum liver tests followed several weeks later by biochemical and sometimes clinical relapse. Hepatitis A is not a cause of chronic hepatitis.

Hepatitis B

Prevention

HBV vaccination decreases the incidence and prevalence of HBV and results in fewer cases of HCC in endemic areas. Hepatitis B vaccine plus HBIG is indicated for postexposure prophylaxis after needle-stick injury and for sexual and household contacts of patients with HBV.

Diagnosis

HBV is transmitted parenterally by exposure to the blood or body fluids of an infected person, including through:

- injection-drug use
- sexual contact with an infected person
- transmission by an infected mother to her infant during delivery

About 30% to 40% of patients with acute hepatitis B have no identifiable risk factors. Symptoms of acute hepatitis B are similar to those of acute hepatitis A. It is not uncommon for persons to have anicteric or subclinical acute infection. Characteristic findings are unexplained increases in serum aminotransferase (AST/ALT) levels; acute liver failure may occur.

There are several stages of hepatitis B but not all patients go through each stage.

- Patients who acquire HBV infection at birth often go through the immune tolerant phase characterized by a normal ALT level despite a positive HBeAg and very high HBV DNA level.
- The inactive carrier is characterized by a normal ALT level and an HBV DNA level <20,000 U/mL.
- Patients in the HBeAg-positive ("immune active") or HBeAg-negative ("immune escape") chronic HBV phases have an elevated ALT level and an HBV DNA level >10,000 U/mL.

When liver biopsy is performed, liver injury and fibrosis are present. Patients with chronic HBV infection should be tested for hepatitis D virus, especially in the presence of an otherwise unexplained acute hepatitis in a patient with chronic hepatitis.

◆ DON'T BE TRICKED

- Chronic hepatitis B may present as membranous GN, polyarteritis nodosa, or cryoglobulinemia.

STUDY TABLE: Interpretation of Hepatitis B Test Results

Clinical Scenario	HBsAg	Anti-HBs	IgM anti-HBc	IgG anti-HBc	HBeAg	Anti-HBe	HBV DNA, U/mL
Acute hepatitis B; occasionally reactivation of chronic hepatitis B	+	–	+	–	+	–	>20,000
Resolved prior infection	–	+	–	+	–	+/–	Undetected
Immunity due to prior vaccination	–	+	–	–	–	–	Undetected
False-positive or resolved prior infection	–	–	–	+	–	–	Undetected
Chronic hepatitis B inactive carrier state	+	–	–	+	–	+	<20,000
HBeAg-positive chronic hepatitis B	+	–	–	+	+	–	>20,000
HBeAg-negative chronic hepatitis B	+	–	–	+	–	+	>10,000

Therapy

Treatment is recommended for those who have:

- acute liver failure
- chronic infection with an elevated ALT level and an HBV DNA level >10,000 U/mL
- immunosuppressive therapy

Treatment usually consists of entecavir or tenofovir.

- Lamivudine, adefovir, and telbivudine are associated with resistance with chronic use.
- Pegylated interferon may be used for patients without cirrhosis who have high ALT levels and relatively low HBV DNA levels

In patients coinfected with HIV and who have not yet been treated for either disease, emtricitabine-tenofovir is typically used as part of ART.

◆ DON'T BE TRICKED

- Do not treat HBV infection in patients in the immune tolerant or inactive carrier phases.
- Interferon alfa should not be used in patients with active autoimmune disorders, severe cytopenias, decompensated cirrhosis, or major depression.

Because 10% of patients taking interferon alfa develop hypothyroidism, check the thyroid status at follow-up visits.

The following characteristics are associated with an increased risk for HCC in patients with HBV and are indications for surveillance with ultrasonography every 6 months:

- cirrhosis
- Asian men >40 years and Asian women >50 years
- black patients >20 years
- elevated ALT level and HBV DNA levels >20,000 U/mL
- family history of HCC

❖ Test Yourself

A 55-year-old woman has a 6-month history of fatigue and malaise. She is taking paroxetine for depression. The serum ALT is 109 U/L. HBsAg, HBeAg, and HBV DNA are positive, and anti-HBV is negative.

ANSWER: The diagnosis is chronic hepatitis B. Begin entecavir or tenofovir; do not select interferon alfa.

Hepatitis C

Screening

Universal screening is recommended for those born between 1945 and 1965.

Diagnosis

HCV is transmitted parenterally and is the most prevalent bloodborne infection in the United States. HCV usually manifests as chronic liver disease because the acute infection is usually asymptomatic. Test for HCV in patients with chronic liver disease, as well as patients with vasculitis, cryoglobulinemia, GN, and porphyria cutanea tarda. Other high-risk groups include injection drug users, recipients of blood transfusions before 1992, and those with HIV or a STI.

Measurement of anti-HCV is the initial diagnostic study. If positive, test for HCV RNA to determine the presence of active infection. HCV genotyping should be performed at the time of diagnosis to help choose a treatment regimen. Patients with spontaneous resolution of acute HCV or who have been treated successfully for HCV will have clearance of HCV RNA but usually remain positive for antibody to HCV.

Chronic HCV infection can cause cirrhosis and is a risk factor for HCC.

◆ DON'T BE TRICKED

- Because normal aminotransferase levels occur in up to 40% of patients with chronic HCV, normal levels cannot exclude a diagnosis of HCV.

Therapy

Treatment regimens based upon genotype. Genotype 1 is the most prominent in the U.S. (70%), and its regimen includes:

- Sofosbuvir and ledipasvir (available as a combination tablet)
- Ombitasvir, paritaprevir, and ritonavir (available as a combination tablet) plus dasabuvir with or without ribavirin
- Sofosbuvir and simeprevir with or without ribavirin

Treatment of patients with HIV coinfection is similar to that for patients with HCV alone. Patients with HCV who have decompensated disease or localized HCC are candidates for liver transplantation.

HCV rarely causes HCC in the absence of cirrhosis. Patients with cirrhosis should undergo sonography surveillance for HCC every 6 months.

Test Yourself

A 45-year-old male injection drug user has a 3-month history of recurrent purpuric lesions on his legs. Skin biopsy shows leukocytoclastic vasculitis. HBsAg is negative.

ANSWER: The probable diagnosis is HCV. Order anti-HCV testing. If positive, test for cryoglobulins and HCV RNA.

Leukocytoclastic Vasculitis: Palpable purpura consistent with HCV-associated leukocytoclastic vasculitis.

Alcoholic Hepatitis

Diagnosis

Hepatic steatosis with inflammation is called alcoholic steatohepatitis. Mild forms of alcoholic steatohepatitis are common, are usually asymptomatic, and are associated with mild elevations in aminotransferase levels. The most severe form of alcoholic steatohepatitis is called AH and is distinguished from alcohol-induced steatosis and steatohepatitis by the presence of symptoms.

AH is a complication of chronic, daily, heavy use of alcohol (>100 g/d) for more than 8 years. Acute alcoholic binges can cause fatty liver. The clinical presentation of patients with acute AH includes jaundice, anorexia, and tender hepatomegaly with or without fever. Findings consistent with portal hypertension may be present. Patients with AH have AST and ALT measurements <300 to 500 U/L, with an AST/ALT ratio ≥2.0.

Therapy

Glucocorticoids or pentoxifylline are indicated for patients with a Maddrey Discriminant Function (MDF) score ≥32, Model for End-Stage Liver Disease (MELD) score ≥18, or encephalopathy and ascites. If the bilirubin level does not improve by day 7, then prednisone should be discontinued.

◆ DON'T BE TRICKED

• Do not use glucocorticoids in patients with AH associated with GI bleeding, infection, pancreatitis, or kidney disease.

Test Yourself

A 46-year-old man has fever and RUQ abdominal pain. He drinks six cans of beer daily. Physical examination discloses ascites. Serum AST is 260 U/L and ALT is 80 U/L. The ascitic fluid leukocyte count is <100/μL.

ANSWER: The diagnosis is alcoholic hepatitis.

Autoimmune Hepatitis

Diagnosis

Autoimmune hepatitis is an inflammatory condition of the liver of unknown cause. It primarily develops in women 20 to 40 years of age. The disease presentation ranges from asymptomatic elevation of aminotransferase levels to acute liver failure. Aminotransferase levels range from mild elevations to >1000 U/L. IgG levels are also elevated. Fifty percent of patients with autoimmune hepatitis have other autoimmune diseases such as thyroiditis, ulcerative colitis, or synovitis. Other findings include a positive ANA and anti–smooth muscle antibody titers, positive p-ANCA, or anti-LKM I antibody. Liver biopsy establishes the diagnosis.

◆ DON'T BE TRICKED

- A high serum total protein and low serum albumin level suggest an elevated serum gamma globulin level and may be the only clue to hypergammaglobulinemia.

Therapy

Patients who have active inflammation on liver biopsy specimen or are symptomatic should be considered for treatment with glucocorticoids and azathioprine. Relapse occurs after stopping treatment in most patients.

Hemochromatosis

Diagnosis

Hereditary hemochromatosis is an autosomal-recessive disorder characterized by increased intestinal absorption of iron and iron deposition in multiple organs.

The most common symptoms are fatigue, erectile dysfunction, destructive arthropathy of the second and third MCP joints characterized by distinctive hook-like osteophytes, and OA involving unusual joints, such as the shoulders, ankles, and elbows. Less commonly patients may have diabetes, HF, hyperpigmentation (skin bronzing), and panhypopituitarism. Patients with cirrhosis due to hereditary hemochromatosis are at increased risk for HCC and periodic screening with ultrasonography is recommended.

The most appropriate screening test for hemochromatosis is fasting serum transferrin saturation. Some guidelines suggest diagnosis when the value is >60% in men or 50% in women, and others suggest >55% for all patients. *C282Y* homozygous or *C282Y/H63D* compound heterozygous *HFE* genotypes are diagnostic of hemochromatosis. Screen for HCC with ultrasonography in patients with cirrhosis every 6 months.

◆ DON'T BE TRICKED

- Advanced liver disease commonly causes an elevated ferritin level, but the iron saturation is usually normal.
- A nondiagnostic *HFE* genotype does not rule out a diagnosis of hemochromatosis.

Hemochromatosis: These hook-like osteophytes are characteristic of hemochromatosis.

Therapy

Patients who are *C282Y* homozygous but have a normal serum ferritin level can be monitored without treatment. Patients with an abnormal ferritin level should be treated with phlebotomy.

A 68-year-old man has increasing pain in the second and third MCP joints of both hands. Medical history is significant for type 2 diabetes mellitus and HF.

ANSWER: The probable diagnosis is hemochromatosis; order transferrin saturation and serum ferritin measurement.

Nonalcoholic Fatty Liver Disease

Diagnosis

NAFLD is the most common cause of abnormal liver test results. Most patients have insulin resistance, obesity, hypertriglyceridemia, and type 2 diabetes mellitus. Approximately 20% of patients with NAFLD have nonalcoholic steatohepatitis (NASH), characterized by hepatic steatosis, inflammation, and often fibrosis.

A presumptive diagnosis of NASH can be made in a patient with:

- mild elevations of aminotransferase levels
- risk factors for NAFLD (diabetes, obesity, and hyperlipidemia)
- hyperechoic pattern on ultrasonography or low-density parenchyma on CT

◆ DON'T BE TRICKED

- Only liver biopsy (not ultrasonography) can confirm or exclude the diagnosis of NASH.

Therapy

Treatment for NAFLD consists of controlling diabetes, obesity, and hyperlipidemia.

◆ DON'T BE TRICKED

- Patients with fatty liver disease and elevated aminotransferase levels **can** be treated with statin therapy.

❖ Test Yourself

A 38-year-old woman with type 2 diabetes mellitus develops abnormal liver chemistry test results. She is obese. She does not use alcohol excessively. Serum AST is 134 U/L and ALT is 147 U/L. Abdominal ultrasonography shows increased echogenicity of the liver.

ANSWER: The diagnosis is probable NASH. Schedule liver biopsy.

Primary Biliary Cirrhosis

Diagnosis

Primary biliary cirrhosis is a chronic progressive autoimmune cholestatic liver disease that occurs predominantly in women between 40 and 60 years of age. Characteristic findings are pruritus, fatigue, weight loss, hyperpigmentation, and/or complications of portal hypertension. Patients may have features of scleroderma, xanthelasma, or xanthomas on physical examination. Approximately 50% of patients are asymptomatic. The diagnostic triad associated with primary biliary cirrhosis includes:

- a cholestatic liver profile
- positive antimitochondrial antibody titer
- granulomatous inflammation centered on the septal bile duct

Patients with primary biliary cirrhosis may have fat-soluble vitamin deficiencies and osteoporosis or osteomalacia.

Biliary ultrasonography is required to exclude extrahepatic bile duct obstruction.

Therapy

Ursodeoxycholic acid is the primary therapeutic agent.

Primary Sclerosing Cholangitis

Diagnosis

PSC is a chronic cholestatic liver disease of unknown cause that is characterized by progressive bile duct destruction and biliary cirrhosis. Eighty percent of patients have an IBD (most often ulcerative colitis). Characteristic findings are:

- pruritus or jaundice
- elevated serum alkaline phosphatase level
- elevated total bilirubin level
- modestly elevated AST and ALT levels

Abdominal ultrasonography is often the initial diagnostic study; if intrahepatic biliary dilation is seen, select MRCP or ERCP to establish the diagnosis (look for the "string of beads" pattern). Patients with PSC are at risk for developing cholangiocarcinoma as well as gallbladder carcinoma and colon cancer (when associated with IBD). The risk of colon cancer in patients with PSC and IBD is high enough that surveillance is recommended, regardless of duration or extent of the IBD. In these patients select annual screening for colon cancer (colonoscopy). Patients with cirrhosis require screening for HCC with ultrasonography every 6 months. No consensus has been reached regarding screening for cholangiocarcinoma and gallbladder cancer.

◆ DON'T BE TRICKED

- Do not confuse PSC with AIDS cholangiopathy (CD4 cell count <100/μL) due to CMV or *Cryptosporidium* infection.

STUDY TABLE: Differentiating Primary Biliary Cirrhosis and Primary Sclerosing Cholangitis		
	Primary Biliary Cirrhosis	**Primary Sclerosing Cholangitis**
Demographic	Women aged 40-60 years	Men aged 20-30 years
Pathology	Cholestatic liver disease of small bile ducts	Cholestatic liver disease of large bile ducts
Associated conditions	Other autoimmune disease	IBD
Look for...	Positive antimitochondrial antibody titer	"String of beads" on MRCP or ERCP
Therapy	Ursodeoxycholic acid	Endoscopic therapy for extrahepatic dominant strictures
		Liver transplantation

Therapy

There is no effective medical therapy for PSC. Pruritus can be treated with cholestyramine; otherwise, patients with a dominant biliary stricture, bile duct stones, or cholangitis may benefit from endoscopic bile duct dilatation/stenting or removal of stones. Liver transplantation is associated with improved quality of life and survival.

❖ Test Yourself

A 45-year-old man with a 15-year history of ulcerative colitis develops fatigue and pruritus. Serum alkaline phosphatase level is 750 U/L, AST is 48 U/L, ALT is 60 U/L, and total bilirubin is 2.0 mg/dL.

ANSWER: The probable diagnosis is PSC. Schedule ultrasonography followed by MRCP or ERCP.

Cirrhosis

Diagnosis

Patients with cirrhosis but no complications have compensated cirrhosis; they may be asymptomatic or have nonspecific symptoms such as fatigue, poor sleep, or itching. Patients with complications of cirrhosis (hepatic encephalopathy, variceal hemorrhage, ascites, spontaneous bacterial peritonitis, hepatorenal syndrome, jaundice, or HCC) have decompensated cirrhosis. Portal hypertension is responsible for the majority of these complications. Portal hypertension also causes splenomegaly and hypersplenism (thrombocytopenia) and loss of hepatic synthetic function (coagulopathy and hypoalbuminemia).

Portal hypertension can be divided into prehepatic, intrahepatic, and posthepatic causes. The most common cause of portal hypertension is cirrhosis, an intrahepatic form. Examples of pre- and posthepatic portal hypertension are portal vein thrombosis and Budd-Chiari syndrome, respectively.

Portal hypertension develops in cirrhosis owing to mechanical factors of fibrosis and regenerative liver nodules as well as increased intrahepatic vascular resistance and increased portal inflow. The high pressure in the portal vein is decompressed through collateral portosystemic shunts that occur in the mucosa of the distal esophagus and proximal stomach.

Select the following options for care of patients with cirrhosis:

- upper endoscopy for all new patients to screen for varices
- ultrasonography to diagnose ascites
- paracentesis for newly discovered ascites and calculation of the serum-ascites albumin gradient (SAAG) to diagnose the cause of ascites
- paracentesis with ascitic fluid granulocyte count and culture for any change in mental status or clinical condition to diagnose spontaneous bacterial peritonitis
- vaccination of nonimmune patients against HAV and HBV as well as other routine vaccinations
- ultrasound screening for HCC every 6 months

STUDY TABLE: Evaluation of Ascites		
Ascitic Fluid Protein	**SAAG >1.1**	**SAAG <1.1**
<2.5 g/dL	Cirrhosis	Nephrotic syndrome
>2.5 g/dL	Right-sided HF, Budd-Chiari syndrome	Malignancy, TB

Ascitic fluid granulocyte count >250/μL confirms spontaneous bacterial peritonitis.

Hepatic encephalopathy is a neuropsychiatric syndrome that develops in patients with hepatic dysfunction. Symptoms range from minimal cognitive changes to coma. The plasma ammonia level can be helpful in cases of diagnostic uncertainty.

Diagnose hepatopulmonary syndrome in patients with:

- dyspnea
- hypoxemia
- cirrhosis
- increased A-a while breathing ambient air

Patients may exhibit platypnea (increased dyspnea sitting up and decreased dyspnea lying flat). The diagnosis of hepatopulmonary syndrome is confirmed by contrast-enhanced TTE with agitated saline administration.

Portopulmonary hypertension is PH in the presence of portal hypertension. Patients without other obvious causes of dyspnea should undergo echocardiography; RV systolic pressure >50 mm Hg requires investigation for causes of PH. Select patients will benefit from liver transplantation.

Hepatorenal syndrome diagnostic criteria consist of:

- an increase in the creatinine to >1.5 mg/dL over days to weeks
- lack of response to an albumin challenge of 1 g/kg/d for 2 days
- exclusion of other causes of AKI

Type 1 hepatorenal syndrome is more severe, with a doubling of the creatinine level in excess of 2.5 mg/dL in <2 weeks.

Type 2 hepatorenal syndrome is less severe, with a more gradual increase in the creatinine level and association with diuretic-refractory ascites.

Hepatic osteodystrophy encompasses osteoporosis, osteopenia, and rarely osteomalacia in the context of liver disease. Standard evaluation includes calcium, phosphate, and vitamin D levels. DEXA scanning is recommended for patients with cirrhosis or primary biliary cirrhosis and before liver transplantation. Osteoporosis should be managed with a bisphosphonate (after vitamin D repletion).

◆ DON'T BE TRICKED

- There is no utility in monitoring serial ammonia values in patients with hepatic encephalopathy.
- Head CT is only warranted in patients with unwitnessed falls, or head trauma.
- Use only IV, not oral, bisphosphonate therapy in patients with esophageal varices.

Therapy

Patients with type 1 hepatorenal syndrome treated in the ICU should receive norepinephrine and albumin, whereas non-ICU patients are treated with midodrine, octreotide, and albumin. Type 1 patients who do not respond to medical therapy should undergo liver transplantation.

STUDY TABLE: Therapy for Cirrhosis	
Indications	**Treatment**
Primary prophylaxis of variceal bleeding	First choice: propranolol or nadolol (must be nonselective β-blockers)
	Second choice: endoscopic band ligation if β-blocker not tolerated or contraindicated
Active variceal bleeding	First choice: octreotide with endoscopic band ligation and prophylactic oral norfloxacin or IV ciprofloxacin
	Second choice: TIPS or shunt surgery if endoscopic therapy is unsuccessful
Transfusion for active bleeding	Hemoglobin transfusion goal 7 g/dL
Ascites not responding to low-sodium diet	Spironolactone with or without furosemide
Diuretic-refractory ascites	Serial large-volume paracentesis (with albumin if >5 L), TIPS, or liver transplantation
Prevention of spontaneous bacterial peritonitis in hospitalized patients with cirrhosis and ascitic fluid protein <1.0 g/dL, variceal bleeding with or without cirrhosis, or previous history of spontaneous bacterial peritonitis and other high-risk categories	Fluoroquinolones chronically if history of spontaneous bacterial peritonitis or otherwise high risk*
	Fluoroquinolones while hospitalized if fluid protein <1 g/dL
	Fluoroquinolones for 7 days if active bleeding
Spontaneous bacterial peritonitis	Cefotaxime and albumin infusion. Administer 1.5 g/kg of albumin on day 1 and 1 g/kg of albumin on day 3 if creatinine is >1 mg/dL, bilirubin >4 mg/dL, or BUN >30 mg/dL
Acute hepatic encephalopathy	Correct precipitating factors, lactulose; add rifaximin if unresponsive
Prevention of hepatic encephalopathy	Lactulose, titrated to 3 stools per day
Hepatic osteodystrophy	Calcium, vitamin D, and IV bisphosphate

*High risk = ascitic total protein <1.5 g/dL and any of the following: serum sodium ≤130 mEq/L, creatinine ≥1.2 mg/dL, BUN ≥25 mg/dL, bilirubin ≥3 mg/dL.

The primary complication of TIPS is portosystemic encephalopathy. Liver transplantation is the definitive treatment for patients with end-stage liver disease and complications such as variceal bleeding, ascites, hepatic encephalopathy, or hepatorenal/hepatopulmonary syndromes.

◆ DON'T BE TRICKED

- Stop ACE inhibitors, ARBs, and NSAIDs in patients with ascites.
- More liberal blood transfusion to hemoglobin >7.0 g/dL leads to increased portal pressures and risk of further bleeding.
- Antimicrobial prophylaxis should be administered during variceal bleeding even if ascites are absent.
- Do not select prophylactic protein restriction to prevent hepatic encephalopathy.
- Do not select neomycin to treat hepatic encephalopathy because of the significant adverse effects of this drug.

❖ Test Yourself

A 55-year-old man with alcoholic cirrhosis is hospitalized with fever and abdominal pain. Paracentesis is performed. The ascitic fluid granulocyte count is 650/μL and the albumin is <1.0 g/dL.

ANSWER: The diagnosis is spontaneous bacterial peritonitis. Begin IV cefotaxime and albumin. Do not wait for results of Gram stain or cultures before beginning therapy.

Acute Liver Injury and Acute Liver Failure

Diagnosis

Acute liver *injury* is associated with a sudden increase in serum AST and ALT levels in a patient without a history of liver disease. Acute liver *failure* refers to acute hepatic injury complicated by encephalopathy and coagulopathy in patients without previous cirrhosis. The most common identifiable causes are acetaminophen hepatotoxicity, idiosyncratic drug reactions, and HBV infection. Other causes include acute HAV infection, hepatic ischemia, mushroom poisoning, Wilson disease, AFLP, HELLP syndrome, and herpes infection.

STUDY TABLE: Differential Diagnosis of Acute Liver Failure		
If you see this...	**Look for this...**	**And choose this...**
Sudden elevation of serum AST and ALT levels up to 20x; normally associated with depression or alcoholism	Acetaminophen overdose, which is the most common cause of acute liver failure Acute liver failure is usually due to acetaminophen ingestion >4 g but can occur with lower doses in patients with alcoholism	Measure serum acetaminophen level and use nomogram to determine if *N*-acetylcysteine is indicated
Outbreaks of acute liver failure associated with foods such as raspberries and scallions	Acute HAV infection	Order serologic studies for HAV
Episode of hypotension	In hospitalized patients, acute elevation of AST to >1000 U/L is most commonly due to hepatic hypoxia	Review hospital course
Acute elevation of liver enzymes and hemolysis in a young patient, or older patient with chronic liver disease, Kayser-Fleischer rings, history of psychiatric disorders, and/or athetoid movements	Wilson disease	Order measurement of serum copper and ceruloplasmin levels and urine copper excretion
Pregnancy, preeclampsia or eclampsia, hemolysis, elevated liver enzymes, and low platelets (thrombocytopenia) in third trimester	HELLP syndrome	Schedule urgent delivery

(Continued on next page)

STUDY TABLE: Differential Diagnosis of Acute Liver Failure (*Continued*)		
If you see this...	**Look for this...**	**And choose this...**
Pregnancy, preeclampsia, eclampsia, thrombocytopenia, and coagulation abnormalities in third trimester	AFLP May be impossible to distinguish from HELLP syndrome, but presence of hypoglycemia or encephalopathy is suggestive of AFLP	Schedule urgent delivery
Mushroom ingestion	*Amanita* poisoning	Obtain history
Herpes (simplex or zoster) infection	AST and ALT >5000 U/L in immunocompromised patient or during pregnancy. Often associated with encephalitis. Rash is not always present.	Clinical history

AFLP = acute fatty liver of pregnancy; HELLP = hemolysis, elevated liver enzyme levels, and a low platelet count.

The cause of acute liver failure is usually determined by a history of toxin or drug exposure, history of ischemic injury, serology for viral or autoimmune hepatitis, or tests for copper overload. Select head CT in patients with altered mental status to rule out intracranial hemorrhage.

Therapy

For patients with acute liver failure, choose:

- immediate contact with liver transplantation center
- chelation with trientine or penicillamine for Wilson disease
- *N*-acetylcysteine for confirmed or suspected acetaminophen poisoning
- penicillin G or silymarin for *Amanita* mushroom poisoning
- acyclovir for herpes hepatitis
- arteriovenous hemofiltration to support kidney function
- FFP to reduce INR in patients with active bleeding or before diagnostic or therapeutic interventions
- lactulose for any degree of encephalopathy

Kayser-Fleischer Ring: A Kayser-Fleischer ring in the cornea is bracketed with arrows.

◆ DON'T BE TRICKED

- Administer mannitol and/or mechanical hyperventilation for elevated intracranial pressure; do not use glucocorticoids.
- *N*-acetylcysteine improves transplant-free survival in non–acetaminophen-related acute liver failure with grades I to II hepatic encephalopathy

❖ Test Yourself

A 24-year-old man has a 1-week history of nausea, jaundice, fatigue, and recent confusion. He is lethargic and unable to recite his telephone number. The INR is 2.3, serum AST is 940 U/L, and total bilirubin is 12.6 mg/dL. HBsAg and IgM anti-HBc are both positive.

ANSWER: The diagnosis is acute liver failure secondary to acute hepatitis B infection. Contact liver transplantation center.

Liver Disease Associated with Pregnancy

Diagnosis

STUDY TABLE: Liver Diseases Unique to Pregnancy						
Disease	**Trimester**	**Clinical Features**	**Laboratory Studies**	**Bilirubin Level**	**Management**	**Recurrence**
Hyperemesis gravidarum	1st	Severe vomiting	ALT elevated in 50% of patients, may be 20x upper limit of normal	Normal	Hydration	Variable
Intrahepatic cholestasis of pregnancy	2nd or 3rd	Pruritus	ALT normal to 10-fold increase, elevated serum bile acids	Usually normal	Ursodiol	45%-70%
Preeclampsia	3rd	Hypertension, edema, and proteinuria	Mild increase in ALT	Normal	Delivery	5%-25%
HELLP syndrome	3rd	Features of preeclampsia	Hemolysis, elevated ALT, thrombocytopenia	Usually normal	Delivery	5%-25%
AFLP	3rd	Features of preeclampsia, features of liver failure	ALT 200-1000 U/L, hemolysis, low platelets, high ammonia	Normal unless severe	Delivery	20%-70%

The onset of intrahepatic cholestasis of pregnancy is typically heralded by the development of intense pruritus, which may precede laboratory abnormalities. Other characteristic findings are markedly elevated serum bilirubin and alkaline phosphatase levels and AST and ALT levels <200 U/L. Patients do not have hemolysis, thrombocytopenia, DIC, evidence of liver failure, or encephalopathy.

Characteristic findings of AFLP are nausea and abdominal pain, elevated AST and ALT levels, and increased PT. The platelet count may be decreased with or without other signs of DIC. About 50% of patients have preeclampsia (hypertension and proteinuria) or eclampsia (preeclampsia plus seizure or coma). Increased hepatic echogenicity is seen on ultrasonography.

The HELLP syndrome is associated with preeclampsia or eclampsia. HELLP syndrome differs from AFLP in that HELLP syndrome is more closely associated with microangiopathic hemolytic anemia and AFLP with more coagulation abnormalities.

Therapy

- Ursodiol is the treatment of choice for intrahepatic cholestasis of pregnancy. Early delivery should be scheduled at the first signs of fetal distress.
- AFLP typically resolves rapidly after delivery of the infant.
- Treatment of HELLP syndrome is delivery of the infant.

Gallstones, Acute Cholecystitis, and Cholangitis

Diagnosis

Biliary pain is the most common cause of upper abdominal pain among patients aged >50 years. Biliary colic is characterized by acute onset of severe, steady epigastric or RUQ pain. Episodes generally last 15 minutes to several hours and are often accompanied by nausea and vomiting. Fever, leukocytosis, and elevated liver enzymes indicate acute cholecystitis or obstruction of the common bile duct. Look for specific syndromes and mimics of biliary disease.

STUDY TABLE: Biliary Disease Syndromes and Mimics

If you see this...	Diagnose this...
Epigastric and RUQ pain; bilirubin <4 mg/dL; AST or ALT may be minimally elevated. Sonography shows thickened gallbladder wall and the presence of pericholecystic fluid	Acute cholecystitis
Biliary colic, cholecystitis, or pancreatitis and no gallstones or bile duct dilation on imaging studies	Biliary crystals (sludge)
RUQ pain, fever, jaundice, or these findings plus shock and mental status changes; bilirubin >4 mg/dL; AST and ALT >1000 U/L	Acute cholangitis
Critically ill, febrile, or septic patient (abdominal pain; Murphy sign may be absent). Sonographic findings compatible with acute cholecystitis	Acute acalculous cholecystitis
Transient elevation of AST or ALT up to 1000 U/L, and cholangitis, or pancreatitis.	Passage of common bile duct stone
Midepigastric pain radiating to the back, nausea, vomiting, elevated amylase and lipase	Acute pancreatitis
Recent significant alcohol intake; RUQ pain, fever, jaundice, AST 2-3x greater than ALT; bilirubin >4 mg/dL	Acute alcoholic hepatitis
RUQ pain, pelvic adnexal tenderness, leukocytosis; cervical smear showing gonococci	Fitz-Hugh–Curtis syndrome (gonococcal or chlamydial perihepatitis)
Impacted gallstone in cystic duct, jaundice, and dilated common bile duct caused by extrinsic compression	Mirizzi syndrome
Biliary colic or cholecystitis with small-bowel obstruction and air in biliary tree	Cholecystenteric fistula (gallstone ileus)
RUQ pain, diarrhea, and obstructive jaundice in advanced HIV	AIDS cholangiopathy (*Cryptosporidium* infection)

Select ultrasonography as the initial imaging modality. Dilatation of the cystic or biliary duct indicates an obstructing stone. In patients with cholecystitis, ultrasonography will show pericholecystic fluid and a thickened gallbladder wall. If ultrasonography is nondiagnostic, select cholescintigraphy (e.g., HIDA scan). Nonvisualization of the gallbladder suggests cystic duct obstruction and cholecystitis. If bile duct stones are suspected, select one of the following:

- magnetic resonance cholangiography
- ERCP

◆ DON'T BE TRICKED

- HIDA scans can be falsely positive in patients with intrinsic liver disease and elevated serum bilirubin levels.

Therapy

Patients with symptoms lasting less than 4 to 6 hours, no fever, and no leukocytosis, have biliary colic. Treat with NSAIDs to decrease the risk of progression to acute cholecystitis.

Broad-spectrum antibiotics are indicated for acute cholecystitis (pain, fever, and leukocytosis) and signs of complications. Appropriate antibiotic regimens include:

- ceftazidime and metronidazole
- monotherapy with piperacillin–tazobactam, ampicillin–sulbactam, or ticarcillin–clavulanic acid

Patients with acute cholecystitis require surgery before hospital discharge. Laparotomy is preferred. Critically ill patients may require percutaneous or endoscopic draining owing to contraindications to cholecystectomy. Common bile duct stones are removed with ERCP.

Select broad-spectrum antibiotics (a fluoroquinolone) and ERCP drainage for acute cholangitis.

◆ DON'T BE TRICKED

- Surgery is not indicated for asymptomatic gallstones.
- Fatty food intolerance is not related to gallbladder disease and does not warrant cholecystectomy.
- Surgery is not indicated for acute cholangitis because surgical procedures are associated with increased mortality.

❖ Test Yourself

A 27-year-old woman is evaluated because of cholecystitis. The serum direct bilirubin level is 5.8 mg/dL. Abdominal ultrasonography shows gallbladder stones. The intrahepatic ducts are dilated. The distal common bile duct is not dilated, and no stones are seen.

ANSWER: The diagnosis is Mirizzi syndrome.

Upper GI Bleeding

Diagnosis

Eighty percent of UGI bleeding is due to 4 causes:

- PUD
- esophagogastric varices
- esophagitis
- Mallory-Weiss tear

PUD caused by *Helicobacter pylori* infection or NSAID use is the most common cause of nonvariceal UGI bleeding. Characteristic findings are hematemesis, melena, or (infrequently) bright-red blood per rectum or a high serum BUN/creatinine ratio. Slow and/or chronic bleeding is suggested by iron deficiency and is typical of erosive disease, tumor, esophageal ulcer, portal hypertensive gastropathy, Cameron lesion (erosions found within large hiatal hernias), and angiodysplasia.

STUDY TABLE: Differential Diagnosis of Upper GI Bleeding	
If you see this...	**Diagnose this...**
Dyspepsia, *H. pylori* infection, NSAID use, anticoagulation, severe medical illness	Peptic ulcer disease
Stigmata of chronic liver disease, evidence of portal hypertension or risk factors for cirrhosis (alcohol use, viral hepatitis)	Variceal bleeding
History of heavy alcohol use and retching before hematemesis, hematemesis following weight lifting, or young woman with bulimia	Mallory-Weiss tear
Heartburn, regurgitation, and dysphagia; usually small-volume or occult bleeding	Esophagitis
Progressive dysphagia, weight loss, early satiety, or abdominal pain; usually small-volume or occult bleeding	Esophageal or gastric cancer
NSAID use, heavy alcohol intake, severe medical illness; usually small-volume or occult bleeding	Gastroduodenal erosions

After the patient is stabilized, upper endoscopy is required to document the source of bleeding. If upper endoscopy shows an ulcer, test for *H. pylori* infection.

◆ DON'T BE TRICKED

- Do not order a barium x-ray because this will interfere with subsequent upper endoscopy or other studies.

Therapy

Risk-stratification tools guide decisions regarding urgent upper endoscopy (within 12 hours), hospital admission and nonurgent upper endoscopy (within 24 hours), and discharge home from the emergency department. The Glasgow-Blatchford score (range 0-23) is particularly useful when the score is 0, which has a nearly 100% negative predictive value for severe GI bleeding and the need for hospital-based intervention.

Pre-endoscopic management:

- IV crystalloids targeting HR <100/min, SBP >100 mm Hg, and no orthostasis
- blood transfusion for hemodynamic instability and ongoing bleeding
- blood transfusion to target hemoglobin level of 7 g/dL
- PPI therapy (stop if no ulcer found on upper endoscopy)
- FFP for INR >1.5
- octreotide and antibiotics before upper endoscopy for suspected variceal bleeding

Upper endoscopy evaluation and treatment:

- upper endoscopy within 24 hours; within 12 hours for suspected variceal bleed
- low-risk ulcers are clean-based or have a nonprotuberant pigmented spot
- treat low-risk ulcers with oral PPI, begin food, early hospital discharge (12-24 hours)
- high-risk ulcers have active arterial spurting or a nonbleeding visible vessel
- treat high-risk ulcers endoscopically (hemoclips, thermal therapy, or injection therapy) and continuous IV PPI infusion for 72 hours
- repeat endoscopic therapy for continued bleeding
- surgery or interventional radiology if endoscopic therapy unsuccessful

Postendoscopic care:

- repeat upper endoscopy is warranted for gastric ulcers after 8 to 12 weeks of PPI therapy if biopsies were not taken during the initial examination or if there is continued concern for malignancy
- test for *H. pylori* and treat if positive, retest if initial test was negative
- resume aspirin within 3 to 5 days for patients with cardiovascular disease
- resume aspirin but temporarily withhold clopidogrel for high-risk ulcers
- resume aspirin and clopidogrel immediately for low-risk ulcers
- provide long-term, daily PPI therapy for patients who must use aspirin and other antiplatelet drugs, NSAIDs, anticoagulants, or glucocorticoids

Re-anticoagulate patients at high thrombotic risk:

- AF with a previous embolic event
- CHADS$_2$ score ≥3
- recent ACS
- mechanical heart valve
- DVT or PE

In these patients begin bridging anticoagulation (LMWH or UFH) and begin oral anticoagulation 7 days after the bleeding event.

◆ DON'T BE TRICKED

- H$_2$-receptor antagonists are not beneficial in managing UGI bleeding.
- Do not select nasogastric tube placement for diagnosis, prognosis, visualization, or therapeutic effect.
- Second-look upper endoscopy is not recommended except for rebleeding.

Lower GI Bleeding

Diagnosis

Acute, painless LGI bleeding in older adult patients is usually due to colonic diverticula or angiodysplasia. Ten percent of rapid rectal bleeding has an UGI source.

Consider outpatient follow-up or early discharge when:

- patient age <60 years
- no hemodynamic instability
- no evidence of gross rectal bleeding
- identification of an obvious anorectal source of bleeding

STUDY TABLE: Differential Diagnosis of Lower GI Bleeding	
If you see this...	**Diagnose this...**
Painless, self-limited, massive hematochezia	Diverticular bleeding (most common overall cause)
Chronic blood loss or acute painless hematochezia in an older adult patient	Angiodysplasia
Stool positive for occult blood in an asymptomatic patient	Colonic polyp or cancer
Risk factors for atherosclerosis and evidence of vascular disease in an older adult patient; typically with LLQ abdominal pain	Ischemic colitis
Aortic stenosis	Angiodysplasia (Heyde Syndrome)
History of bloody diarrhea, tenesmus, abdominal pain, fever	IBD
Rapid UGI bleeding	Dieulafoy lesion (large, tortuous, submucosal arteriole)
Large hiatal hernia	Cameron lesion (mucosal erosions)
Recent liver or biliary procedure	Hemobilia
Necrotizing pancreatitis	Hemosuccus pancreaticus (bleeding from pancreas)
Aortic aneurysm repair	Aortoenteric fistula
Painless hematochezia in a young patient and normal upper endoscopy and colonoscopy	Meckel diverticulum
Mucocutaneous telangiectasias	Hereditary hemorrhagic telangiectasia

Therapy

According to expert opinion, the blood transfusion threshold for patients with colonic bleeding is a hemoglobin value <9 g/dL (note this is different for the evidence-based threshold for UGI bleeding). If the patient is hemodynamically unstable, resuscitate the patient before diagnostic studies are performed. Most episodes of LGI bleeding resolve spontaneously. Colonoscopy is recommended early, usually within the first 48 hours of admission, and endoscopic therapy is used to control continued bleeding. If colonoscopy does not identify a discrete lesion or endoscopic therapy does not control the bleeding, interventional angiography or surgery may be indicated. Patients with angiodysplasia in the setting of AS (Heyde Syndrome) may benefit from valve replacement surgery.

Bleeding of Obscure Origin

Diagnosis

Obscure GI bleeding is recurrent blood loss without an identified source of bleeding despite upper endoscopy and colonoscopy. Patients aged ≤50 years are more likely to have tumors (leiomyomas, carcinoid, adenocarcinoma, or lymphoma), Dieulafoy lesion, or Crohn disease. Older patients are more likely to have vascular lesions, such as angiodysplasia. Angiodysplasia is the most common cause of obscure GI bleeding overall (40% of all cases). Patients may present with either melena or hematochezia or positive FOBT. The first step is to repeat upper endoscopy and/or colonoscopy, which is diagnostic in approximately 40% of cases.

For patients with obscure **active** GI bleeding:

- perform nuclear studies (technetium 99m-labeled erythrocyte or sulfur colloid nuclear scan) first, followed by angiography
- if unrevealing, consider push enteroscopy or balloon-assisted enteroscopy (deep enteroscopy)
- surgery and intraoperative enteroscopy is a last diagnostic option

For patients with occult GI bleeding:

- capsule endoscopy (first choice) or deep enteroscopy
- if unrevealing, repeat endoscopic examinations (upper endoscopy, colonoscopy, capsule endoscopy), or deep enteroscopy

◆ DON'T BE TRICKED

- Do not order small bowel x-ray as a first-line study in the evaluation of obscure GI bleeding.
- Do not use capsule endoscopy in the setting of obstruction or strictures (severe Crohn disease).

General Internal Medicine

Biostatistics

Sensitivity, Specificity, Predictive Values, Likelihood Ratios and ROC Curves

Sensitivity is the ability of a test to detect a disease when it is truly present. Specificity is the ability of a test to exclude disease when it is truly absent.

A ROC curve is a graph of the sensitivity vs. (1 – specificity). In medicine, a ROC analysis helps select tests with optimal performance characteristics. The cut-point with the best combined sensitivity and specificity will be closest to the upper left corner of the graph. When comparing two or more tests, the test with the greatest overall accuracy will have the largest area under the ROC graph.

Receiver Operator Characteristic (ROC) Curve

Receiver Operating Characteristic Curve: ROC curve showing sensitivity (true-positive rate) vs. (1 − specificity) (false-positive rate).

◆ **DON'T BE TRICKED**

- As the prevalence of a condition increases, the positive predictive value increases and the negative predictive value decreases.
- Changes in prevalence do not alter the sensitivity or specificity but do alter the predictive values.

The likelihood ratio (LR) is a measurement of the odds of having a disease independent of the disease prevalence. Separate LRs are calculated for use when a test result is positive (LR+) or when the test result is negative (LR–):

- LR+ = Sensitivity/(1 – Specificity)
- LR– = (1 – Sensitivity)/Specificity
- LR+ of 2, 5, and 10 increase the probability of disease by approximately 15%, 30%, and 45%, respectively.
- LR– of 0.5, 0.2, and 0.1 decrease the probability of disease by approximately 15%, 30%, and 45%, respectively.

Study Designs

It is important to recognize the characteristics of various study designs and their evidence-based medicine "strength."

STUDY TABLE: Study Designs

Type	Characteristics
Cross-section	The presence of the presumed risk factor and presence of the outcome are measured at the same time in a population
Retrospective (case control)	Subjects are divided into groups based on the presence or absence of the outcome of interest, and then the frequency of risk factors in each group is compared
Prospective (cohort)	Subjects are divided into groups based on the presence or absence of the presumed risk factor and followed for a period of time
	At the end of the study, the frequency of the outcome is compared
Randomized controlled trial	Subjects are randomly divided into groups; one group receives the intervention (patients and researchers may be blinded to treatment) and followed forward in time
	At the end of the study, the frequency of the outcome is compared
	This study design reduces the effect of unmeasured (confounding) variables that may influence outcomes of a study
Systematic review	Usually, multiple clinical trials using similar randomization techniques and interventions can be combined into one large analysis to address very precise clinical questions
	The results may be analyzed using the technique of meta-analysis

STUDY TABLE: Evidence-based Medicine Strength of Research Designs in Descending Order (Strongest to Weakest)

Description
Evidence from RCT including systematic reviews of RCTs
Evidence from RCT without randomization
Evidence from case-control or cohort study
Evidence from many points in time, with or without intervention
Evidence based on experience, descriptive studies, or expert opinion

Risk Estimates

STUDY TABLE: Common Calculations Used in Clinical Research

Term	Definition	Calculation	Notes
Absolute risk	The probability of an event occurring in a group during a specified time period	AR = patients with event in group / total patients in group	Also known as *event rate*. Often, an EER is compared with a CER
Relative risk	The ratio of the probability of developing a disease with a risk factor present to the probability of developing the disease without the risk factor present	RR = EER / CER	Used in cohort studies and RCTs

(Continued on next page)

STUDY TABLE: Common Calculations Used in Clinical Research *(Continued)*			
Term	**Definition**	**Calculation**	**Notes**
Absolute risk reduction	The *absolute difference* in rates of events between experimental group and control group	ARR = | EER − CER |	
Relative risk reduction	The *ratio* of AR reduction to the event rate among controls	RRR = | EER − CER | / CER	
Number needed to treat	Number of patients needed to receive a treatment for one additional patient to benefit	NNT = 1 / ARR	A good estimate of the effect size
Number needed to harm	Number of patients needed to receive a treatment for one additional patient to be harmed	NNH = 1 / ARR	

AR = absolute risk; ARR = absolute risk reduction; CER = control event rate; EER = experimental event rate; NNH = number needed to harm; NNT = number needed to treat; RCT = randomized controlled trial; RR = relative risk; RRR = relative risk reduction.

An odds ratio (OR) estimates the odds of having or not having a particular outcome. When comparing therapeutic outcomes, in most cases OR can be substituted for RR as an equivalent measurement.

AR, RR, and OR are estimates of the cumulative risk over time, usually defined as at the end of the study.

A hazard ratio (HR) is a type of RR and calculates the risk of an outcome in a group exposed to a risk compared with a control group not exposed to the risk. The difference between an HR and RR is that an HR calculates the risk of an event occurring at a particular instantaneous point in time, whereas the RR calculates the cumulative risk of an event occurring over the entire duration of the study period.

◆ DON'T BE TRICKED

- A disadvantage of RR is the potential for exaggeration. For example, interventions that reduce the rate of a disease from 40% to 20% and 4% to 2% each have a RR reduction of 50%, but the ARR for the first case is 20% and the ARR for the second case is only 2%. Based upon the ARR, the NNT can be calculated. In the first case the NNT is 5 (1/0.2) whereas the NNT for the second case is 50 (1/0.02).

Confidence Interval

CI provides boundaries within which exists a high probability (95% by convention) of finding the "true" value. For example, if the measured mean difference between two groups is 2.4, and the 95% CI is 1.9-3.0, the probability that the true value lies between 1.9 and 3.0 is 95%.

When used in association with RR, if the CI includes the number 1, there is no risk or benefit; the outcomes for the control and experimental groups are the same.

P Values, Type I and Type II Errors in Clinical Research

The *P* value indicates the likelihood of the study result being caused by chance alone. A *P* value of less than 0.05 represents a 1 in 20 chance of obtaining the observed results by chance.

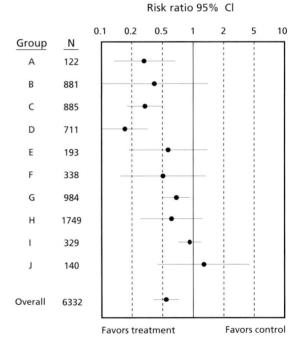

Standard Meta-Analysis: This figure shows a standard meta-analysis plot of the ratio for the risk of an outcome comparing an active treatment to placebo (or, it could be another treatment). The dots show the point estimates for the RR of each study and the pooled point estimate, and the horizontal lines show the CIs. Any CI that crosses the centerline denotes a study whose result is not significant. N is the number of subjects in each study. As a standard convention, an RR of less than 1 denotes a reduction of the event that is being studied compared with the control group or other active treatment. Note that the smaller the study, the larger the CI. Finally, although one study does not favor the intervention (J) and some CIs overlap 1 (B, E, F, H), suggesting no reduction in risk, overall this analysis suggests the intervention is associated with a reduction in risk.

A type I error is incorrectly concluding that a statistically significant difference exists between the experimental and control groups. If the study's P value is <0.05, then a <5% chance exists that a type I error has occurred. A type II error is incorrectly concluding no difference exists between the experimental and control groups. Studies with small numbers of subjects may not have the statistical "power" to detect true differences between groups and may be subject to type II errors.

◆ **DON'T BE TRICKED**

- Do not confuse statistical significance with clinical importance; a study that reports statistically significant P values may not be clinically relevant if there is a small effect size (absolute difference between outcomes is small).

❖ **Test Yourself**

A 19-year-old woman with RLQ abdominal pain and fever has an estimated pretest probability of acute appendicitis of 50%. An appendiceal CT scan shows inflammation and a thickened appendiceal wall. This finding is associated with an LR of 13.3 for acute appendicitis. What is the posttest likelihood of acute appendicitis?

ANSWER: >95% (50% plus 45% = 95%). The key to this question is remembering that a LR+ of 10 increases the posttest likelihood of the diagnosis by 45%.

The mortality rate after cardiogenic shock managed with standard care is 72%, but the rate for patients receiving a new medication is 67%. How many patients with cardiogenic shock must be treated with the new medication to save one life?

ANSWER: The NNT is $[1/(0.72 - 0.67)] = 1/0.05 = 20$.

Screening and Prevention

STUDY TABLE: Summary of Vaccination Recommendations for Adults		
Disease	**Vaccine Type**	**ACIP Recommendation**
Influenza	Inactivated, live attenuated, recombinant	One dose annually for all persons ≥6 months of age
Tetanus, diphtheria, and pertussis	Inactivated	Td booster every 10 y for all adults (replace one time with Tdap); primary series for unvaccinated adults; all pregnant women between 27-36 weeks' gestation, every pregnancy
Varicella	Live attenuated	Two doses given at interval of ≥4 weeks for all persons lacking immunity
Herpes zoster	Live attenuated	All nonimmunocompromised persons age ≥60 y
Pneumococcal	Inactivated	All adults age ≥65 y; adults ages 19-64 y with risk factors (see Pneumococcal Immunization table, below)
HPV	Inactivated	Females 11-26 y (bivalent or quadrivalent vaccine); men 11-26 y (quadrivalent vaccine)
MMR	Live attenuated	Adults born in 1957 or later without evidence of vaccination or immunity
Meningococcal	Inactivated	One dose indicated for first-year college students residing in dormitories (unless vaccinated at age ≥16 y), travelers to endemic areas, military recruits, and exposed persons; asplenia or complement deficiencies
Hepatitis A	Inactivated	Any adult requesting immunization and those at high risk
Hepatitis B	Inactivated	Any adult requesting immunization and those at high risk

ACIP = Advisory Committee on Immunization Practices.

◆ **DON'T BE TRICKED**

- For pregnant women, do not select live vaccines, including MMR, intranasal influenza, yellow fever, varicella, and zoster vaccines.

STUDY TABLE: Pneumococcal Immunization

Risk Group	PCV13	PPSV23	
	Recommended	Recommended	Revaccination with PPSV23 at 5 years after first dose
Immunocompetent adults age >65 y	×	×	Only if originally immunized before age 65 y
Immunocompetent persons with chronic heart, lung, or liver disease, diabetes mellitus, alcoholism, cigarette smoking		×	×
Persons with functional (sickle cell disease, hemoglobinopathies) or anatomic asplenia	×	×	×
Immunocompromised persons with HIV, chronic renal failure, nephrotic syndrome, leukemia, lymphoma, Hodgkin disease, multiple myeloma, generalized malignancy, on immunosuppressant drugs, congenital immunodeficiencies, solid organ transplant	×	×	×
CSF leaks or cochlear implants	×	×	

Travel Immunizations

Routine vaccines are recommended for a patient whose vaccines are not up to date, including influenza, pneumococcal, varicella (chickenpox and zoster for age >60 y), MMR, hepatitis B, and Tdap booster. Select the following vaccinations when appropriate:

- polio, hepatitis A and/or immune globulin, and typhoid for travelers to all developing countries
- yellow fever for travelers to Africa and South America
- meningococcal for travelers to sub-Saharan Africa
- rabies for extended-stay travelers or those who will have difficulty accessing postexposure treatment in endemic areas, including Asia, Africa, and South and Central America

❖ **Test Yourself**

An 18-year-old woman has completed her primary vaccination series for HPV, Tdap, polio, MMR, and varicella. What vaccination is needed before she travels through Western Europe?

ANSWER: She needs the hepatitis B vaccination.

STUDY TABLE: USPSTF-Recommended Screening

Condition	Screening Recommendation
Chronic Diseases	
Abdominal aortic aneurysm	One-time abdominal ultrasonography in all men ages 65-76 y who have ever smoked; selectively screen men ages 65-75 y who have never smoked
Depression	All adults, when staff-assisted depression care support is available
Diabetes mellitus	Age >45 y; all adults BP >135/80 mm Hg; PCOS; first-degree relative with diabetes mellitus; history of gestational diabetes; high-risk ethnic group (African Americans, American Indians/Alaska Natives, Asian Americans, Hispanics/Latinos, and Native Hawaiians/Pacific Islanders)
Hypertension	All adults
Lipid disorders	All men age ≥35 y; all women age ≥45 y; start at age 20 y for adults at increased cardiovascular risk
Obesity	All adults
Osteoporosis	Women age ≥65 y; women <65 y of age when 10-year fracture risk is ≥9.3%

(Continued on next page)

STUDY TABLE: USPSTF-Recommended Screening (*Continued*)

Condition	Screening Recommendation
Infectious Diseases	
Chlamydia	All sexually active women age ≤24 y; all sexually active women at increased risk of infection
Gonorrhea	All sexually active women at increased risk of infection
HCV	One-time screening for adults born between 1945-1965; all adults at high risk
HIV infection	One-time screening for all adults ages 15-65 y; repeated screening for adults at high risk
Syphilis	All adults at increased risk for syphilis infection
Tuberculosis	Screening of high-risk individuals
Substance Abuse	
Alcohol misuse	All adults
Tobacco use	All adults
Cancer	
Breast cancer	Biennial screening mammography for women ages 50-74 y; initiation of screening before age 50 y should be individualized
Cervical cancer	Women ages 21-65 y with cytology (Pap smear) every 3 y; in women ages 30-65 y who want to lengthen screening, screen with cytology and HPV testing every 5 y
Colon cancer	All adults ages 50-75 y using annual FOBT, flexible sigmoidoscopy every 5 y with FOBT every 3 y, or colonoscopy every 10 y
Lung cancer	Annual low-dose CT scan in high-risk patients (adults ages 55-80 y with a 30 pack-year smoking history, including former smokers who have quit in the last 15 years)

Smoking Cessation

Smoking cessation reduces all-cause mortality by up to 50%; when it appears as a potential answer to a test question, it is always correct.

Therapy

The Five A's and the 5 R's are two motivational interviewing techniques to use when counseling for behavior change, including smoking cessation, at-risk drinking, and other substance abuse.

STUDY TABLE: Behavioral Interventions

Five A's	Five R's
Ask about tobacco use.	Encourage patient to think of **R**elevance of quitting smoking to their lives.
Advise to quit.	Assist patient in identifying the **R**isks of smoking.
Assess willingness to quit.	Assist the patient in identifying the **R**ewards of smoking cessation.
Assist in attempt to quit.	Discuss with the patient **R**oadblocks or barriers to attempting cessation.
Arrange follow-up.	**R**epeat the motivational intervention at all visits.

STUDY TABLE: Pharmacologic Therapies for Smoking Cessation

Agent	Notes
Nicotine gum, patch, spray, inhaler, lozenges	Increases smoking cessation 1.5 times more than control. Avoid with recent MI, arrhythmia, and unstable angina.
Bupropion	Increases smoking cessation rates about 2 times more than control. Avoid with seizure disorder and eating disorder. May be associated with suicidal ideation. Safety in pregnancy is unclear.
Varenicline	Increases smoking cessation rates about 3.5 times more than control and almost 2 times more than bupropion. Associated with suicidal ideation and increased risk of cardiovascular events.

Combination therapy is more effective than monotherapy:

- behavioral intervention and pharmacotherapy are more effective than either therapy used alone
- bupropion and varenicline can be used with long-acting (nicotine patches) or short-acting (nicotine gum, lozenges, inhalers, nasal spray) nicotine replacement
- combination nicotine replacement therapy (long- and short-acting nicotine replacement) is more effective than nicotine monotherapy

◆ DON'T BE TRICKED

- SSRIs show no significant benefit for smoking cessation.

Alcohol Use Disorder

Screening

Ask all patients about their level of alcohol consumption and follow up with screening tests as appropriate. Patients with AUDIT-C scores >6 or a CAGE questionnaire score >1 are candidates for further evaluation and intervention.

Diagnosis

Look for alcoholism in patients with selected conditions, including repeated trauma, hypertension, AF, HF, pancreatitis, AH, and cirrhosis. Laboratory clues such as an elevated MCV, γ-glutamyltransferase level, and AST-ALT ratio >2 are suggestive but not diagnostic.

STUDY TABLE: Categories and Patterns of Alcohol Use	
Categories	**Patterns**
At-risk drinking	Men: >14 drinks per week or >4 drinks per occasion
	Women and adults age ≥ 65 y: >7 drinks per week or >3 drinks per occasion
Alcohol use disorder	Alcohol use leading to significant impairment or distress, as manifested by multiple psychosocial, behavioral, or physiologic features

In patients undergoing alcohol withdrawal, look for:

- tremor, anxiety, diaphoresis, and palpitations 6 to 36 hours after the last drink
- visual, auditory, and tactile hallucinations 12 to 48 hours after the last drink
- generalized tonic-clonic seizure within 6-24 hours after the last drink
- delirium tremens (hallucinations, delirium, agitation, fever, palpitations, and hypertension) 48 to 96 hours after the last drink

◆ DON'T BE TRICKED

- Alcohol misuse screening begins with quantifying amount of alcohol consumed, not CAGE or AUDIT-C questions.
- Multiple seizures (>1) are not consistent with alcohol withdrawal syndrome and should prompt an evaluation for another disorder.

Therapy

For management of alcohol use disorder, the USPSTF recommends referral for specialty treatment.

For at-risk drinking, brief behavioral counseling (such as the five A's and the five R's, listed above) may be useful.

Use naltrexone to prevent relapse of alcohol abuse and dependence and in patients who are actively drinking. Naltrexone is contraindicated in patients receiving or withdrawing from any opioid and in those with liver failure or hepatitis. Acamprosate enhances abstinence but is contraindicated in kidney insufficiency. Disulfiram leads to the accumulation of acetaldehyde if alcohol is consumed, resulting in flushing, headache, emesis, and the need to avoid all additional alcohol-containing items.

Hospitalize patients with moderate to severe alcohol withdrawal or another compelling need for hospitalization.

Long-acting benzodiazepines are indicated for:

- patients with previous alcohol-related seizures or delirium tremens
- significant withdrawal symptoms
- pregnant patients
- patients with acute medical or surgical illnesses

Use a symptom-triggered regimen to treat alcohol withdrawal. Adjunctive therapy with β-blockers and clonidine may help control tachycardia and hypertension but are not used as monotherapy.

◆ DON'T BE TRICKED

- Give thiamine replacement before administering glucose.
- Do not prescribe antipsychotic medications because these agents lower the seizure threshold.
- No evidence supports that continuous infusion therapy with short-acting benzodiazepines provides better outcomes than oral therapy for acute alcohol withdrawal.
- Not all heavy drinkers who stop abruptly experience withdrawal, and treatment with benzodiazepines is not always needed.
- Standing orders for benzodiazepines for alcohol withdrawal in patients with cirrhosis can precipitate hepatic encephalopathy.

❖ Test Yourself

A 36-year-old man with a history of heavy alcohol use is evaluated within 24 hours of his last drink. BP is 172/98 mm Hg, and pulse rate is 120/min. He is tremulous and having visual hallucinations.

ANSWER: The diagnosis is alcohol withdrawal syndrome. Hospitalize the patient, and treat him with benzodiazepines using a symptom-triggered protocol.

Intimate Partner Violence

Screening

USPSTF recommends screening for intimate partner violence (IPV) in women of childbearing age (14 to 46 years old).

Diagnosis

Physical and psychological IPV are associated with significant mental and physical health consequences for both male and female victims. Abuse frequently starts or increases during pregnancy.

Characteristic findings:

- exacerbations or poor control of chronic medical conditions
- seeming nonadherence to medications
- chronic abdominal pain

- sleep or appetite disturbances, fatigue, reduced concentration
- depression, anxiety, acute or posttraumatic stress, somatization, and eating disorders
- suicide attempts and substance abuse
- frequent appointment changes
- STIs, HIV, unplanned pregnancies
- visible bruises or injuries
- partner unwilling to leave during examination

Assess the risk of homicide, suicide, or serious injury. Inquire about:

- escalating threats or abuse and escalating level of fear
- stalking
- weapons, especially firearms, in the home
- sexual assault and abuse during pregnancy
- recent separation or abuser's awareness of impending separation

Therapy

Initiate safety planning. Determine if the patient wants to leave home, return home, or have the abuser removed from his or her household. Refer the patient to a domestic violence advocate.

Patient Safety

Diagnostic Errors

Reasoning errors can lead to diagnostic errors.

STUDY TABLE: Reasoning Errors	
Heuristic	**Definition**
Availability	Clinician has encountered a similar presentation and jumps to the conclusion that the current diagnosis must be the same as the previous
Anchoring	Clinician accepts at face value a previous diagnosis made by another clinician
Blind obedience	Acceptance of a diagnosis or plan made by another of higher authority
Premature closure	Full differential diagnosis is not considered

Error Analysis

Root-cause analysis is an exercise used to determine the contributors to an adverse event. Often, a cause-effect "fishbone" diagram is used to illustrate causation, beginning with a problem or error at the fish's head. Working back down the spine, the team is asked repetitively, "And what contributed to this?" This continues until as many prime factors as possible are identified. An average of 6 system-related or cognitive factors contribute to medical error in a single case. This is conceptualized as the "Swiss cheese" model of error, in that there must be a breakdown of several layers in a system to actually cause an injury.

Quality Improvement

A common methodology to improve quality is the Plan-Do-Study-Act (PDSA) cycle. The clinician might *plan* a test of quality improvement, *do* the test by trying the new protocol on a limited number of patients, *study* the results, and *act* by refining the protocol based on what was learned and planning the next test.

Patient Handoffs

The best practice for handoff includes person-to-person communication, providing an opportunity to ask and respond to questions, and providing information that is accurate and concise (including name, location, history, diagnoses, severity of illness, medication and problem lists, status, recent procedures, a "to do" list that has "if/then" statements, and contingency plans).

Medical Ethics and Professionalism

Patient Privacy

With the advent of the HIPAA regulations, patients must have control over who has access to their personal health information, especially with regard to family members. The preservation of confidentiality is not absolute. Safeguarding the individual or public from harm or honoring the law prevails over protecting confidentiality.

> ❖ **Test Yourself**
>
> A 78-year-old man is admitted with GI bleeding. Colonoscopy reveals metastatic colon cancer. His daughter wishes to know the results of the colonoscopy.
>
> **ANSWER:** The information cannot be released unless approved by the patient.

Advance Planning

Advance care planning is a process in which the patient articulates and documents his or her values, goals, and preferences for future health care. Advance care planning includes completion of an advance directive, which contains written instructions for health care that are used in the event that the patient loses decision-making capacity.

Advance directives include:

- the living will, in which the patient lists preferences regarding specific treatments and pain control preferences during terminal illness
- the health care power of attorney, in which the patient designates a surrogate decision-maker
- the combined advance directive, which has features of both a living will and health care power of attorney

◆ **DON'T BE TRICKED**
- The surrogate named by the patient in his or her advance directive is the legal decision-maker regardless of the surrogate's relationship with the patient.
- If a surrogate is not specifically named and the patient is incapacitated, then the order of decision making is spouse, adult child, parent, adult sibling.

Decision-Making Capacity

The physician must assess the patient's decision-making abilities to decide whether a surrogate decision-maker should be enlisted. To make their own decisions, patients need a set of values and goals, the ability to communicate and understand information, and the ability to reason and deliberate about options. The core components of decisional capacity are (1) understanding the situation at hand, (2) understanding the risks and benefits of the decision being made, and (3) being able to communicate a decision.

◆ **DON'T BE TRICKED**
- Minors, who are not living independently of their parents, not married, or not in the armed forces cannot legally make their own decisions.
- Any physician can determine if a patient has decision-making capacity.

"Competence" is a legal term; only the courts can determine competence. If a patient is incapable of medical decision making, a surrogate decision-maker is identified. Surrogates can use one of two standards for decision making:

- Substituted judgment standard: The surrogate makes the decision that he or she believes the patient would have made.
- Best interests standard: The surrogate selects the medical treatment that he or she personally feels is best for the patient.

❖ **Test Yourself**

An 82-year-old woman is hospitalized for the fourth time in 12 months. She lives alone and is unable to take her medications properly. She cannot articulate a plan to manage her disease.

ANSWER: Seek guardianship, because the patient cannot describe realistic plans for living home alone.

Withholding or Withdrawing Treatment

Withdrawing treatment is reasonable if, from the patient's perspective, the expected benefits of treatment no longer outweigh its burdens. Do-not-resuscitate orders must be documented in the medical record, along with notes and orders that describe the affirmative goals of continued care and how they will be met. Patients who have do-not-resuscitate orders are still eligible to receive other therapeutic life-prolonging or palliative measures.

Physicians are not obligated to administer interventions that are physiologically futile. Physicians may also disagree with a patient's legitimate choice of care if it violates their ethical principles. If consensus about treatment cannot be reached, options include transfer of the patient to another physician and review by a hospital ethics committee. Administration of nutrients and fluids by artificial means is a life-prolonging measure, guided by the same principles for decision making that are applied to other treatments.

Physician-Assisted Death

In physician-assisted suicide, death occurs when the physician provides a means for the patient to terminate his or her life (lethal prescription). In euthanasia, the physician directly terminates the patient's life (for example, by lethal injection).

In caring for patients at the end of life, there may be circumstances in which an intervention may unintentionally hasten death (for example, IV narcotic analgesics). Using such interventions is ethical if:

- the action itself is good or indifferent (for example, pain control)
- the good effect (pain control), not the bad effect (death), is intended
- the good effect is not achieved by means of the bad effect
- there is a proportionally serious reason (refractory pain due to widely metastatic cancer) for risking the bad effect

Disclosing Medical Errors

When patients are injured as a consequence of medical care, whether or not error is involved, they should be informed promptly about what has occurred. An apology should be given if it was due to error or system failure. Data does not support concerns that disclosure of an error promotes litigation.

The Impaired Physician

Physicians are ethically—and in some states, legally—bound to protect patients from impaired colleagues by reporting such physicians to appropriate authorities, including chiefs of service, chiefs of staff, institutional committees, or state medical boards.

Conflict of Interest

A conflict of interest exists when physicians' primary duty to their patients conflicts or appears to conflict with a secondary interest, which may consist of another important professional responsibility, a contractual obligation, or personal gain.

Physicians are obligated to avoid significant conflicts of interest whenever possible. For less serious or unavoidable conflicts of interest, disclosure is appropriate. Even small gifts may affect clinical judgment and heighten the perception (or the reality) of a conflict of interest. The acceptance of gifts, hospitality, trips, and subsidies of all types from those in the health care industry is strongly discouraged.

Palliative Care

Palliative care may be provided concurrently with life-prolonging therapies or with therapies with curative intent. Hospice, on the other hand, is a specialized type of palliative care that is reserved for patients in the terminal phase of their disease, arbitrarily defined as the last 6 months of life.

Pain

Pharmacologic management of pain progresses in a stepwise fashion. The World Health Organization pain ladder has proven efficacious in managing pain.

- Use acetaminophen, aspirin, or NSAIDs for mild to moderate pain.
- If pain persists or increases, add a low-dose or low-potency opioid (e.g., oxycodone).
- Increase opioid potency (e.g., morphine) or add higher doses for persistent or moderate to severe pain at onset.
- Add adjuvant agents at any step (tricyclic antidepressants, anticonvulsants).
- Prescribe around-the-clock analgesics for persistent, chronic pain rather than as needed.

Opioids do not have an analgesic efficacy ceiling and can be titrated upward as needed, until limiting side effects appear. Common side effects of opioids include constipation, sedation, nausea, and itching (not from an allergy).

Warnings about opioid use:

- fentanyl should only be used in opioid-tolerant patients
- meperidine is not recommended for pain due to increased risk of seizure
- tramadol has significant drug interactions
- methadone should only be initiated and titrated by experts

In the administration of opioids, oral routes are preferred (do not use IM).

- Subcutaneous administration is preferred for patients unable to use an oral route.
- Long-acting formulations are no more effective than short-acting formulations.

Neuropathic pain is characterized by burning, tingling, or lancinating pain. Add tricyclic antidepressants, SNRIs (venlafaxine, duloxetine), and antiepileptic medications (gabapentin, pregabalin, carbamazepine) to pain regimen.

Treat bone pain with anti-inflammatory medications (NSAIDs or glucocorticoids) or bisphosphonates (pamidronate, zoledronate).

All patients on scheduled opioids should be on a scheduled bowel program to prevent constipation, in this order:

- stimulant laxative with or without docusate
- osmotic agent (PEG, sorbitol, or lactulose)
- methylnaltrexone

Dyspnea

Treat reversible causes of dyspnea, such as pleural effusions, infection, and anemia. Systemic opioids are the standard of care for refractory dyspnea in advanced disease.

- Oxygen supplementation is helpful if the patient is hypoxic but is otherwise ineffective.
- Fans are effective in reducing the symptom of dyspnea in nonhypoxic patients.

Depression and Anxiety

It is difficult to distinguish grief from depression. Helplessness, hopelessness, worthlessness, guilt, and anhedonia are signs of depression rather than normal grief.

Depression will respond to typical pharmacologic and nonpharmacologic therapy. If prognosis is less than 6 weeks, use a psychostimulant with a faster onset, such as methylphenidate. Benzodiazepines can help reduce anxiety in a palliative care setting.

Anorexia

Artificial nutrition in cachexia of advanced disease does not improve morbidity or mortality. Medications used to stimulate appetite (progesterones, dronabinol, glucocorticoids) do not improve morbidity or mortality.

Chronic Noncancer Pain

Diagnosis

Psychological screening for depression, anxiety, and somatization are important adjuncts to a thorough history and physical examination.

Therapy

Evidence-based nondrug therapy includes:

- exercise
- massage
- cognitive behavioral therapy

Drug therapy for neuropathic pain includes:

- capsaicin cream or a lidocaine patch or cream
- gabapentin and pregabalin
- tricyclic antidepressants (increased drug interactions, poor side effect profile, and potential cardiac toxicities)
- SNRIs (duloxetine and venlafaxine)

Drug therapy for nociceptive pain includes:

- acetaminophen
- NSAIDs (if there is an inflammatory component)

There is no evidence to support the efficacy of long-term opioids in managing chronic pain. If opioids are used, an assessment is performed to assess risk of abuse and diversion.

Despite the lack of evidence, written treatment agreements, adherence monitoring (urine drug screens), and surveillance using prescription monitoring programs are recommended by most guidelines.

◆ **DON'T BE TRICKED**
- Do not concurrently prescribe both opioids and sedative-hypnotics.

Chronic Cough

Diagnosis

Chronic cough lasts ≥8 weeks. Upper airways cough syndrome (UACS) due to postnasal drip, asthma, and GERD are responsible for approximately 90% of cases of chronic cough but are responsible for 99% in patients who are nonsmokers, have a normal chest x-ray, and are not taking an ACE inhibitor.

All patients should undergo chest x-ray. Smoking cessation and discontinuation of ACE inhibitors is indicated for 4 weeks before additional evaluation.

STUDY TABLE: Causes and Therapy of Chronic Cough		
If you see this...	**Diagnose this...**	**Choose this...**
Postnasal drainage, frequent throat clearing, nasal discharge, cobblestone appearance of the oropharyngeal mucosa, or mucus dripping down the oropharynx	UACS	1st generation antihistamine-decongestant combination or intranasal glucocorticoid (for allergic rhinitis)
Asthma, cough with exercise or exposure to cold	Cough-variant asthma	Methacholine or exercise challenge if diagnosis is uncertain
		Standard asthma therapy; may take 6 weeks to respond
GERD symptoms (GERD may be silent)	GERD-related cough	Empiric PPI therapy without testing; may take 3 months to respond
Taking ACE inhibitor	ACE-inhibitor cough	Stop ACE inhibitor, substitute ARB; takes approximately 1 month to respond
Voluminous sputum production with purulent exacerbations	Bronchiectasis	CT to show thickened bronchial walls in a tram-line pattern
		Treat with chest physiotherapy and treat acute exacerbations with antibiotics
Normal chest x-ray findings, normal spirometry, and negative methacholine challenge test	Possible nonasthmatic eosinophilic bronchitis	Sputum induction or bronchial wash for eosinophils
		Treat with inhaled glucocorticoids, avoidance of sensitizer
Paroxysms of cough with gagging and posttussive vomiting	Pertussis	Nasopharyngeal culture for *Bordetella pertussis*
		Treat with a macrolide antibiotic

Chronic Fatigue

Diagnosis

Chronic fatigue, also called systemic exertion intolerance disease (SEID), is defined as unexplained fatigue lasting more than 6 consecutive months that impairs the ability to perform desired activities.

Extensive diagnostic evaluation is not needed in patients with typical symptoms and with normal physical examination and basic laboratory study results.

Therapy

Chronic fatigue typically improves with treatment of the underlying medical cause.

Establishing goals of therapy and managing patient expectations are key treatment components of SEID. Focus treatment on minimizing the impact of fatigue through nonpharmacological interventions (cognitive behavioral therapy and graded exercise), which are beneficial in improving, but not curing, symptoms. No specific class of medication has been shown to be effective in SEID.

DON'T BE TRICKED

- Do not obtain multiple viral titers to evaluate chronic fatigue.
- Do not treat chronic fatigue empirically with antibiotics.

Vertigo

Diagnosis

Vertigo is the illusion of either personal or environmental movement (head spinning). Once vertigo is suspected, the next important step is to distinguish central from peripheral causes with the Dix-Hallpike maneuver.

STUDY TABLE: Interpretation of Dix-Halpike Maneuver

Characteristic	Peripheral Disease (benign positional vertigo, vestibular neuronitis, labyrinthitis)	Central Disease (brainstem or cerebellar stroke or tumor, MS)
Latency of nystagmus (lag time between maneuver and onset of nystagmus)	2-40 s	None
Duration of nystagmus	<1 min	>1 min
Severity of symptoms	Severe	Less severe
Fatigability (findings diminish with repetition)	Yes	No
Direction of nystagmus	Horizontal with rotational component; never vertical	Can be vertical, horizontal, or torsional

STUDY TABLE: Diagnosing Common Causes of Peripheral Vertigo

Cause	Findings
Benign paroxysmal positional vertigo	Brief vertigo (10-30 s) and nausea associated with abrupt head movement (turning over in bed). Treat with Epley maneuver (canalith repositioning procedure)
Vestibular neuronitis	Severe and longer lasting vertigo (days), nausea and often vomiting
Labyrinthitis	Similar to vestibular neuronitis but with hearing loss

Less common causes of peripheral vertigo are Meniere disease (vertigo, hearing loss, tinnitus), perilymphatic fistula (vertigo and hearing loss with history of straining or trauma), acoustic neuroma (hearing loss, tinnitus, unsteadiness, facial nerve involvement), aminoglycoside toxicity, herpes zoster (Ramsey Hunt syndrome), and migraine.

Diseases associated with central vertigo may be life threatening. Vertebrobasilar stroke is usually, but not always, accompanied by dysarthria, dysphagia, diplopia, weakness, ataxia or gait instability, or numbness. MS is suggested by relapsing and remitting neurologic abnormalities. Obtain an MRI for suspected central vertigo.

Therapy

Pharmacologic therapies of peripheral vertigo are not curative but may provide symptom relief: glucocorticoids, centrally-acting antihistamines (meclizine), vestibular suppressants (benzodiazepines), and antiemetic drugs.

DON'T BE TRICKED

- The Epley maneuver is the primary treatment of benign paroxysmal positional vertigo, not drugs.

Insomnia

Diagnosis

Insomnia includes problems of sleep initiation, sleep maintenance, early morning waking, or nonrestorative and poor-quality sleep. Insomnia may be associated with shift work and an irregular sleep schedule, obesity, sleep apnea, and restless legs syndrome. Obtain polysomnography for suspected sleep apnea or periodic limb movement disorder.

STUDY TABLE: Differential Diagnosis of Insomnia and Daytime Sleepiness	
Condition	**Characteristics**
Restless legs syndrome	An uncomfortable or restless feeling in the legs most prominent at night and at rest, associated with an urge to move and alleviated by movement
	Look for iron deficiency
	Associated with periodic limb movement disorder in most patients
Periodic limb movement disorder	Repetitive stereotypic leg movement during sleep and during quiet wakefulness
Central sleep apnea syndrome	Repetitive pauses in breathing during sleep without upper airway occlusion
	Associated history of HF or CNS disease
Obstructive sleep apnea syndrome	Upper airway obstruction during inspiration in sleep
	History of snoring, witnessed pauses in respiration, large shirt collar size, and daytime sleepiness
Shift-work sleep disorder	History of insomnia associated with shift work (permanent night shifts)
Sleep deprivation	Six hours or less of sleep is associated with daytime sleepiness and performance deficits
Narcolepsy	Daytime sleepiness with cataplexy, hypnagogic hallucinations, and sleep paralysis frequently coexisting with other sleep disorders

Therapy

Nondrug therapy of insomnia includes:

- sleep hygiene practices (regular bedtimes and waking times; spending no more than 8 hours in bed, using bed only for sleep)
- avoiding caffeine, nicotine, alcohol, and electronic device use prior to sleep
- cognitive behavioral therapy
- melatonin for short-term insomnia due to travel or shift work

Benzodiazepines (flurazepam, triazolam, temazepam, oxazepam, lorazepam, diazepam) are associated with tolerance, daytime somnolence, falls, rebound insomnia, cognitive impairment, anterograde amnesia, and potential for dependence.

Nonbenzodiazepines (zolpidem, zaleplon, eszopiclone) have fewer side effects but sedation, disorientation, and agitation may occur as well as (rarely) sleep driving, sleep walking, and sleep eating.

Restless legs syndrome is treated with dopaminergic agents (pramipexole or ropinirole) or with levodopa-carbidopa. Prescribe supplemental iron for patients with restless legs syndrome when the serum ferritin level is <50 ng/mL. Treatments for narcolepsy include modafinil, methylphenidate, or an amphetamine. These stimulants may cause serious cardiovascular and psychiatric side effects.

◆ DON'T BE TRICKED

- Do not select antidepressants for insomnia unless the patient is depressed.
- Do not select an antihistamine for insomnia.
- Do not prescribe benzodiazepines for the treatment of insomnia in the elderly (risk of delirium, falls, fractures, cognitive impairment, and motor vehicle accidents).

Syncope

Diagnosis

An uncomplicated faint (vasovagal or neurocardiogenic syncope) is common and can be diagnosed by the history and absence of any suggestion of heart disease from the physical examination and ECG. Look for the 4 P's:

- previous history
- posture (prolonged standing)
- provoking factors (blood draw, pain, emotion)
- prodromal symptoms (sweating, nausea, feeling warm)

A history of heart disease, chest pain prior to syncope, significant cardiac risk factors, or exertional syncope suggests structural cardiac disease or arrhythmias as the cause of syncope.

STUDY TABLE: Causes of Syncope	
If you see this...	**Diagnose this...**
A prodrome of nausea, diaphoresis, pallor, and brief loss of consciousness (<1 min) with rapid recovery and absence of postsyncopal confusion	Uncomplicated faint (vasovagal or neurocardiogenic syncope)
Preceding pressure on the carotid sinus (tight collar, sudden turning of head)	Carotid sinus hypersensitivity
Association with specific activities (urination, cough, swallowing, defecation)	Situational syncope (neurocardiogenic)
Upon assuming an upright position	Orthostatic hypotension caused by hypovolemia, pharmacologic agents, or autonomic nervous system disorders (e.g., parkinsonism, diabetes)
Brainstem neurologic signs and symptoms	Posterior circulation vascular disease; consider subclavian steal syndrome if preceded by upper extremity exercise
Witnessed "seizure"	Syncope can cause tonic-clonic jerking of extremities; primary seizure is unlikely if findings of diaphoresis or nausea before the event, a brief episode of unconsciousness, and immediate postsyncopal orientation are present
Related to exercise or associated with angina	Obstruction to LV outflow: AS, HCM, PE, and PH
Syncope with sudden loss of consciousness without prodrome	Arrhythmia, sinoatrial and AV node dysfunction (ischemic heart disease and associated with use of β-blockers, calcium channel blockers, and antiarrhythmic drugs)
Syncope following a meal	Postprandial syncope, often in older adult patients

Patients with uncomplicated faint can be discharged home without additional evaluation. Patients with suspected cardiac causes of syncope should be admitted to the hospital.

Consider the appropriate indications for the following diagnostic tests:

- ECG: Done in all cases. The finding of an arrhythmia and conduction block may establish the diagnosis, but a normal ECG does not rule out a cardiac etiology.
- Echocardiography: Obtain if structural heart disease is suspected.
- Ambulatory ECG recording: Indicated if cardiac arrhythmia is suspected or the cause is unclear. The choice of the recording device is determined by the frequency of the patient's symptoms (see Cardiovascular Medicine, Palpitations and Syncope).
- Stress testing: Indicated for patients with exercise-associated syncope or those with significant risks for ischemic heart disease.
- Carotid sinus massage: For suspected carotid sinus syncope or for unexplained syncope in those aged >60 years.
- Tilt-table testing: Hardly ever indicated, almost always the incorrect answer. Reserved for presumed neurocardiogenic syncope only if it is recurrent or represents high risk for injury and to assess whether it is associated with asystole.
- Electrophysiologic testing: Rarely helpful and almost always the incorrect answer.

◆ DON'T BE TRICKED

- Do not order carotid vascular studies to diagnose cause of syncope.
- Do not order brain imaging, cardiac enzymes, or EEG to evaluate syncope.

Therapy

Treatment of structural cardiac disease and arrhythmias is covered in the Cardiovascular Medicine section. For hypovolemia or orthostatic syncope, eliminate α- and β-blockers and anticholinergic agents, if possible. Increase fluid and sodium intake and consider compression stockings. As a last resort, add mineralocorticoids and α-adrenergic receptor agonists. For recurrent neurocardiogenic syncope, choose β-blockers.

✧ Test Yourself

An 18-year-old woman fainted while standing in line to purchase concert tickets. She felt "woozy" and became pale and sweaty before fainting. Friends observed jerking motions of her face and fingers.

ANSWER: Diagnose neurocardiogenic syncope (uncomplicated faint).

Musculoskeletal Pain

Elbow

Olecranon bursitis is inflammation of a bursa that lies in the posterior aspect of the elbow and presents as a fluid-filled mass. This condition can result from repetitive trauma, infection, or systemic inflammatory conditions. Olecranon bursitis does not cause restriction or pain with range of motion of the elbow whereas joint pathology will cause pain and restricted movement.

Aspirate a bursa if tender or warm to analyze fluid for crystals and infection. NSAIDs and rest (if noninfectious) are first-line treatments.

Epicondylitis involves pain and tenderness at either the insertion of the extensor radii tendons (lateral epicondylitis) or the flexor carpi radialis tendons (medial epicondylitis). Lateral epicondylitis ("tennis elbow") is caused by overuse that involves pronation and supination with the wrist flexed. First-line treatment is stretching and strengthening exercises and avoidance of activities that cause pain. Braces may be useful when exacerbating activities cannot be avoided. Oral and topical NSAIDs provide short-term relief. Do not inject glucocorticoids.

◆ DON'T BE TRICKED

- Do not obtain imaging studies in patients with findings compatible with epicondylitis.

Back

Patients with low back pain can be grouped into one of three broad categories:

- nonspecific pain (85%)
- radiculopathy or spinal stenosis (7%)
- specific spine disorder such as cancer, fracture, infection, or ankylosing spondylitis (8%)

Look for the "red flags" related to malignancy, spinal infection, fracture, and cauda equina syndrome and need for early imaging.

The "red flags" of cauda equina syndrome include:

- urinary retention or incontinence
- diminished perineal sensation
- bilateral motor deficits

Also perform diagnostic imaging and testing for patients with low back pain when severe or progressive neurologic deficits are present.

Look for a herniated disk when acute back pain radiates down the leg and is associated with:

- positive straight leg raising
- weakness of the ankle and great toe dorsiflexion (L5)
- loss of ankle reflexes (S1)
- less commonly, loss of knee reflex (L4)

Spinal stenosis usually occurs in older adults and is characterized by neurogenic claudication—radiating back pain and lower extremity numbness—that is exacerbated by walking and spinal extension but improved by sitting and leaning forward. A wide-based gait and abnormal Romberg test are highly specific (>90%) for spinal stenosis. MRI establishes the diagnosis.

Recovery is generally quick for acute, nonspecific low back pain regardless of the intervention used. The first step is self-care (remain active, application of superficial heat). Other interventions include:

- pharmacologic (acetaminophen, NSAIDs)
- spinal manipulation
- massage

Collapsed Vertebral Body: Unenhanced T2-weighted MRI of the thoracic spine shows collapse of the vertebral body and compression of the spinal cord from posteriorly displaced bony fragments in a patient with metastatic breast cancer.

Muscle relaxants and benzodiazepines may be modestly beneficial for pain relief but dizziness and sedation limit their usefulness. Systemic glucocorticoids or epidural injections have not been shown to be effective in the treatment of low back pain.

Sciatica can be treated conservatively, and most are substantially improved within 1 to 3 months. Patients with sciatica assigned to early surgery and those assigned to conservative treatment have similar 1-year outcomes. Patients with spinal stenosis treated surgically have greater improvement in pain and function at 2 years compared with patients treated nonsurgically.

Neoplastic epidural spinal cord compression, including the cauda equina syndrome, is a surgical emergency. Begin management by administering dexamethasone and obtaining immediate MRI of the entire spine.

◆ DON'T BE TRICKED

- Do not obtain imaging for patients with nonspecific low back pain.

Knee

The most common cause of knee pain in patients aged <45 years, especially women, is the patellofemoral pain syndrome. The pain is peripatellar and exacerbated by overuse (running), descending stairs, or prolonged sitting. Diagnosis is confirmed by firmly compressing the patella against the femur and moving it up and down along the groove of the femur, reproducing pain. The condition is self-limited. Minimizing high-impact activity, performing quadriceps strengthening exercises, and treatment with NSAIDs improve symptoms.

Prepatellar bursitis is associated with anterior knee pain and swelling anterior to the patella and is often caused by trauma or repetitive kneeling. Perform a joint aspiration to rule out infection if warmth and erythema are present.

The anserine bursa, which is located medially about 6 cm below the joint line, can cause knee pain that is worse with activity and at night. Anserine bursitis is common in patients with OA.

In general, bursitis treatment includes:

- rest
- ice
- NSAIDs
- local glucocorticoid injection for persistent symptoms

Iliotibial band syndrome is a common cause of knife-like lateral knee pain that occurs with vigorous flexion-extension activities of the knee (running). Treat with rest and stretching exercises.

Trauma may result in a ligament tear, which produces a noticeable "popping" sensation in 50% of patients. Typically, a large effusion collects rapidly. Check for stability of major ligaments by stressing the ligament; normal knees will have minimal give.

Meniscal tears present with pain, locking, and clicking. Tenderness usually localizes to the joint line on the affected side and with tibial rotation as the leg is extended. No physical examination maneuver reliably establishes or excludes the diagnosis. Initial therapy for acute meniscal tears includes rest, ice, and physical therapy. Surgery for acute meniscal tears is reserved for mechanical symptoms that persist beyond 4 weeks. MRI is reserved for patients in whom surgery is being considered and in patients with persistent locking and catching despite appropriate initial management.

Hip

Most patients with chronic hip pain have degenerative arthritis associated with other large-joint arthritis symptoms.

Look for trochanteric bursitis, characterized by lateral point tenderness and full range of motion except for painful resisted abduction. Manage with local glucocorticoid injection and stretching exercises.

Risk factors for osteonecrosis include sickle cell disease, SLE, and prolonged glucocorticoid use. Diagnose early osteonecrosis with hip MRI. Advanced disease will show flattening of the femoral head on x-ray. Treatment of osteonecrosis is often hip replacement for recalcitrant pain and disability.

Consider bone metastases to the hip in patients with a history of cancer.

◆ **DON'T BE TRICKED**
- **True hip joint pain usually presents as groin pain.**

Ankle

Look for ecchymoses around the joint, suggesting bleeding in the region of a torn ligament, and any swelling or obvious deformity. Ability to bear weight rules out fracture or severe sprain.

Look for Achilles tendon rupture (a snapping sound followed by posterior ankle pain and inability to plantarflex). Rarely this can occur in older men who are taking a fluoroquinolone antibiotic.

◆ **DON'T BE TRICKED**
- **Select ankle x-ray following trauma only if the patient cannot bear weight or if bone pain is localized to the lateral or medial malleolus, base of the fifth metatarsal, or the navicular bone.**

Foot

Plantar fasciitis, the most common cause of inferior heel pain, is characterized by pain that worsens with walking, especially with the first steps in the morning or after resting, in addition to localized tenderness along the plantar fascia or the calcaneal insertion site. Manage with stretching exercises.

Symptoms of a Morton neuroma include pain, numbness, and tingling in the forefoot, usually between the third and fourth toes, aggravated by walking on hard surfaces and wearing tight or high-heeled shoes. Compressing the forefoot or space between the third and fourth toes reproduces the symptoms. Initial therapy includes wearing wider shoes and arch support.

- Do not order heel radiography for plantar fasciitis.

Hand

De Quervain tenosynovitis is typically seen in young women with pain on the radial side of the wrist during pinch grasping or during thumb and wrist movement. The diagnosis is established with a positive Finkelstein test, in which the patient folds fingers over thumb to make a fist, and the examiner rotates the hand, stretching the thumb tendons, which produces pain.

Consider carpal tunnel syndrome for pain and paresthesias, particularly at night, localized to the thumb, first two fingers, and the radial half of the ring finger. Keep in mind secondary causes of carpal tunnel syndrome, especially in patients with bilateral symptoms, such as hypothyroidism, diabetes mellitus, pregnancy, paraproteinemias, and RA of the wrist. Splinting at night plus NSAIDs is first-line therapy for carpal tunnel syndrome. Carpal tunnel release surgery is indicated for severe carpal tunnel syndrome (muscle weakness or EMG evidence of nerve injury) and has an excellent outcome in more than 90% of patients.

Shoulder

Patients with rotator cuff tendinitis and subacromial bursitis typically have gradually worsening pain, especially with overhead activity that limits range of motion. The pain is worse at night and may extend down the arm but rarely below the elbow. Consider the following:

- pain without weakness is consistent with tendinitis
- pain with weakness is consistent with a tendon tear
- severe pain and frank weakness (inability to maintain the arm at 90 degrees of abduction) suggests complete rupture of the rotator cuff tendon

MRI is the best imaging modality for complete or partial rotator cuff tears, although ultrasonography is more cost effective.

Consider other causes of shoulder pain:

- impingement syndrome when lateral deltoid pain is aggravated by reaching
- frozen shoulder when an impingement pain pattern is accompanied by stiffness and loss of active and passive external rotation or abduction
- causes of anterior shoulder pain (acromioclavicular joint, glenohumeral joint, or long head of the biceps)

Acromioclavicular joint pain is localized to the distal end of the clavicle most pronounced when the patient reaches across their body to the opposite shoulder. Glenohumeral joint pain is aggravated by any shoulder movement. Pain due to biceps tendinitis is aggravated by lifting and wrist supination.

Rupture of the biceps tendon is often associated with a traumatic event or may be spontaneous. Physical examination findings include a visible or palpable mass near the elbow or mid arm ("Popeye sign") and ecchymosis.

Conservative therapy is indicated for patients with suspected rotator cuff tendinitis, incomplete tears and subacromial bursitis. NSAIDs and exercises that strengthen the rotator cuff muscles and improve flexibility are effective in improving pain.

Immediate surgery is indicated for an acute full-thickness tear in younger patients. Full-thickness tears are frequently managed conservatively in older patients.

Biceps Tendon Rupture: Biceps tendon rupture showing a visible mass ("Popeye sign") at the mid arm with associated ecchymoses.

◆ **DON'T BE TRICKED**

- Constant shoulder pain with normal shoulder examination suggests referred pain (e.g., Pancoast tumor) or neuropathic pain (e.g., cervical spine radiculopathy).

Dyslipidemia

Diagnosis

In a marked change from previous guidelines, the 2013 ACC/AHA Guideline for the Treatment of Blood Cholesterol to Reduce Atherosclerotic Cardiovascular Risk in Adults does not focus on LDL cholesterol treatment targets, but rather on a person's overall risk of developing ASCVD.

◆ **DON'T BE TRICKED**

- Do not obtain lipoprotein(a), apolipoprotein B, and LDL particles in the evaluation of dyslipidemia.

Therapy

All patients should be treated with a heart-healthy diet, avoid tobacco, maintain a healthy weight, and regularly engage in physical exercise.

The ACC/AHA guideline on the treatment of cholesterol identifies four patient groups in which statin therapy is beneficial:

- established clinical ASCVD (CAD, PAD, cerebrovascular disease)
- LDL cholesterol level of ≥190 mg/dL
- diabetes, age 40-75 years, LDL cholesterol 70-189 mg/dL, and no ASCVD
- no ASCVD or diabetes and 10-year ASCVD risk ≥7.5% as estimated by the Pooled Cohort Equations

High-intensity statin therapy is indicated for:

- patients with ASCVD, age ≤75 years
- patients age >20 years with an LDL cholesterol of ≥190 mg/dL
- patients 40-75 years of age with diabetes and an LDL cholesterol level of 70 to 189 mg/dL and 10-year ASCVD risk ≥7.5%

Moderate-intensity statin therapy is indicated for:

- patients 40-75 years of age with diabetes and an LDL cholesterol level of 70 to 189 mg/dL and 10-year ASCVD risk <7.5%
- patients with ASCVD and age >75 years, impaired renal or hepatic function, muscle disorders, and use of drugs affecting statin metabolism (calcium channel blockers, fibrates, protease inhibitors, amiodarone, macrolide antibiotics)
- Patients with no history of ASCVD or diabetes and an LDL cholesterol level of 70-189 mg/dL, and 10-year ASCVD risk ≥7.5% are treated with either high- or moderate-intensity statin therapy.

STUDY TABLE: High- and Moderate-Intensity Statins	
High Intensity	**Moderate Intensity**
Atorvastatin 40-80 mg	Atorvastatin 10-20 mg
Rosuvastatin 20-40 mg	Rosuvastatin 5-10 mg
	Simvastatin 20-40 mg
	Pravastatin 40-80 mg
	Lovastatin 40 mg
	Fluvastatin 40 mg

◆ DON'T BE TRICKED

- Simvastatin 80 mg/d is not recommended by the FDA because of the increased risk of rhabdomyolysis.

Baseline labs and monitoring:

- baseline fasting lipid panel ALT level
- monitor ALT and CK only if a patient develops symptoms of hepatic or muscle disease

Patients with a fasting triglyceride ≥500 mg/dL are treated to prevent pancreatitis. Fibrates are the most potent triglyceride-lowering agents.

Obesity

Diagnosis

STUDY TABLE: Obesity Definitions	
Diagnosis	**BMI**
Overweight	25-29.9
Obese	
Class I	30-34.9
Class II	35-39.9
Class III	≥40

Therapy

A reasonable initial goal is weight loss of 0.5 kg to 1.0 kg/week to achieve a total weight loss of 10%.

A specific daily calorie limit should be prescribed (typically, 1500-1800 kcal/d for men and 1200-1500 kcal/d for women). All diets are equally effective. Exercise is helpful as an adjunct to diet change but not effective as monotherapy.

Pharmacologic therapy may be used as an adjunctive therapy in patients with a BMI ≥30 or in patients with a BMI ≥27 and weight-associated comorbidities.

STUDY TABLE: Drugs for Weight Loss		
Drug	**Expected Weight Loss**	**Cautions and Contraindications**
Orlistat (inhibitor of gastric and pancreatic lipases)	3 kg	Diarrhea, oily stools; must replace fat soluble vitamins
Combination phentermine (sympathomimetic) and low-dose topiramate (anticonvulsant)	8-10 kg	Contraindications: pregnancy, glaucoma, hyperthyroidism, and MAOI use
Lorcaserin (brain serotonin 2C receptor agonist)	4 kg	Caution in patients taking medications that increase serotonin levels
Combination sustained-release bupropion (norepinephrine-dopamine reuptake inhibitor) and sustained-release naltrexone (opioid receptor antagonist)	2-6 kg	Contraindications: epilepsy, uncontrolled hypertension, and opioid or opioid agonist use

Bariatric surgery is considered for patients with a BMI >40 and also for BMI >35 with serious obesity-related comorbidities (severe sleep apnea, diabetes, severe joint disease).

Bariatric surgery outcomes are associated with:

- improved control or remission of type 2 diabetes
- improved quality of life

- reduced medication use
- reduced mortality

Commonly performed bariatric procedures include laparoscopic adjustable gastric banding, Roux-en-Y gastric bypass, and sleeve gastrectomy.

STUDY TABLE: Bariatric Surgery Complications	
Surgery	**Complications**
Banding procedures	Intractable nausea and vomiting
	Marginal ulcers, stomal obstruction
Gastric bypass	Stomal stenosis
	Cholelithiasis
	Nephrolithiasis
	Dumping syndrome
	Anatomic stricture or ulceration
	Bacterial overgrowth
	Micronutrient deficiencies: B_1; B_6; folate; B_{12}; vitamins C, A, D, E, and K; iron; zinc; selenium; and copper
Sleeve gastrectomy	Staple-line bleeding, stenosis (dysphagia and vomiting), and staple-line leakage

❖ **Test Yourself**

A 41-year-old woman is evaluated for persistent nausea and vomiting after laparoscopic gastric bypass surgery 6 weeks ago for morbid obesity.

ANSWER: Select upper endoscopy to diagnose stomal stenosis or marginal ulcer.

Male Sexual Dysfunction

Diagnosis

Testosterone deficiency, hyperprolactinemia, diabetes, and thyroid disorders can cause erectile dysfunction. Rapid onset of sexual dysfunction suggests psychogenic causes or medication effects, whereas a more gradual onset suggests the presence of medical illnesses. Decreased libido suggests hormonal deficiencies, psychogenic causes, or medication effects. Look for:

- vascular, neurogenic, and endocrine (assess for signs of hypogonadism) disorders
- perineal, pelvic, or nervous system trauma and radiation or surgery to the pelvis or retroperitoneum
- interpersonal relationship problems and affective disorders
- antihypertensive, antidepressant, anticonvulsant, or antiandrogen and NSAID use
- alcohol, tobacco, cocaine, opiate, and marijuana use

The role of routine hormonal evaluation is not clear. If pursued, 8:00 AM total testosterone is the most appropriate study (See Endocrinology and Metabolism, Male Hypogonadism).

Suspect androgen steroid abuse in patients with infertility, muscular hypertrophy, testicular atrophy, and acne; laboratory data show elevated hemoglobin, suppressed LH and FSH levels.

Therapy

First-line therapy for erectile dysfunction is oral PDE-5 inhibitors (sildenafil, vardenafil, or tadalafil). These drugs are contraindicated in men who receive nitrate therapy in any form and in men with a history of nonarteritic anterior ischemic optic neuropathy and used with caution in men taking α-blockers.

Intraurethral or intracavernous alprostadil are second-line therapies for men who cannot take PDE-5 inhibitors.

A 72-year-old man cannot maintain an erection. He has diabetes mellitus, peripheral vascular disease, and CAD with stable angina, for which he takes aspirin, atenolol, isosorbide dinitrate, and glipizide.

ANSWER: Begin intraurethral or intracavernous alprostadil.

Benign Prostatic Hyperplasia

Diagnosis

BPH leads to irritative symptoms (urinary urgency, frequency, and nocturia) and obstructive symptoms (decreased urinary stream, intermittency, incomplete emptying, and straining). BPH is diagnosed primarily by medical history and digital rectal examination. When a diagnosis of BPH has been established, the American Urological Association Symptom Index quantifies symptom severity and guides treatment decisions.

Therapy

For most patients, conservative treatment is sufficient (reduce fluid intake, stop contributing medications [diuretics, anticholinergics]). The two major BPH drug classes include:

- α-adrenergic blockers (terazosin, tamsulosin, doxazosin, alfuzosin, and prazosin)
- 5-α reductase inhibitors (finasteride, dutasteride)

α-Adrenergic blockers are superior to 5-α reductase inhibitors. α-Adrenergic blockers plus finasteride are more effective than either drug alone but are associated with increased adverse effects.

Transurethral resection of the prostate (TURP) or transurethral needled ablation (TUNA) is indicated in patients with severe urinary symptoms, urinary retention, persistent hematuria, recurrent UTIs, or renal insufficiency clearly attributable to BPH.

Acute Scrotal Pain

Diagnosis

Patients with testicular torsion have severe acute pain and may have nausea and vomiting. Absence of the cremasteric reflex on the affected side is nearly 99% sensitive for torsion. The testis is usually high within the scrotum and may lie transversely. Doppler flow ultrasonography demonstrates diminished blood flow to the affected testicle. Testicular elevation will not relieve pain.

Epididymitis causes pain localizing to the posterior and superior aspects of the testicle. Pain onset is subacute and may be accompanied by dysuria, pyuria, and fever. The scrotum may be edematous and erythematous. Pain may decrease with testicular elevation.

Orchitis is usually caused by viral infection (mumps) or extension of a bacterial infection from epididymitis or UTI. The testicle is diffusely tender. In both epididymitis and orchitis, ultrasonography demonstrates normal or increased blood flow to the testicle and epididymis.

Therapy

Treatment of testicular torsion is immediate surgical exploration and reduction.

In men younger than 35 years with epididymitis or men who engage in anal intercourse, treat for gonorrhea and chlamydial infection (ceftriaxone and doxycycline). In men older than 35 years, treat with an oral fluoroquinolone.

Acute Prostatitis

Diagnosis

Symptoms of acute prostatitis include fevers, chills, dysuria, pelvic pain, cloudy urine, obstructive symptoms, and blood in the semen. Some men may present in septic shock. The diagnosis is established by finding a tender prostate on physical examination and a positive urine culture.

Therapy

Begin empiric antibiotics that cover gram-negative organisms (trimethoprim-sulfamethoxazole, fluoroquinolone) for 4 to 6 weeks. For patients who appear toxic, hospitalize and add gentamicin to a fluoroquinolone.

Female Sexual Dysfunction

Diagnosis

Female sexual dysfunction describes sexual difficulties that are persistent and distressing to the patient. Screening for concurrent depression is indicated, as sexual dysfunction and depression often coexist.

A pelvic examination is helpful in identifying specific areas of pain or tenderness, vulvovaginal atrophy, decreased lubrication, or tissue friability. Laboratory testing is recommended only if an underlying disorder is suspected.

Abnormalities in female sexual response fall into three categories:

- sexual interest/arousal disorder (lack of sexual interest and responsiveness)
- orgasmic disorder (absence of orgasm following normal excitement phase)
- genitopelvic pain/penetration disorder (difficulty or pain with penetration)

Therapy

There are currently no FDA-approved pharmacologic agents for treatment of sexual dysfunction in women. Keep this approach in mind:

- treat underlying contributing causes (e.g., vaginitis, interstitial cystitis, pelvic adhesions, infections, or endometriosis)
- use vaginal or systemic hormone therapy to alleviate dyspareunia
- cognitive behavioral therapy for depression or anxiety

◆ **DON'T BE TRICKED**
- Do not treat with low-dose testosterone or phosphodiesterase inhibitors.

Breast Cancer Prevention and Screening

Prevention

The Gail Model Risk Assessment Tool is used to estimate any woman's 5-year and lifetime breast cancer risk. Women age >35 years with a 5-year breast cancer risk of ≥1.7% or with lobular carcinoma in situ are candidates for breast cancer prophylaxis:

- tamoxifen prior to menopause
- tamoxifen and raloxifene, or exemestane after menopause

Expert opinion recommends women with *BRCA1/2* mutations should undergo:

- breast cancer screening with MRI beginning at age 25 then mammography beginning at age 40
- ovarian cancer screening with pelvic examinations, ultrasonography, and CA-125 measurement

Surgical prophylaxis options for carriers of *BRCA1/2* mutations include prophylactic bilateral mastectomy and prophylactic bilateral salpingo-oophorectomy (after childbearing).

◆ **DON'T BE TRICKED**

- Testing for the *BRCA* gene is recommended only for women whose family history suggests increased risk for mutations in the *BRCA1* or *BRCA2* gene (first-degree relative, or two second-degree relatives on the same side of the family, with breast or ovarian cancer).

Screening

The USPSTF recommends biennial screening mammography for average-risk women beginning at age 50 years. Individualize screening decisions in women aged 75 or older, based on breast cancer risk, overall prognosis and comorbid conditions, and personal patient preferences.

Breast Mass

Diagnosis

A dominant breast mass is defined as a lump or suspicious change in the breast texture is discrete and distinctly different from the rest of the surrounding breast tissue. Most breast lumps are benign, but clinical examination cannot distinguish between benign and malignant.

STUDY TABLE: Evaluation of Breast Mass	
Breast Finding	**Diagnostic Testing**
Palpable lump or mass and age <30 years	Consider observation to assess resolution within 1 or 2 menstrual cycles
	If persistent, choose ultrasonography
	If simple cyst on ultrasound, aspirate and repeat clinical breast examination in 4-6 weeks
	If complex cyst on ultrasound, perform mammography and fine-needle aspiration or core-needle biopsy
	If aspirate fluid is bloody or a mass persists following aspiration, choose mammography and biopsy
	If solid on ultrasonography, choose mammography and obtain tissue diagnosis (core biopsy or surgical excision)
Palpable lump or mass and age ≥30 years	Mammography: If BI-RADS category 1-3 (benign or close follow-up recommended), obtain ultrasonography and follow protocol above; if BI-RADS category 4-5 (suspicious or highly suspicious), obtain tissue diagnosis.
Nipple discharge, no mass, any age	Bilateral, milky: Pregnancy test (if negative, choose endocrine evaluation)
	Persistent, spontaneous, unilateral, one duct, or serous/bloody: Cytology is optional; choose mammography and surgical referral for duct exploration
Skin changes (erythema, peau d'orange, scaling, nipple excoriation, eczema) and age <30 years	Consider mastitis and treat with antibiotics if appropriate and reevaluate in 2 weeks. Otherwise, evaluate as below
Skin changes (erythema, peau d'orange, scaling, nipple excoriation, eczema) and age ≥30 years	Perform bilateral mammography: If normal, obtain skin biopsy; if abnormal or indeterminate, obtain needle biopsy or excision (also consider skin punch biopsy)
BI-RADS = Breast Imaging Reporting and Data System.	

◆ **DON'T BE TRICKED**

- Do not stop the evaluation of a breast mass if mammogram is normal.
- On mammography, an irregular mass with microcalcifications or spiculation is suspicious for malignant disease, and biopsy is mandatory.

Cervical Cancer Screening

Screening

The USPSTF recommends cervical cancer screening in women aged 21 to 65 years with cytology (Pap test) every 3 years. The screening interval can be increased to every 5 years in women aged 30 to 65 years by combining cytology and HPV testing.

The USPSTF recommends against routine screening in women younger than 21 years and in women older than 65 years (provided normal results obtained on previous screenings and not otherwise at high risk).

- If the cytology results are negative but high-risk HPV DNA testing is positive, both tests should be repeated in 6-12 months.
- If HPV DNA test remains persistently positive, refer for colposcopy.
- If the cytology result is atypical squamous cells of undetermined significance (ASUS), test for HPV infection (alternatively, repeat Pap test at 6 and 12 months and refer for colposcopy if results are grade ASUS or higher).
- If the cytology is positive for high-grade squamous intraepithelial lesions, SCC, or atypical glandular cells, refer for colposcopy regardless of HPV results.

◆ **DON'T BE TRICKED**

- Do not screen women following a hysterectomy for benign disease (e.g., fibroids).
- HPV vaccine does not protect against all HPV infections and does not treat existing HPV.
- HPV vaccine can be given to patients who are HIV-positive and otherwise immunosuppressed.

Contraception

Available contraceptive methods include:

- hormonal contraception including intrauterine devices
- barrier contraceptives
- sterilization

STUDY TABLE: Comparison of Contraceptive Options

Agent	Advantages	Disadvantages
Combination estrogen-progestin preparations (oral, patch, vaginal ring)	Decreased incidence of endometrial, ovarian cancers	Increased risk of cancers of the cervix, liver, breast
	Decreased dysmenorrhea, menorrhagia, symptomatic ovarian cysts	Increased risk of MI, ischemic stroke, VTE, hypertension
	Less iron-deficiency anemia	Breakthrough bleeding
Progestin-only preparations (mini-pill)	Use when estrogen is contraindicated	Irregular bleeding, breakthrough bleeding
		Must maintain precise daily dosing schedule

(Continued on next page)

STUDY TABLE: Comparison of Contraceptive Options *(Continued)*		
Agent	**Advantages**	**Disadvantages**
Long-acting reversible preparations (depot medroxyprogesterone [IM or SQ], progestin implants)	Decreased risk of endometrial cancer, PID Improves endometriosis Decreased menstrual frequency	Irregular bleeding, amenorrhea, decreased bone mineral density (especially in adolescents) Delayed return to ovulation (10 months)
Intrauterine devices (copper, levonorgestrel)	Least dependence on user adherence Nonhormonal Effective for 5 to10 years	Bleeding, pain, expulsion (rare) No protection from STIs
Barrier methods (cervical cap, diaphragm, male condom, female condom, vaginal sponge)	Only use when needed Protection from STIs	Most dependent on user adherence May require use of spermicide
Sterilization		
Female (tubal ligation)	May reduce ovarian cancer risk	Surgical complications Regret
Male (vasectomy)	Lower costs, more effective than tubal ligation	Surgical complications
SQ = subcutaneous.		

Contraindications to combination hormonal products include:

- uncontrolled hypertension
- breast cancer
- venous thromboembolism
- liver disease
- migraine with aura

Estrogen-containing preparations are contraindicated in women older than 35 years who smoke more than 15 cigarettes per day.

Emergency contraception is postcoital hormonal contraception used to prevent pregnancy after inadequately protected coitus. Options include:

- over-the-counter levonorgestrel
- prescription ulipristal

Menopause

Diagnosis

Menopause describes the cessation of menses and fertility and is definitive once a woman has experienced amenorrhea for 12 months. The average age of experiencing natural menopause is 51 years. Irregular menstrual cycles, sometimes associated with vasomotor symptoms, are characteristic findings.

◆ DON'T BE TRICKED

- Do not order hormone levels to diagnose menopause.

Therapy

Symptoms generally resolve spontaneously within a few years, and treatment should be based on symptom severity. The most effective treatment is systemic hormone therapy and can be used in healthy women <60 years and within 10 years of menopause. Keep these treatment points in mind when using estrogen:

- contraceptive needs must be addressed during perimenopause
- transdermal estrogen may be associated with less VTE risk than oral estrogen
- all women with an intact uterus must receive progesterone
- duration of treatment >5 years is associated with increased risk of breast cancer
- the need for continued treatment should be reevaluated annually

In the absence of systemic estrogen therapy, genital symptoms can be treated with vaginal lubricants or local estrogen (estrogen creams, vaginal estradiol tablets, estradiol vaginal ring) which have minimal systemic estrogen absorption.

Nonhormonal options for women with contraindications to hormone therapy include low-dose antidepressant agents (venlafaxine, desvenlafaxine, paroxetine, citalopram, and escitalopram) and gabapentin.

◆ DON'T BE TRICKED

- Data regarding black cohosh are inconclusive, as are studies of other herbs, soy, and other phytoestrogens.

Abnormal Uterine Bleeding

Diagnosis

Bleeding is excessive, scanty, or occurs outside the normal menstrual cycle. Uterine fibroids are the most common cause of menorrhagia. Anovulatory cycles are the most common cause of unpredictable bleeding.

Perimenarche and perimenopause are frequently characterized by abnormal bleeding patterns and typically do not require evaluation. The perimenopausal transition begins with changes in the interval between menstrual periods and ends 1 year after the last period; it is highly variable, lasting between 4 to 8 years. Transvaginal ultrasonography is indicated for women >35 years with abnormal uterine bleeding, or refractory bleeding to assess endometrial stripe thickness. An endometrial stripe ≥5 mm (increased) warrants endometrial biopsy.

◆ DON'T BE TRICKED

- Pregnancy should always be considered in the differential diagnosis of abnormal uterine bleeding.
- Postmenopausal bleeding is always abnormal and requires evaluation.

STUDY TABLE: Selected Causes of Abnormal Uterine Bleeding		
Disorder	**Characteristics**	**Evaluation**
Anatomic lesions	Endometrial polyps, uterine fibroids (leiomyomata), and endometrial hyperplasia or carcinoma	Pelvic examination, Pap test, and a bimanual examination Ultrasonographic imaging Endometrial biopsy if endometrium is ≥5 mm in thickness or is heterogeneous
von Willebrand disease	20% of adolescents with menorrhagia	Bleeding time, aPTT, and functional and quantitative measurement of vWF
Kidney failure	Interferes with estrogen clearance Associated with abnormalities in platelet function	Serum creatinine level
Cirrhosis	Reduced ability to metabolize estrogen	Liver chemistry tests
Thyroid disease	Scanty or heavy menstrual bleeding	TSH level

Therapy

Combination oral contraceptives can regularize anovulatory bleeding in women who do not wish to become pregnant. Medroxyprogesterone acetate may be used to promote withdrawal bleeding and regulate cycles for women who wish to become pregnant. NSAIDs inhibit endometrial prostaglandins and decrease blood flow.

Surgery is indicated when bleeding is excessive and/or unresponsive to medical therapy or when a cervical or endometrial polyp, cancer, or fibroid is present.

Dysmenorrhea

Diagnosis

Symptoms of dysmenorrhea include abdominal cramps, backache, headache, nausea, vomiting, and diarrhea. Symptoms coincide with the onset of menses and last 2 to 3 days.

Dysmenorrhea is classified as primary or secondary. Primary dysmenorrhea, which occurs in 90% of patients, is associated with normal ovulatory cycles and no pelvic pathology.

A secondary cause, such as endometriosis, fibroids, or uterine pathology, is found in 10% of patients.

Dysmenorrhea is sometimes associated with other cyclic symptom complexes such as PMS and PMDD. These disorders include physical and psychological symptoms that begin approximately 1 week before menses and cease with menstruation. PMDD is characterized by significant depressive symptoms that interfere with daily activities.

Initial evaluation includes a thorough history, with attention to risks for infection and possible physical, sexual, or emotional abuse.

Therapy

Primary dysmenorrhea is treated symptomatically without further testing with NSAIDs and cyclooxygenase-2 inhibitors. Second-line therapy includes combined hormonal contraceptive therapy.

Fluoxetine, sertraline, and paroxetine are effective first-line treatments for PMS and PMDD.

Pelvic Pain

Diagnosis

Endometriosis is characterized by ectopic endometrial implants, usually in the pelvis, but they can be found anywhere and cause cyclic bleeding, such as in the lungs (hemoptysis), CNS (catamenial headache), and rectum (rectal bleeding during menses). It is a common cause of chronic pelvic pain that is worse just before and during menses and is associated with dysmenorrhea.

Physical examination findings may be normal or may include abdominal masses and tenderness and abnormalities of the cervix, uterus, and adnexa. Also look for abnormalities of uterosacral ligaments on bimanual examination.

The lesions can be visualized by laparoscopy, the gold standard for diagnosis, but it is not required for medical treatment when other causes of pelvic pain have been ruled out. Cervical culture or DNA probe is indicated for patients at risk for *Chlamydia* infection and gonorrhea.

◆ DON'T BE TRICKED

- All patients with chronic pelvic pain require a urine pregnancy test and transvaginal ultrasonography.

STUDY TABLE: Differential Diagnosis of Pelvic Pain	
If you see this...	**Diagnose this...**
Acute pelvic or abdominal pain, vaginal discharge, and fever	PID, usually caused by *Chlamydia* infection or gonorrhea
Pelvic heaviness, abnormal uterine bleeding, infertility, and enlarged uterus on bimanual examination or ultrasonography	Uterine fibroids
History of sexual abuse and normal physical examination and ultrasonography	Chronic pelvic pain syndrome
Adolescents with dysmenorrhea	Primary dysmenorrhea
Urinary frequency, urgency, nocturia, and dysuria; suprapubic pain possibly relieved with voiding; and examination that shows vestibular and suprapubic tenderness	Interstitial cystitis

◆ DON'T BE TRICKED

- Endometriosis does not cause fever or vaginal discharge.

Therapy

NSAIDs are first-line therapy for endometriosis, followed by oral contraceptives (if pregnancy is not desired) if NSAIDs are ineffective. Counseling is important for abused women with chronic pelvic pain syndrome.

Vaginitis

Diagnosis

Vaginitis is characterized by vaginal irritation, pruritus, pain, malodor, or unusual discharge. The three most common infectious causes of acute vaginitis are bacterial vaginosis, vulvovaginal candidiasis, and *Trichomonas*. Trichomoniasis is the only cause of vaginitis that is sexually transmitted.

STUDY TABLE: Diagnosis of Vaginitis	
Test	**Characteristics**
Physical examination	Bacterial vaginosis: Thin, white discharge with "fishy" odor but without irritation or pain
	Candidiasis: External and internal erythema with itching and irritation; nonodorous; white, curd-like discharge
	Trichomoniasis: Frothy, yellow discharge; erythema of the vagina and cervix ("strawberry cervix")
Vaginal pH (normal <4.5)	Bacterial vaginosis and trichomoniasis: >4.5
	Candidiasis: <4.5
"Whiff" test	Bacterial vaginosis: "Fishy" odor after adding KOH
Microscopic examination of vaginal fluid	Bacterial vaginosis: Squamous epithelial cells covered with bacteria that obscure edges ("clue cells")
	Candidiasis: Budding yeast and pseudohyphae
	Trichomoniasis: Motile trichomonads
Other point-of-care testing	Nucleic acid testing is available for bacterial vaginosis and trichomoniasis (gold standard for trichomoniasis)

◆ DON'T BE TRICKED

- Do not order vaginal cultures to diagnose the cause of vaginitis.
- Treatment of vulvovaginal candidiasis can be initiated empirically if symptoms are accompanied by characteristic findings.

Candida albicans: A KOH wet mount shows budding yeast and pseudohyphae, indicating *Candida albicans.*

Clue Cell: An epithelial cell with borders that are studded by bacteria (clue cell) indicates bacterial vaginosis.

Therapy

STUDY TABLE: Treating Vaginitis	
If the diagnosis is...	**Treat with...**
Vaginal candidiasis	Topical (e.g., fluconazole, miconazole, clotrimazole)
	Single dose of oral fluconazole (contraindicated during pregnancy); less effective in complicated conditions (e.g., diabetes, HIV infection)
Recurrent vaginal candidiasis	Combination topical therapy and oral fluconazole. Suppressive therapy with weekly oral fluconazole for 6 months (correct any underlying precipitating factor, such as uncontrolled hyperglycemia) for multiple recurrences
Bacterial vaginosis	Oral or topical metronidazole or clindamycin (safe during pregnancy)
Trichomoniasis	Oral metronidazole and also for male partner (safe during pregnancy)

◆ DON'T BE TRICKED

- Because vaginal yeast is found in 10% to 20% of healthy women, the identification of *Candida* species in patients without symptoms does not require treatment.

❖ Test Yourself

A 21-year-old woman has a vaginal discharge and odor. Pelvic examination shows a thin, white homogeneous vaginal discharge with a normal cervix and normal vaginal mucosa. Wet mount is negative for *Trichomonas* and *Candida*. Vaginal pH is 6.0.

ANSWER: The diagnosis is bacterial vaginosis.

Eye Disorders

Red Eye

Red eye consists of categories of entities with or without ocular pain and/or visual loss. The combination of red eye, ocular pain, and visual loss warrants emergent referral to an ophthalmologist. Select Snellen visual acuity testing for all patients.

STUDY TABLE: Causes and Treatment of Red Eye

If you see this...	Diagnose this...	Do this...
Unilateral then bilateral purulent discharge without pain or visual disturbance	Bacterial conjunctivitis	Topical fluoroquinolones or bacitracin-polymyxin; culture not needed
Conjunctivitis associated with herpes zoster rash involving ophthalmic division of 5th cranial nerve	Herpes zoster conjunctivitis	Emergency ophthalmology referral
Acute hyperpurulent discharge in a sexually active adult	*Neisseria gonorrhoeae* conjunctivitis	Topical and systemic antibiotics and emergency ophthalmology referral
Giant papillary conjunctivitis with itching and watery discharge, preauricular lymphadenopathy	Chlamydial conjunctivitis	Oral treatment with tetracycline, erythromycin, or doxycycline
Unilateral then bilateral conjunctivitis with morning crusting of the eye and daytime watery or mucoid discharge	Viral conjunctivitis	Supportive care
Itching and tearing of the eyes, nasal congestion	Allergic conjunctivitis	Topical vasoconstrictors, NSAIDs, ocular antihistamines, cromolyn
Pain, photophobia, inflammation confined to corneal limbus, corneal irregularity, edema	Iridocyclitis or keratitis	Consider associated spondyloarthropathies, sarcoidosis, and herpes zoster; emergency ophthalmology referral
Unilateral deep ocular pain, nausea, vomiting, fixed nonreactive pupil, shallow anterior chamber	Acute angle-closure glaucoma	Emergency ophthalmology referral
Severe ocular pain that worsens with eye movement and light exposure; a raised hyperemic lesion that may be localized or diffuse and obscures the underlying vasculature	Scleritis	Commonly associated with collagen vascular and rheumatoid diseases; emergency ophthalmology referral
Nonpainful red, flat, superficial lesion that allows visualization of the underlying vasculature	Episcleritis	Self-limited; no treatment required
Red eye with scales and crusts around the eyelashes or dandruff-like skin changes and greasy scales around the eyelashes	Blepharitis	*Staphylococcus* (crusting) or seborrheic dermatitis (greasy scales, dandruff); warm compresses, washing with mild detergent, topical antibiotics

◆ **DON'T BE TRICKED**

- Do not treat a red eye with topical glucocorticoids.

Episcleritis: The nontender, prominent, superficial dilated blood vessels of episcleritis are shown.

Herpes Zoster: Herpes zoster infection involving the forehead, and top of the head and eye, with evident hyperemic conjunctivitis. Corneal ulceration, episcleritis, and lid droop can occur.

Viral Conjunctivitis: Acute adenovirus conjunctivitis is characterized by diffuse injection of the palpebral and bulbar conjunctivae and pseudomembrane formation involving the palpebral conjunctiva.

Allergic Conjunctivitis: Allergic conjunctivitis with prominent cobblestoning of the palpebral conjunctiva is shown.

Bacterial Conjunctivitis: The conjunctiva is diffusely erythematous with mucopurulent discharge consistent with bacterial conjunctivitis. Consider gonorrhea in sexually active adult.

Iritis: Intense ciliary flush around the corneal-scleral junction and an irregularly shaped pupil characteristic of iritis are shown.

❖ **Test Yourself**

A 39-year-old man has bilateral red eyes and pain for 2 days. He has arthritis and chronic low back pain. Visual acuity is 20/40 bilaterally. Eyes are intensely injected, with prominent circumcorneal erythema.

ANSWER: Diagnose acute iritis associated with ankylosing spondylitis and select emergent referral to an ophthalmologist.

Age-Related Macular Degeneration

Dry AMD involves the deposition of extracellular material (drusen) in the macular region of one or both eyes and may cause diminished visual acuity. Smoking cessation is imperative. Progression of advanced dry AMD may be slowed with the use of zinc or antioxidants supplements.

A small percentage of patients with dry AMD will progress to develop new vessel growth under the retina (wet AMD). Bleeding and exudation results in sudden (or rapid onset over weeks), painless blurring or warping of central vision. Laser photocoagulation and intraocular injection of VEGF is recommended for wet AMD.

Retinal Detachment

Retinal detachment occurs mainly in myopic patients. Symptoms are floaters, flashes of light (photopsias), and squiggly lines, followed by a sudden, peripheral visual field defect that resembles a black curtain and progresses across the entire visual field. Emergent ophthalmology referral is crucial, as prognosis depends on the time to surgical treatment.

Central Retinal Artery Occlusion

CRAO is caused by thrombi or emboli. Patients are usually elderly and present with profound and sudden painless vision loss.

Funduscopic examination reveals an afferent pupillary defect and cherry red fovea that is accentuated by a pale retinal background. Treatment may include measures to lower the intraocular pressure and emergent ophthalmology consultation.

Central Retinal Vein Occlusion

CRVO is usually caused by occlusion of the central retinal vein by a thrombus. Patients with CRVO present with sudden, painless, unilateral visual loss. Funduscopic examination may reveal afferent pupillary defect, congested retinal veins, scattered retinal hemorrhages, and cotton wool spots in the region of occlusion. Immediate ophthalmological consultation is necessary.

Hearing Loss

Diagnosis

Appropriate initial tests for healing loss include the whispered voice test and finger rub test. The Weber and Rinne tests help distinguish conductive from sensorineural hearing loss.

STUDY TABLE: Conductive and Sensorineural Hearing Loss			
Condition	Weber Test Result (Tuning fork to forehead)	Rinne Test Result (Tuning fork to mastoid then in front of ear)	Differential Diagnoses
Conductive hearing loss	Louder in the affected ear	Bone conduction > air conduction	Cerumen impaction, foreign body, otitis media, otosclerosis, perforated tympanic membrane
Sensorineural hearing loss	Louder in the good ear	As loud or louder in the bad ear	Presbyacusis, Meniere disease, acoustic neuroma, sudden sensorineural hearing loss

In patients with a conductive hearing loss, a nonmobile tympanic membrane may indicate fluid or a mass in the middle ear or retraction from negative middle ear pressure.

Select audiography for all patients with unexplained hearing loss. For patients with progressive asymmetric sensorineural hearing loss, select MRI or CT to evaluate for acoustic neuroma.

Sudden sensorineural hearing loss occurs acutely, usually within 12 hours of onset, and is unilateral in 90% of cases. It has many etiologies, including viral, vascular, autoimmune, and most commonly idiopathic.

Therapy

Treat otitis or cerumen impaction if present. Select urgent referral to an ENT specialist for sudden, unexplained hearing loss. The evidence for treatment with glucocorticoids is weak but frequently provided. For presbyacusis, hearing aids that amplify sound are often helpful.

A 35-year-old previously healthy man has had difficulty hearing in his right ear since last night. He has rhinorrhea and nasal congestion. His external auditory canals and tympanic membranes are normal; a 512-Hz tuning fork is placed on his forehead, and he hears the tone louder in his left ear than in his right ear.

ANSWER: Choose sudden sensorineural hearing loss and emergent ENT referral.

Otitis Media

Diagnosis

Acute otitis media is characterized by fluid and inflammation in the middle ear accompanied by symptoms of infection. Many patients first present with viral URI symptoms. If the tympanic membrane ruptures, purulent drainage from the ear canal may be present. Otitis media with effusion is characterized by fluid in the middle ear without signs of infection.

Therapy

Evidence on treatment in adults is lacking, however, analgesic therapy and decongestants are the mainstays of treatment. There is no evidence that favors one antibiotic over another; amoxicillin is often selected. Complications include hearing loss, tympanic membrane perforation, meningitis, and mastoiditis.

External Otitis

Diagnosis

Patients with typical external otitis present with otalgia, ear discharge, pruritus, and conductive hearing loss. Be aware of the several other varieties of external otitis:

- Malignant external otitis is characterized by systemic toxicity and evidence of infection spread beyond the ear canal (mastoid bone, cellulitis) and is typically found in elderly patients with type 2 diabetes or patients who are immunocompromised. Most commonly caused by *Pseudomonas aeruginosa*.
- Ramsay Hunt syndrome is caused by varicella zoster viral infection and characterized by facial nerve paralysis, sensorineural hearing loss, and vesicular lesions on and in the ear canal.

Drug Therapy

Select combination antibiotic and glucocorticoid drops for typical external otitis, systemic antipseudomonal antibiotics and hospitalization for malignant external otitis, and antiviral agents for Ramsay Hunt syndrome.

Ramsay Hunt Syndrome: Image shows vesicular lesions on and in the ear canal characteristic of the Ramsay Hunt syndrome caused by varicella zoster virus infection.

A 70-year-old man with type 2 diabetes mellitus has had a severe left earache since yesterday. He has a fever and tachycardia, and his left external ear canal is swollen. Moist white debris and granulation tissue are visible.

ANSWER: Diagnose malignant external otitis and select hospitalization and IV ciprofloxacin.

Sinusitis

Diagnosis

Viral infection causes most cases of sinusitis. Bacterial sinusitis is more likely if the following are present:

- persistent symptoms (lasting >10 days)
- severe symptoms or fever (lasting 3-4 days)
- "double-sickness" characterized by worsening symptoms following a period of improvement over 3-4 days

Imaging, including CT, should be considered in patients with AIDS or in other immunocompromised patients to evaluate for fungal infection or other atypical infections, but is not otherwise indicated.

Complications of acute sinusitis are unusual but deadly. Patients with cavernous sinus thrombosis have fever, nausea, vomiting, headache, orbital edema, or cranial nerve involvement. Other complications include brain abscess, bacterial meningitis, and osteomyelitis.

Drug Therapy

The first-line choice for suspected bacterial sinusitis is amoxicillin-clavulanate. Doxycycline is recommended for patients allergic to penicillin.

Allergic Rhinitis

Diagnosis

Rhinitis is an inflammation of the nasal mucosal membranes that causes rhinorrhea, nasal itching, sneezing, nasal congestion, and postnasal drainage.

Allergic rhinitis can be seasonal or perennial. Diagnosis of allergic rhinitis is usually made by history and confirmed with empiric treatment. If empiric treatment fails, diagnostic allergy testing may be appropriate to guide allergen avoidance or immunotherapy. Allergy skin testing is preferred to in vitro specific IgE antibody assay (or RAST).

In allergic rhinitis, the nasal mucosa is edematous and pale.

STUDY TABLE: Mimics of Allergic Rhinitis	
Look for...	**Diagnose...**
Systemic illness with saddle nose deformity, nasal ulceration, or chronic sinusitis	Granulomatosis with polyarteritis
Nasal polyposis, asthma, eosinophilia, mononeuritis, petechial skin lesions	Eosinophilic granulomatosis with polyangiitis (formerly Churg-Strauss)
Young person, nasal polyposis, chronic sinusitis, malnourishment, infertility, and chronic or recurrent bronchitis	Cystic fibrosis
Nonseasonal rhinitis with negative skin tests	Chronic nonallergic rhinitis (vasomotor rhinitis)
Refractory congestion after chronic use of topical nasal decongestants	Rhinitis medicamentosa
Nasal congestion in the last 6 or more weeks of pregnancy	Pregnancy rhinitis
Rhinitis, nasal polyps, asthma, and aspirin intolerance (respiratory symptoms)	Aspirin sensitivity (triad asthma or Samter syndrome)

Therapy

Therapy includes the select removal of animals and carpet; allergy encasements for bedding; and small-particle filters for air conditioning.

Intranasal glucocorticoids are first-line therapy. Second-line agents include: intranasal antihistamines, oral combination anti-histamines/decongestants, oral montelukast, or intranasal cromolyn. Ipratropium bromide is effective for severe rhinorrhea.

Choose skin testing and allergen immunotherapy if symptoms are not well controlled by intranasal glucocorticoids with supplemental antihistamines or decongestants.

The most consistently effective treatments for chronic nonallergic rhinitis are topical intranasal glucocorticoids, topical intranasal antihistamines, and topical ipratropium bromide. Patients with chronic rhinitis, nasal polyps, asthma, and aspirin intolerance may improve following aspirin desensitization.

◆ DON'T BE TRICKED

- Do not refer patients with allergic rhinitis for skin testing/immunotherapy without a trial of empiric therapy.

❖ Test Yourself

For the past 2 months, a 30-year-old man has had nasal congestion that began with rhinorrhea, coughing, and sore throat. He has used oxymetazoline nasal spray since his symptoms started.

ANSWER: The diagnosis is rhinitis medicamentosa. Stop the topical decongestant and select a short course of prednisone or intranasal glucocorticoid.

Pharyngitis

Diagnosis

Use the 4-point Centor criteria to stratify adult patients according to risk of group A streptococcal pharyngitis:

- fever (subjective)
- absence of cough
- tender anterior cervical lymphadenopathy
- tonsillar exudates

Management is based on number of Centor criteria present:

- 0 or 1: neither test nor treat with antibiotics
- 2 or 3: obtain a rapid antigen detection test (RADT) or culture (not both); management is based on results
- 4: treat without testing

Fusobacterium necrophorum infection should be considered in adolescents and young adults with a negative RADT and an unusually prolonged and severe pharyngitis. *F. necrophorum* is the causative agent of Lemierre syndrome, septic thrombophlebitis of the internal jugular vein resulting in metastatic pulmonary infections.

Drug Therapy

Select oral penicillin for 10 days. Choose a macrolide for patients allergic to penicillin. *F. necrophorum* is treated with ampicillin-sulbactam.

Depression

Screening

Routine screening is recommended for all adults, including postpartum women and the elderly, utilizing the two-question model:

- "Over the past 2 weeks, have you felt down, depressed, hopeless?"
- "Over the past 2 weeks, have you felt little interest or pleasure in doing things?"

Diagnosis

Major depressive disorder is diagnosed when at least 5 of the following symptoms are consistently present during the same 2-week period, at least 1 of which is depressed mood or loss of interest or pleasure:

- depressed mood
- loss of interest in daily activities
- weight loss or gain
- insomnia or hypersomnia
- psychomotor agitation or retardation
- fatigue
- feelings of worthlessness or guilt
- diminished ability to concentrate
- recurrent thoughts of death or suicide

Refer patients with a suicide plan or psychotic features to a psychiatrist, and hospitalize any patient (even against the patient's wishes) who is in imminent danger of harming himself or herself or others.

◆ DON'T BE TRICKED

- **Select bipolar disorder if depression is accompanied by previous or current manic symptoms.**

Mimics of major depressive disorder:

- Situational adjustment reaction with depressed mood: depression with a clear precipitant. Usually resolves without medication following resolution of the acute stressor.
- Bipolar disorder: one or more manic or mixed manic and depressive episodes, usually accompanied by major depressive disorder.
- Seasonal affective disorder: a subtype of major depression, with onset during fall or winter and seasonal remission. Responds to phototherapy and SSRIs.
- Grief reaction: transient major depression may be present, but sadness without complete depression is more common. Pervasive and generalized guilt and persistent vegetative signs and symptoms are not consistent with normal grief. Loss of self-esteem is a symptom of depression rather than grief.
- PMDD: characterized by the cyclical recurrence of ≥5 symptoms of depression, anxiety, and emotional lability with onset within 1 week before menstruation and resolution within 1 week after menstruation.
- Medical conditions: consider substance abuse, hypothyroidism, Cushing syndrome, Parkinson disease, and medications (interferon, glucocorticoids). Routine laboratory testing for these conditions is not warranted unless suggested by history and physical examination findings.

Therapy

Begin psychotherapy, pharmacologic therapy, or both for mild to moderate depression. Combine psychotherapy and antidepressants for severe depression. Any second-generation antidepressant medication can be used to treat major depressive disorder. Guide selection of an antidepressant by differences in side-effect profiles and personal or family history of response to a specific agent. Commonly tested treatment principles include:

- sertraline is safe for patients with cardiovascular disease
- bupropion has fewer effects on sexual function and weight gain
- mirtazapine causes sedation and weight gain (useful for patients with insomnia or weight loss)
- paroxetine is classified as pregnancy category D (don't use)

For patients in whom treatment with a single SSRI is unsuccessful, response does not differ whether patients receive a different SSRI, a non-SSRI antidepressant, a combination of two antidepressants, augmentation with lithium, or cognitive therapy. Therefore, in nonresponding patients, modify treatment (increase dose, switch, or add another drug) if the patient does not have ≥50% reduction in symptom score to pharmacotherapy within 6 to 8 weeks.

STUDY TABLE: Managing Duration of Antidepressant Therapy	
Indications	**Therapy**
First episode of depression	Initiate treatment and continue at the dosage required to achieve remission for an additional 4 to 9 months.
First recurrence of depression	Increase maintenance treatment to one to two times the inter-episode interval (for example, choose 18 to 36 months if the second episode occurs 18 months after the first episode).
Three or more recurrences of depression, recurrence within 1 year of successful treatment, or suicide attempt	Select lifetime maintenance therapy

Be alert for serotonin syndrome in patients taking SSRIs, particularly with concurrent use of other SSRIs, MAOIs, St. John's wort, trazodone, dextromethorphan, linezolid, tramadol, and buspirone. Mild symptoms include nausea, vomiting, flushing, and diaphoresis. Severe symptoms include hyperreflexia, myoclonus, muscular rigidity, and hyperthermia.

◆ DON'T BE TRICKED
- Always ask about episodes of mania or hypomania before starting antidepressant therapy.
- Antidepressant drugs should not be stopped abruptly.
- Bereavement does not usually require pharmacologic treatment.

Bipolar Disorder

Diagnosis

Bipolar disorder features episodes of depression as well as periods of mania or hypomania. Manic findings include elevated, expansive, or irritable mood; hypersexuality; spending sprees; grandiosity; decreased need for sleep; and disruption of social or occupational functioning. Mimics of bipolar disorder include thyrotoxicosis, partial-complex seizures, SLE, and glucocorticoid side effects.

Therapy

Lithium is the most effective mood stabilizer, but long-term therapy carries significant side effects, including kidney insufficiency, hypothyroidism, and DI. Anticonvulsants and second-generation antipsychotics are alternative first-line treatments. Monotherapy with SSRIs can unmask mania in patients with untreated bipolar disorder.

A 27-year-old woman requests thyroid medication to make her "stronger" because she wants to run for the senatorial position for the state of California. She is sleeping 2 to 3 hours per night and has not been eating. She spends her time writing her political action plan and shopping and has exceeded the limit on her credit card.

ANSWER: The diagnosis is mania.

Generalized Anxiety Disorder

Diagnosis

Generalized anxiety disorder is characterized by pervasive and excessive anxiety about a variety of events or activities, restlessness, difficulty concentrating, irritability, functional impairment, and sleep disturbance. Patients commonly have a comorbid psychiatric disorder.

Therapy

Cognitive behavioral therapy, with or without pharmacologic therapy, is first-line treatment for generalized anxiety disorder. SSRIs and SNRIs are effective. Benzodiazepines are acceptable for short-term use while titrating antidepressant doses, but dependence and tolerance complicate long-term use. Benzodiazepines should be avoided in patients with a history of substance abuse.

Social Anxiety Disorder

Diagnosis

Diagnostic criteria for social anxiety disorder include severe fear of social or performance situations, resulting in symptoms such as blushing, dyspnea, palpitations, and emotional distress. Anxiety may be generalized or specific to a single activity.

Therapy

Treat social anxiety disorder with cognitive behavioral therapy and SSRIs.

Panic Disorder

Diagnosis

Diagnose panic attacks when ≥4 of the following are present:

- palpitations, sweating, and shortness of breath
- fear of dying
- chest pain
- nausea or abdominal distress
- unsteadiness, lightheadedness, faintness, paresthesias
- self-detached feeling

Panic disorder involves recurrent, unexpected attacks and persistent worry about future attacks.

Therapy

Cognitive behavioral therapy and SSRIs are first-line treatment. Long-acting benzodiazepines can be used as short-term therapy for disabling disorders until first-line treatments become effective.

◆ DON'T BE TRICKED

- Do not prescribe benzodiazepines as first-line, long-term treatment for panic disorder.

Somatic Symptom and Related Disorders

Diagnosis

Diagnostic criteria for somatic symptom disorder are as follows:

- at least one somatic symptom causing distress or interference with daily life
- excessive thoughts, behaviors, and feelings related to the somatic symptom(s)
- persistent somatic symptoms for at least 6 months

Patients attribute their symptoms to an undiagnosed disorder despite multiple negative evaluations and are often not reassured despite repeated evaluations.

Therapy

The principles of therapy include regular office appointments with one physician. The patient should be reassured that life-threatening conditions have been ruled out and should be given a plausible explanation for the symptoms. Among all treatments, cognitive behavioral therapy has the broadest evidence of benefit.

◆ DON'T BE TRICKED

- Choose malingering if a patient adopts a physical symptom for the purpose of gain.
- Choose factitious disorder if a patient adopts symptoms to remain in the sick role.
- Choose conversion disorder if a patient has abnormal sensation or motor function (such as limb weakness) that are not explained by a medical condition and are inconsistent with physical examination findings.
- Choose illness anxiety disorder (previously hypochondriasis) if the patient has excessive worry about general health and preoccupation with health-related activities.

Posttraumatic Stress Disorder

Diagnosis

Indicators suggesting PTSD include 1) history of exposure to trauma, 2) persistent re-experiencing of the traumatic event, 3) avoidance of stimuli associated with the trauma, and 4) increased arousal. Assess for coexisting psychiatric disorders and domestic abuse.

Therapy

Cognitive behavioral therapy is the treatment of choice for PTSD. Sertraline and paroxetine are FDA-approved, adjuvant treatments. Benzodiazepines have not been shown to be effective.

◆ DON'T BE TRICKED

- Do not prescribe benzodiazepines for PTSD.

Obsessive-Compulsive Disorder

Diagnosis

Obsessions are defined as persistent ideas, thoughts, impulses, or images that are intrusive and inappropriate and associated with significant anxiety or distress.

Compulsions are repetitive behaviors (handwashing, checking, and ordering) or mental acts (counting or repeating words silently) performed to try to decrease the anxiety or stress associated with the obsessions. The person must recognize that the obsessions or compulsions are excessive or unreasonable.

Therapy

Obsessive-compulsive disorder is treated with cognitive behavioral therapy and often with an SSRI.

Eating Disorders

Diagnosis

Two types:

- restricting, in which patients restrict intake (anorexia nervosa)
- binge eating/purging, in which patients binge and purge to control weight (bulimia nervosa)

Diagnostic clues for the restricting type of anorexia include:

- low BMI
- fear of weight gain
- distorted body image
- amenorrhea or lack of onset of menstruation

The medical complications include anemia, osteopenia, hypotension, electrolyte abnormalities, and arrhythmias. During the first few weeks of eating, patients are at risk for the refeeding syndrome, which can include cardiac arrest and delirium caused by exacerbation of hypophosphatemia and hypokalemia.

Diagnostic clues for bulimia nervosa are episodes of binging with loss of control followed by purging (vomiting, diuretic or laxative abuse), fasting, or excessive exercise. Patients usually have normal weight. Medical complications may be the presenting problem and can include acid-induced dental disease, esophageal tears, electrolyte derangements (low chloride and potassium), and metabolic alkalosis.

Therapy

For anorexia nervosa, daily supplementation with calcium and vitamin D is used to treat osteopenia. Cognitive behavioral therapy is considered first-line treatment. Psychotropic drugs do not work.

Patients with bulimia respond to cognitive behavioral therapy and antidepressants (fluoxetine or imipramine).

◆ DON'T BE TRICKED
- Do not choose bupropion for eating disorders because of the increased incidence of tonic-clonic seizures.

A 24-year-old woman has reflux esophagitis, recurrent sore throat, and a dry cough. She exercises regularly and is "always dieting" because of her "weight problem." BMI is 25. On physical examination, the posterior pharynx and soft palate are injected without exudate. The tooth enamel is eroded.

ANSWER: The diagnosis is bulimia nervosa. Begin cognitive behavioral therapy and fluoxetine.

Schizophrenia

Diagnosis

The following usually begin in mid to late adolescence:

- unusual perceptual experiences
- false beliefs
- illogical thoughts
- disorganized speech, such as frequent derailment or incoherence
- grossly disorganized or catatonic behavior
- negative symptoms, such as affective flattening, alogia (concrete replies to questions and restricted spontaneous speech), or avolition (inability to initiate and persist in goal-directed activities)

Therapy

Begin a second-generation antipsychotic agent (olanzapine, risperidone, quetiapine, aripiprazole).

Attention-Deficit/Hyperactivity Disorder

Diagnosis

ADHD usually first manifests in childhood and is characterized by inattention, hyperactivity, and impulsivity with functional impairment in at least two settings (home, work, school). ADHD is more prevalent in patients with mood disorders and substance abuse.

Therapy

Treat ADHD with stimulants (e.g., amphetamine or methylphenidate) but beware of the potential for abuse and use with caution in patients with hypertension or cardiovascular disease. Atomoxetine is an SNRI approved for treatment of ADHD in adults. Cognitive behavioral therapy may be used as an adjunctive therapy.

Autism Spectrum Disorders

Diagnosis

Autism is defined as impairment in social interaction and communication, and repetitive patterns of behavior, interests, or activities plus delay in communication, social interaction, or play, with onset before 3 years of age.

Therapy

Autism spectrum disorders are treated with a combination of behavioral therapy and environmental modifications.

Falls

Diagnosis

Patients with a history of one fall in the last year should be evaluated for balance or gait disturbance with a Timed Up and Go test. A time of longer than 20 s is abnormal, and the patient should be referred for full fall evaluation. Medications associated with fall risk (psychotropics, sedative/hypnotics) should be removed if possible.

Therapy

Multidisciplinary treatment programs that include assessment for risk factors (review of medications, sensory deficits), physical therapy, and risk factor modification are the most effective nonpharmacologic interventions for older patients.

Specific interventions for community-dwelling older adults:

- prescribe exercise programs that emphasize balance, gait, and strength training (physical therapy or tai chi)
- prescribe vitamin D, 800 U/d (regardless of vitamin D level)
- prescribe appropriate adaptive equipment (canes, walkers)
- reduce polypharmacy (particularly psychoactive medications)
- treat orthostasis

◆ **DON'T BE TRICKED**

- Modification of the home environment in isolation is ineffective in reducing falls but is part of a multi-modal approach.
- Hip protectors in older people who fall are ineffective in preventing hip fractures.

❖ **Test Yourself**

An 80-year-old woman presents after a mechanical fall at home. Her medications are calcium, clonazepam, amlodipine, levothyroxine, and pantoprazole.

ANSWER: Discontinue clonazepam. Start vitamin D and risk factor modification.

Urinary Incontinence

STUDY TABLE: Diagnosis and Treatment of Urinary Incontinence		
If you see this...	Diagnose this...	Choose this...
Daytime frequency, nocturia, bothersome urgency	Urge incontinence	First-line therapy is bladder training; second-line therapy is anticholinergic drugs (oxybutynin, tolterodine)
Involuntary release of urine secondary to effort or exertion (sneezing, coughing, physical exertion)	Stress incontinence	First-line therapy is pelvic floor muscle training for women (Kegel exercises)
Urgency and involuntary release of urine	Mixed incontinence (urge and stress incontinence)	Bladder training and pelvic floor muscle training
		(Continued on next page)

STUDY TABLE: Diagnosis and Treatment of Urinary Incontinence (*Continued*)

If you see this...	Diagnose this...	Choose this...
Unable to get to bathroom on time because of mental or physical limitations	Functional incontinence	Portable commode, regular prompted urination with physical assistance to commode, treatment of underlying disorders
Nearly constant dribbling of urine, incomplete emptying of bladder, high postvoiding residual urine	Overflow incontinence	Timed urination, intermittent bladder catheterization

Obese women with either urge or stress incontinence will benefit from weight loss and exercise.

◆ **DON'T BE TRICKED**

- Do not prescribe systemic estrogen-progestin therapy because it can worsen stress and urge incontinence.
- Do not order urodynamic testing because outcomes are no better than those associated with management based on clinical evaluation alone.

❖ **Test Yourself**

A 78-year-old woman has urinary urgency, nocturia, and urine loss with coughing and sneezing. Her medical history includes HF and glaucoma.

ANSWER: The diagnosis is mixed incontinence. Begin pelvic muscle exercises and bladder training techniques.

Chronic Venous Insufficiency

Diagnosis

Characteristic symptoms and findings of chronic venous insufficiency include:

- leg heaviness, tiredness
- dependent leg edema
- hyperpigmentation, especially at medial ankle
- pruritus and eczema
- venous ulceration
- varicose or reticular veins

Therapy

First-line therapy includes compression (stockings, wraps, pumps) and leg elevation. Emollients are used for dry, itchy skin; topical glucocorticoids can be added for eczema.

Venous ablation therapy (chemical, surgical, and thermal) should be reserved for patients who have failed conservative therapy and who have documented retrograde valvular flow on duplex ultrasonography.

Pressure Ulcers

Diagnosis

Pressure ulcers are ischemic soft tissue injuries resulting from pressure, usually over bony prominences. The external appearance of a pressure ulcer may underestimate the extent of injury.

Therapy

Advanced static mattresses and overlays (such as foam, gel, or air mattresses/overlays) help prevent pressure ulcers in at-risk individuals.

STUDY TABLE: Pressure Ulcer Staging and Therapy	
Ulcer Stage	**Therapy**
Stage 1: The skin is intact with nonblanchable redness	For all ulcer stages: positioning and support to minimize tissue pressure
Stage 2: Shallow ulcer with a red-pink wound bed or serum-filled blister	Occlusive or semipermeable dressing that will maintain a moist wound environment
Stage 3: Subcutaneous fat may be visible	Pain control, correction of identified nutritional deficiencies (supplements, tube feeding, or hyperalimentation if necessary), debridement, topical or systemic antibiotics
Stage 4: Exposed bone, tendon, or muscle	Same as Stage 3

Basic rules for treating pressure ulcers:

- air-fluidized beds enhance healing of pressure ulcers compared to standard hospital mattresses
- dressings should maintain a moist wound environment and manage exudates
- restrict systemic antibiotics for cellulitis treatment (surrounding erythema, warmth, pain)
- débride eschars and nonviable tissue

◆ DON'T BE TRICKED

- Nutritional supplementation to enhance wound healing remains controversial.
- Hyperbaric oxygen therapy is not effective in the treatment of pressure ulcers.
- Always consider the possibility of underlying osteomyelitis.

Involuntary Weight Loss

Diagnosis

Causes of involuntary weight loss vary according to age (malignancy is most common in the young) and venue (depression, medications, dehydration, and issues related to dementia are most common in extended care facilities). Other causes include:

- endocrine disorders (especially thyroid disorders and diabetes)
- late-stage HF or COPD
- TB
- HIV disease
- medications

Weight loss is commonly associated with depression and dementia. Socioeconomic and functional problems, such as difficulty obtaining food, lack of financial resources, and social isolation, cause or exacerbate weight loss. Initial diagnostic testing is limited to basic studies unless the history and physical examination suggest a specific cause. In patients with GI symptoms or abnormalities in blood counts or liver tests, obtain an upper GI series, abdominal ultrasonography, abdominal CT, or EGD, as appropriate.

◆ DON'T BE TRICKED

- Imaging of the thorax and abdomen with CT or MRI in the absence of supporting history, physical examination, or laboratory findings is not helpful.

Therapy

Treat the specific underlying disorder. The proven benefit of oral nutritional supplementation for weight loss is limited. Appetite stimulants have been shown to promote weight gain, but a survival benefit has never been demonstrated.

STUDY TABLE: Selected Nutritional Deficiencies	
Finding	**Deficiency**
Hair loss, brittle hair	Biotin, protein, vitamin B_{12}, and folate
Coiled, corkscrew hair	Vitamins A and C
Skin desquamation	Riboflavin
Petechiae, perifollicular hemorrhage, gingival bleeding	Vitamin C
Ecchymosis	Vitamins C and K
Skin pigmentation, cracking, and crusting	Niacin
Acro-orificial dermatitis (erythematous, vesiculobullous, and pustular)	Zinc
Angular stomatitis and cheilosis	Vitamin B complex, iron, and protein
Glossitis	Niacin, folate, and vitamin B_{12}
Ophthalmoplegia and foot drop	Thiamine
Paresthesia	Thiamine, vitamin B_{12}, and biotin
Depressed vibratory and position senses	Vitamin B_{12}
Memory disturbance	Vitamin B_{12}
Wernicke-Korsakoff syndrome	Severe thiamine deficiency

Perioperative Medicine

Preoperative Testing

Routine diagnostic testing is not indicated preoperatively. Do not obtain:

- routine preoperative laboratory studies in healthy patients undergoing elective or low-risk surgery
- preoperative chest radiography in the absence of cardiopulmonary symptoms
- repeat laboratory studies within 6 months of surgery in the absence of a clinical change

Cardiovascular Risk Assessment

For patients with an elevated risk of a major adverse cardiac event (≥1%) and an estimated functional capacity of <4 METs should undergo pharmacologic stress testing if the results will change management.

Activities requiring the equivalent of ≥4 METs:

- climbing a flight of stairs
- walking up a hill without stopping
- running a short distance
- lifting or moving heavy furniture
- participating in moderate-exertion sporting activities such as bowling or golf

Obtain an ECG within 1-3 months of surgery (except low-risk surgery) in any patient with:

- CAD
- significant arrhythmias
- cerebrovascular disease (stroke or TIA)
- PAD

◆ DON'T BE TRICKED

- Patients with a functional capacity ≥4 METS can undergo surgery.
- If a patient has no history, symptoms, or risk factors for CAD, no preoperative coronary evaluation is necessary, including ECG.
- Low-risk surgeries (cataract extraction, carpal tunnel release, breast biopsy, inguinal hernia repair) do not require cardiac testing even if a calculated risk score is elevated.
- Do not obtain troponin and BNP levels or CTA to assess cardiac risk.
- There is no survival benefit associated with revascularization in stable patients with CAD unless they otherwise met the general requirements for revascularization.

Cardiovascular Risk Management

Patients with a known recent major adverse cardiac event should not undergo surgery within:

- 60 days of an MI
- 30 days of bare-metal coronary stent implantation
- 6 months of a drug-eluting coronary stent placement

Continue perioperative β-blockade in patients who are already on a β-blocker.

Continue statins to reduce perioperative cardiac risk reduction.

◆ DON'T BE TRICKED

- Do not recommend routine postoperative surveillance with ECG or cardiac biomarkers unless symptoms of an ACS are present.

Pulmonary Perioperative Management

Screen all surgical patients for OSA with a validated tool such as the STOP-BANG survey. Obtain polysomnography for patients with presumed OSA and initiate CPAP for patients with severe OSA undergoing high-risk elective surgical procedures.

The greatest benefit from smoking cessation comes from quitting >8 weeks before surgery.

Select lung expansion maneuvers (deep breathing exercises, incentive spirometry, intermittent positive pressure breathing, CPAP) to prevent pulmonary complications.

◆ DON'T BE TRICKED

- Do not order spirometry for risk assessment in the absence of dyspnea or hypoxia of uncertain cause.

Perioperative Management of Anticoagulant Therapy

Anticoagulation must be stopped for most surgical procedures except those with minimal expected blood loss (cataract surgery, dermatologic procedures, endoscopic procedures without biopsy).

- Stop warfarin 5 days prior to surgery.
- Stop apixaban, rivaroxaban, dabigatran 1-2 days prior to surgery if eGFR >50 mL/min/1.73 m². Stop earlier if eGFR is lower.

Bridging anticoagulation is providing heparin during the perioperative period until an oral anticoagulant is resumed.

- Low-risk patients do not receive bridging anticoagulation (bileaflet mechanical aortic valve, AF with CHADS$_2$ score <2, VTE >12 months ago).
- High-risk patients receive bridging anticoagulation (mitral or caged ball valve or aortic tilting disc aortic mechanical valve, AF with CHADS$_2$ score >4, rheumatic heart disease, recent CVA or TIA, VTE within the past 3 months).

Stopping and restarting perioperative anticoagulation:

- start heparin 36 hours after the last dose of warfarin
- stop UFH 4 to 6 hours before surgery
- stop LMWH 12 hours before surgery
- restart heparin 24 hours after surgery
- restart warfarin 12 to 24 hours after surgery
- restart dabigatran, rivaroxaban, and apixaban 24 hours after surgery

Hematology

Aplastic Anemia and Paroxysmal Nocturnal Hemoglobinuria

Diagnosis

Aplastic anemia is a disorder in which hematopoietic stem cells are severely diminished, resulting in hypocellular bone marrow and pancytopenia. All cell lines are involved. No cause is identified in 50% of patients. Autoimmune attack on stem cells is the most common identifiable cause. Other causes include toxins, ionizing radiation, drugs, nutritional deficiencies, and infections. Some patients have an associated thymoma. Patients with aplastic anemia are at increased risk of developing acute leukemia and MDS.

Aplastic anemia, PNH, and MDS are all acquired defects of hematopoietic stem cells, so clinical overlap is considerable. PNH results from a genetic mutation of membrane proteins that ameliorate complement-mediated destruction of erythrocytes. PNH is characterized by:

- chronic hemolytic anemia
- iron deficiency through urinary losses
- venous thrombosis (including abdominal venous thrombosis resulting in Budd-Chiari syndrome)
- pancytopenia

The basic evaluation of patients presenting with pancytopenia includes:

- bone marrow aspirate and biopsy (hypocellular with increased fat content)
- cytogenetic analysis to exclude other bone marrow disorders (e.g., MDS)
- PNH screen flow cytometry from CD55 and CD59
- B_{12} and folate levels, liver chemistry tests, hepatitis serologies, and HIV testing

Aplastic Anemia: The bone marrow is profoundly hypocellular, with the marrow space composed mostly of fat cells and marrow stroma.

Therapy

Initial treatment of aplastic anemia involves withdrawal of any potentially causative agents. Immunosuppression with cyclosporine and antithymocyte globulin is first-line therapy and leads to disease control in 70% of adult patients. Allogeneic HSCT is a potentially curative therapy and should be considered for those younger than 50 years who have compatible donors.

Treatment of PNH in the absence of hemolysis is generally not indicated. In symptomatic patients, eculizumab reduces intravascular hemolysis, hemoglobinuria, and the need for transfusion. Allogeneic HSCT can lead to long-term survival. Prophylactic anticoagulation and supplementation with iron and folic acid are indicated in all patients.

◆ DON'T BE TRICKED

- Treatment of aplastic anemia with hematopoietic growth factors is ineffective.
- PNH may present as a Coombs-negative hemolytic anemia or as aplastic anemia

Pure Red Cell Aplasia

Diagnosis

Acquired chronic pure red cell aplasia is characterized by the absence or a marked decrease of erythrocyte production with normal leukocyte and platelet counts. The cause is predominately T cell autoimmunity (pregnancy, thymoma, malignancy) or direct toxicity to erythrocyte precursors (viral infection, drug toxicity). Bone marrow shows profound erythroid hypoplasia. Clonal CD57 positive T cells consistent with large granular lymphocytosis are often found. It is diagnosed by peripheral blood smear showing large granular lymphocytes and CD57 positivity on flow cytometry.

The basic evaluation of pure red cell aplasia is similar to that for pancytopenia but includes CT of the chest to rule out thymoma.

Therapy

Patients with pure red cell aplasia are treated with:

- transfusion support and immunosuppressive drugs (prednisone, cyclosporine, antithymocyte globulin)
- thymectomy for thymoma
- IV immune globulin for patients with AIDS and chronic parvovirus B19 infection
- methotrexate or cyclosporin for large granular lymphocytosis

Neutropenia

Diagnosis

Isolated neutropenia usually has a hereditary, infectious, toxic, or immune cause

- acute HIV, CMV, EBV
- Rickettsial infection
- cytotoxic chemotherapies
- NSAIDs, carbamazepine, phenytoin, propylthiouracil, cephalosporins, trimethoprim-sulfamethoxazole
- SLE, RA

Large granular lymphocytes may be identified in Felty syndrome (RA, splenomegaly, neutropenia).

Therapy

Remove offending drug. Granulocyte colony-stimulating factor can shorten the duration of neutropenia associated with chemotherapy. Treat immune-associated neutropenia (e.g., Felty syndrome) with immunosuppressive therapy (prednisone, cyclosporine, antithymocyte globulin).

Myelodysplastic Syndromes

Diagnosis

MDS are clonal disorders of the hematopoietic stem cells that occur predominantly in patients older than 60 years and are characterized by ineffective hematopoiesis and peripheral cytopenias; bone marrow findings show a hypercellular marrow with dyserythropoiesis. Look for cytopenia in at least 2 lines (anemia, leukopenia, thrombocytopenia) and morphologic abnormalities of erythrocytes (macrocytosis with nucleated erythrocytes and teardrop cells). Half of patients may present only with anemia, an elevated MCV, and normal vitamin B_{12} and folate levels. Detection of clonal abnormalities commonly involving chromosomes 3, 5, 7, 8, and 17 supports the diagnosis. Look for 5q- syndrome, a subtype of MDS that has a specific therapy. The differential diagnosis includes vitamin B_{12} and folate deficiency, alcohol- or drug-induced cytopenias, acute leukemia, and myeloproliferative syndromes. Most patients eventually progress to acute leukemic syndromes or die of complications of bone marrow failure. The revised International Prognostic Scoring System (IPSS-R) is used to determine prognosis and inform therapy.

Therapy

Many patients with low-risk MDS (by IPSS-R score) require no treatment at all or infrequent transfusions. In patients needing frequent transfusions, erythropoiesis-stimulating agents (ESAs) can decrease transfusion burden in some patients.

Patients considered high or very high risk by IPSS-R criteria require treatment to prevent AML. Allogeneic HSCT is offered to fit, younger patients, and azacytidine and decitabine to persons at high or very high risk for AML transformation who are not bone marrow transplant candidates.

Use lenalidomide for the specific treatment of 5q- syndrome, because more than two thirds of patients with this syndrome will respond.

❖ **Test Yourself**

> A 74-year-old man has a hemoglobin concentration of 7.5 g/dL, leukocyte count of 2200/μL, and platelet count of 87,000/μL. The peripheral blood smear shows a few nucleated erythrocytes. Bone marrow shows hypolobulated neutrophils.
>
> **ANSWER:** The diagnosis is MDS.

Myeloproliferative Neoplasms

The MPNs are caused by acquired genetic defects in myeloid stem cells and are characterized by deregulated production of leukocytes, eosinophils, erythrocytes, or platelets. Although each disorder is named according to the dominant cell line affected (CML, PV, essential thrombocythemia, primary myelofibrosis), all can cause an elevation in several cell lines.

The MPNs may present with unusual thromboses; massive splenomegaly; or fevers, chills, weight loss, and drenching night sweats. Each has a chronic phase that may progress to AML.

Chronic Myeloid Leukemia

CML is a clonal hematopoietic stem cell disorder characterized by myeloid proliferation associated with a t(9;22) translocation (the Philadelphia chromosome). Patients usually present in the chronic phase. CML may transform into acute leukemia (myeloid in two thirds of patients, lymphoid in one third of patients). The transformation may be recognized as an accelerated phase or as blast crisis (AML).

Characteristic findings in asymptomatic patients are splenomegaly, an elevated leukocyte count, and increased number of granulocytic cells in all phases of maturation on the peripheral blood smear. Very immature cells or blasts represent 1% to 5% of the granulocytes, with increasing numbers of promyelocytes, myelocytes, and metamyelocytes. When blasts represent more than 10% of the leukocytes, accelerated (10%-20%) or blast phase (>20%) should be considered.

The diagnosis is confirmed by the presence of the Philadelphia chromosome in molecular testing for *BCR-ABL* in the peripheral blood or cytogenetic analysis of the bone marrow. The *BCR-ABL* gene produces a mutant, activated tyrosine kinase that leads to constant downstream proliferative signaling.

STUDY TABLE: Therapy for CML	
Treatment	**Goal**
Hydroxyurea	Palliative, only to alleviate leukocytosis and splenomegaly
Tyrosine kinase inhibitors: imatinib mesylate, dasatinib, and nilotinib	Disease control with lifelong treatment; eradicating the Philadelphia chromosome and achieving molecular remission in patients with chronic-phase CML
Allogeneic HSCT	Potential cure for some patients with accelerated disease or blast crisis

◆ **DON'T BE TRICKED**

- All tyrosine kinase inhibitors can prolong the QT interval and periodic ECG monitoring is recommended.
- Dasatinib has a unique association with pericardial and pleural effusions and pulmonary artery hypertension.

❖ **Test Yourself**

An asymptomatic 54-year-old man has an enlarged spleen. The hemoglobin concentration is 13.0 g/dL, platelet count is 470,000/µL, and leukocyte count is 170,000/µL, with mostly segmented and band neutrophils and circulating metamyelocytes and myelocytes. Eosinophilia and basophilia are present.

ANSWER: The probable diagnosis is CML. Order cytogenetic analysis of bone marrow cells or *BCR-ABL* gene detection in the peripheral blood. The presence of eosinophilia and basophilia helps separate this diagnosis from secondary leukocytosis.

Essential Thrombocythemia

Essential thrombocythemia, the most common MPN, occurs in middle-aged and older adults and is characterized by thrombotic and hemorrhagic complications. It is a stem cell disorder marked by a predominant increase in megakaryocytes and platelet counts greater than 600,000/µL in the absence of secondary thrombocytosis. Symptoms include:

- vasomotor disturbances such as erythromelalgia (red and painful hands or feet with warmth and swelling)
- livedo reticularis
- headache
- vision symptoms
- arterial or venous thromboses

Splenomegaly (up to 50%) may be present. The *JAK2* mutation is found in about half of cases and may help distinguish essential thrombocythemia from secondary thrombocythemia due to bleeding, iron deficiency, chronic inflammatory diseases, and cancer.

Low-risk patients may be treated with low-dose aspirin, which reduces vasomotor symptoms. Low-risk patients have all of the following characteristics:

- age <60 years
- no previous thrombosis
- leukocyte count <11,000/µL

High-risk nonpregnant patients are treated with hydroxyurea. High-risk pregnant patients can be treated with interferon alfa. Plateletpheresis is used when the platelet count must be reduced quickly in life-threatening situations such as TIA, stroke, MI, or GI bleeding.

◆ **DON'T BE TRICKED**

- The most common causes of thrombocytosis are iron deficiency anemia and infection and will improve within a couple of weeks following iron replacement or resolution of the infection, respectively.
- A negative *JAK2* test does not exclude the diagnosis of essential thrombocythemia.

A 67-year-old man is evaluated because of red, warm, and painful feet and a platelet count of 975,000/μL.

ANSWER: The diagnosis is essential thrombocythemia. Prescribe hydroxyurea. Low-dose aspirin can be used to treat the erythromelalgia.

Polycythemia Vera

PV is a disorder of the myeloid/erythroid stem cell that causes erythropoietin-independent (low erythropoietin level) proliferation of erythrocytes. An activating mutation of JAK2 is present in 97% of PV. PV is suspected when hemoglobin level is >18.5 g/dL in men or >16.5 g/dL in women after secondary causes are excluded. Most causes of secondary erythrocytosis are associated with an elevated erythropoietin level. Causes of secondary polycythemia include hypoxemia (most common), volume contraction due to diuretics, use of androgens, and secretion of erythropoietin by kidney or liver carcinoma.

Characteristic findings are thrombosis or bleeding, facial plethora, erythromelalgia, pruritus exacerbated by bathing in hot water, and splenomegaly. Serious complications may include TIA, MI or stroke, DVT, and Budd-Chiari syndrome.

◆ **DON'T BE TRICKED**

- Hepatic vein thrombosis (the Budd-Chiari syndrome) or portal vein thrombosis should prompt consideration of PV.

Therapeutic phlebotomy should be instituted with the goal of lowering the hematocrit level to <45%. Low-dose aspirin is indicated unless there are strong contraindications. Hyperuricemia is treated with allopurinol, and patients with pruritus are given antihistamines. Hydroxyurea in addition to phlebotomy is often the treatment of choice for patients at high risk for thrombosis (e.g., >60 years, previous thrombosis, leukocytosis).

◆ **DON'T BE TRICKED**

- Do not prescribe high-dose aspirin, which may cause increased bleeding.

A 67-year-old man has intolerable pruritus. He does not smoke and takes no medications. The hematocrit value is 60%, and he has splenomegaly.

ANSWER: The probable diagnosis is PV. Order PCR for *JAK2* mutation and measure the erythropoietin level.

Primary Myelofibrosis

Primary myelofibrosis is the result of clonal proliferation of abnormal hematopoietic stem cells that release fibrosis-promoting cytokines in the bone marrow. The disorder is characterized by massive splenomegaly, normocytic anemia, circulating erythroblasts and myeloid precursors, giant platelets, teardrop erythrocytes, and bone marrow fibrosis. Splenomegaly and hepatomegaly result from extramedullary hematopoiesis, and patients can develop portal hypertension. Death commonly results from bone marrow failure, transformation to acute leukemia, or portal hypertension complications.

Therapy is usually supportive. Hydroxyurea and ruxolitinib (a *JAK2* inhibitor) may alleviate splenomegaly and constitutional symptoms. Allogeneic HSCT is indicated for patients <60 years of age.

Myelofibrosis: Peripheral blood smear showing teardrop erythrocytes, nucleated erythrocytes, and giant platelets characteristic of myelofibrosis.

◆ **DON'T BE TRICKED**

- Splenectomy is avoided in most patients because it is associated with hemorrhagic and thrombotic complications, increased risk of progression to leukemia, and no impact on survival.

Eosinophilia and Hypereosinophilic Syndromes

HES are diseases characterized by eosinophil counts greater than 1500/μL and eosinophilic infiltrates of the liver, spleen, heart, and lymph nodes, and systemic symptoms such as fevers, chills, night sweats, and weight loss. HES may have a reactive or primary cause. Primary HES is a MPN with molecular activation of platelet-derived growth factor receptor (PDGFR) α or β.

For patients with activating mutations of PDGFR α or β, imatinib leads to durable responses. Otherwise glucocorticoid therapy is used.

STUDY TABLE: Causes of Eosinophilia (CHINA)
Collagen vascular disease
Helminthic (parasitic worm) infection
Idiopathic HES (no cause after extensive investigation)
Neoplasia (lymphomas most common)
Allergy, atopy, asthma

Acute Lymphoblastic Leukemia

Diagnosis

ALL is an extremely aggressive disease of precursor T or B cells. The usual presenting clinical features include rapidly rising blast cells in the blood and bone marrow, bulky lymphadenopathy (especially in the mediastinum), a younger age at onset, and cytopenia secondary to bone marrow involvement. Up to 30% of patients with ALL have CNS involvement.

Therapy

Induction therapy involves intensive combination chemotherapy often followed by allogeneic HSCT consolidation. CNS prophylaxis (intrathecal chemotherapy with or without radiation) is also indicated. Patients who are positive for the Philadelphia chromosome [t(9;22)] can be treated with the tyrosine kinase inhibitor dasatinib in addition to chemotherapy and allogenic HSCT.

Acute Myeloblastic Leukemia

Diagnosis

AML is a malignant clonal proliferation of myeloid cells that do not fully mature. AML can appear de novo; arise after exposure to radiation, benzene, or chemotherapy; or occur as a result of transformation of a MPN, such as CML or PV. MDS may also transform into AML.

AML presents with fatigue, pallor, and easy bleeding. Of all the leukemias, AML will most likely involve significant thrombocytopenia with bleeding, bruising, petechiae, and with infection. Patients with AML seldom develop lymphadenopathy or hepatosplenomegaly; if present, these findings suggest an alternative or concomitant diagnosis. When the leukocyte count is very high, patients may present with leukostasis syndrome characterized by tissue hypoxia because of reduced blood flow.

The diagnosis of AML is suggested by:

- an elevated leukocyte count
- anemia
- thrombocytopenia
- blasts on the peripheral blood smear

Gingival hypertrophy and leukemia cutis (violaceous, nontender cutaneous plaques) are commonly encountered. Pathognomonic Auer rods may be seen on a peripheral blood smear. The diagnosis is confirmed by bone marrow aspiration and biopsy showing >20% myeloblasts. Cytogenetic studies can classify patients into risk (for relapse) and prognostic categories:

- favorable risk: t(8;21), inv(16), t(15;17)
- high risk: complex genetic abnormalities (≥5 abnormalities); -5, -7, del(5q), or 3q abnormalities

Acute promyelocytic leukemia is a special case marked by the t(15;17) translocation, which disturbs a retinoic acid receptor. Patients with acute promyelocytic leukemia have significant bleeding because of fibrinolysis and DIC.

Tumor lysis syndrome may develop in treated patients and causes a release of intracellular metabolites (urate, potassium, and phosphorus).

◆ **DON'T BE TRICKED**

- In older patients, acute leukemia may present with pancytopenia but bone marrow examination will demonstrate a hypercellular marrow with 20% or more blasts.

Therapy

Platelet transfusion is indicated for patients with hemorrhage or a platelet count <10,000/μL. Only leukocyte reduced and irradiated blood products should be used.

Drug therapy and indications are as follows:

- vigorous hydration and allopurinol or rasburicase (if urate particularly high) before chemotherapy to prevent tumor lysis syndrome
- hemodialysis for acute kidney failure related to tumor lysis syndrome
- ATRA is the backbone for acute promyelocytic leukemia
- chemotherapy for non–promyelocytic leukemia (e.g., cytarabine and an anthracycline, azacitidine, or decitabine for older and frail patients)
- leukapheresis for leukostasis syndrome (usually WBC >50,000/μL); symptoms include CNS manifestations, hypoxia, and diffuse infiltrates on chest x-ray
- allogeneic and autologous HSCT for high-risk patients in first complete remission, first relapse, or second complete remission

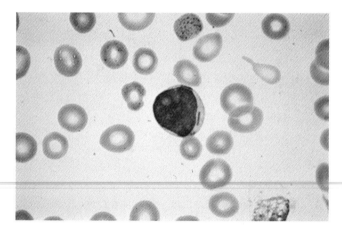

Auer Rod: This myeloblast has findings associated with AML: a large nucleus, displaced nuclear chromatin, azurophile cytoplasmic granules, and a rod-shaped inclusion (Auer rod).

Patients taking ATRA or arsenic trioxide are at risk for developing differentiation syndrome. Characteristic findings are fever, pulmonary infiltrates, hypoxemia, and, occasionally, hyperleukocytosis. Treatment is dexamethasone.

Plasma Cell Dyscrasias

Diagnosis

Plasma cell dyscrasias consist of abnormal clonal proliferation of immune globulin–secreting differentiated B lymphocytes and plasma cells. Multiple myeloma is the most common malignant plasma cell dyscrasia. Other plasma cell dyscrasias include monoclonal gammopathy of undetermined significance (MGUS), Waldenström macroglobulinemia, and light-chain–associated amyloidosis (AL amyloidosis). Characteristic findings for multiple myeloma include:

- low anion gap
- anemia (with rouleaux formation)
- kidney disease
- hypercalcemia
- vertebral compression fractures, osteoporosis, osteopenia, and lytic bone lesions
- (rarely) hyperviscosity syndrome (IgM monoclonal gammopathy: blurred vision, fatigue, mucosal bleeding, HF, head-ache, and altered mentation)

Diagnostic tests in patients include a CBC; serum chemistries; SPEP; 24-hour UPEP; serum and urine immunofixation assays; serum free light chain testing; and serum IgG, IgA, and IgM measurements.

For non-IgM gammopathies, a skeletal survey (plain x-rays of the skeleton) is performed to assess for the presence of lytic bone lesions or osteopenia. IgM gammopathies are more likely associated with B-cell lymphomas, and CT scans of the chest, abdomen, and pelvis should be performed in patients with unexplained fevers or weight loss, drenching sweats, lymphadenopathy, or hepatosplenomegaly.

STUDY TABLE: Diagnosis of Multiple Myeloma and MGUS	
Multiple Myeloma/MGUS	**Findings**
MGUS	Serum monoclonal protein <3 g
	Bone marrow clonal plasma cells <10%
	No end-organ damage
Asymptomatic (smoldering) multiple myeloma	Serum monoclonal protein >3 g
	Bone marrow clonal plasma cells ≥10%
	No end-organ damage
Multiple myeloma	Serum monoclonal protein present
	Bone marrow clonal plasma cells ≥10%
	End-organ damage present (see CRAB mnemonic)

Patients with MGUS are periodically reassessed after initial diagnosis for development of asymptomatic myeloma, multiple myeloma, or AL amyloidosis.

STUDY TABLE: CRAB Mnemonic for Myeloma-related Signs and Symptoms	
Hyper**C**alcemia	Serum calcium >10.5 mg/dL
Renal failure	Serum creatinine >2 mg/dL
Anemia	Hemoglobin <10 g/dL or 2 g/dL below the lower limit of normal
Bone disease	Lytic bone lesions or osteoporosis

Most asymptomatic multiple myeloma progresses to symptomatic multiple myeloma or AL amyloidosis. Patients with multiple myeloma may have leukopenia and suppressed immunoglobulin production, leading to frequent infections.

◆ DON'T BE TRICKED

- In patients with back pain, a MRI should also be performed to assess for spinal cord impingement.
- Do not select bone scans in patients with suspected myeloma as they are not as sensitive as a skeletal survey.

AL amyloidosis is found in 10% of patients with multiple myeloma.

Clues to the presence of AL amyloidosis:

- nephrotic syndrome and enlarged kidneys on ultrasonography
- delayed gastric emptying, intestinal pseudo-obstruction, malabsorption
- hepatomegaly and portal hypertension
- distal sensorimotor polyneuropathy
- restrictive cardiomyopathy with granular appearance on echocardiography, low voltage ECG
- bleeding diathesis, periorbital purpura, factor X deficiency with prolonged PT and aPTT
- macroglossia

Confirmation of AL amyloidosis requires:

- abdominal fat pad aspirate or bone marrow biopsy demonstrating apple green birefringence under polarized light with Congo red staining
- typing of amyloidosis with κ/λ light-chain immunohistochemistry, immunofluorescence of a biopsy sample, or mass spectroscopy-based protein sequencing
- presence of an M protein on serum or urine testing or clonal plasma cells in the marrow

Waldenström macroglobulinemia is a neoplastic infiltrate consisting of:

- clonal lymphocytes, plasmacytoid lymphocytes, plasma cells, and immunoblasts comprising ≥10% of the bone marrow cellularity *or*
- M-protein level ≥3 g/dL *and*
- presence of disease-related signs, symptoms, or organ dysfunction

Lymphadenopathy, hepatomegaly, and splenomegaly are found on physical examination. One third of patients will have hyperviscosity symptoms including headache, blurred vision, hearing loss, dizziness, altered mental status, and nasal and mucosal bleeding. Funduscopic evaluation may reveal hyperviscosity-related findings, including dilated retinal veins, papilledema, and flame hemorrhages.

Therapy

Treat symptomatic multiple myeloma with induction chemotherapy, including some combination of:

- a proteasome inhibitor (bortezomib)
- an immunomodulatory agent (thalidomide or lenalidomide)
- a glucocorticoid (prednisone or dexamethasone)
- an alkylating agent (melphalan or cyclophosphamide) for nontransplant candidates

Following induction chemotherapy, autologous HSCT followed by high-dose melphalan may be considered.

Supportive care includes:

- plasmapheresis for patients with hyperviscosity syndrome
- glucocorticoids and radiation therapy to treat spinal cord compression
- surgical stabilization for impending fractures
- palliative radiation therapy for symptomatic bone disease
- pamidronate or zoledronate to reduce the risk of a skeletal event
- erythropoietin to help improve anemia and quality of life (risk of thrombosis)
- prophylactic immunizations for pneumonia (both 13- and 23-valent vaccines) and annual influenza
- immune globulin infusion for hypogammaglobulinemia to treat recurrent bacterial infections

- varicella zoster vaccine for patients receiving bortezomib
- IV fluids and chemotherapy for myeloma cast nephropathy
- IV fluids and bisphosphonates for hypercalcemia

Treatment algorithms for AL amyloidosis are similar to those for multiple myeloma.

Waldenström macroglobulinemia hyperviscosity syndrome is a medical emergency treated with plasmapheresis.

◆ **DON'T BE TRICKED**

- Do not treat MGUS.
- Do not use melphalan induction therapy in candidates for HSCT.
- Bortezomib and thalidomide are associated with a high risk of peripheral neuropathy.
- Patients taking thalidomide, lenalidomide, or pomalidomide are at increased risk of VTE.

Normocytic Anemia

Diagnosis

Normocytic anemia is associated with a normal MCV of 80 to 100 fL. The reticulocyte count can help differentiate the cause. An appropriately increased reticulocyte count (>100,000/μL) almost always reflects either erythrocyte loss (bleeding or hemolysis) or response to appropriate therapy (iron, folate, or cobalamin). A lower-than-expected reticulocyte count indicates underproduction anemia, including any of the following:

- deficient erythropoietin
- nutritional deficiencies (iron, folate, cobalamin)
- hypometabolism (hypothyroidism, testosterone deficiency)
- inflammatory block
- a primary hematopoietic disorder (red cell aplasia or myelodysplasia)

The most frequent cause of normocytic anemia is inflammatory anemia. Iron deficiency and inflammatory anemia are often confused. Both disorders are associated with a decreased serum iron concentration; however, iron deficiency is more likely in a patient with an elevated serum TIBC and a low transferrin saturation (serum iron transferrin <10%). A serum ferritin level >100 ng/mL rules out iron deficiency, even in patients with inflammation. Inflammatory anemia is usually not severe and rarely requires therapy.

STUDY TABLE: Differentiating Iron Deficiency and Inflammatory Anemia

Test	Iron Deficiency Anemia	Inflammatory Anemia
Serum iron	Low	Low
Ferritin	Low	High
TIBC	High	Low
Transferrin saturation	Low	Low/Normal

Recommended diagnostic studies:

- FOBT for all patients (33% of patients with iron deficiency have a normal MCV)
- peripheral blood smear to detect spherocytes, fragmented erythrocytes (schistocytes), or blister cells associated with hemolysis
- direct antiglobulin (Coombs) test if spherocytes are found on a peripheral blood smear
- hemoglobin electrophoresis if target or sickle cells are found on a peripheral blood smear

- lead level if basophilic stippling is found on a peripheral blood smear
- bone marrow aspiration and biopsy if leukopenia, thrombocytopenia, myelocytes, or nucleated erythrocytes (in normocytic, microcytic, and macrocytic anemias) are found on peripheral smear
- bone marrow aspiration and biopsy if lymphadenopathy or splenomegaly are present

Spherocytes: This peripheral blood smear shows small erythrocytes with loss of usual central pallor. Consider acquired immune hemolytic anemia and hereditary spherocytosis.

Erythrocyte Fragmentation: The erythrocytes show marked anisocytosis and poikilocytosis with prominent fragmentation. Consider DIC, TTP, mechanical heart valve, or malignant hypertension.

Microcytic Anemia

Diagnosis

Microcytic anemia is associated with an MCV of <80 fL. The most common cause of microcytic anemia is iron deficiency, usually related to menstrual or GI blood loss or malabsorption syndromes (celiac disease). The hallmark of iron deficiency is a microcytic hypochromic anemia but anemia tends to precede morphologic changes in the cells, and abnormalities in iron studies typically precede the anemia. As hemoglobin levels decline, erythrocytes become heterogeneous in size (anisocytosis) and shape (poikilocytosis). An elevated platelet count (usually not >1 million/μL) may be found in early disease. Serum ferritin levels are the most useful test in the diagnosis of iron deficiency. However, because ferritin is an acute-phase reactant, it has less diagnostic value in patients with infection or inflammatory disorders. Virtually all patients with serum ferritin levels <10 to 15 ng/mL are iron deficient. Signs and symptoms of iron deficiency include restless legs syndrome, hair loss, and spoon nails (koilonychia). Other causes of microcytic anemia include:

- inflammatory disorders
- lead intoxication
- thalassemia

Patients with microcytic anemia since childhood should be evaluated for the thalassemia trait, other hemoglobinopathies, or ineffective erythropoiesis (hereditary sideroblastic anemia).

Recommended diagnostic studies:

- serum iron and ferritin levels and TIBC in most patients
- hemoglobin electrophoresis if iron studies are normal
- endoscopy studies, starting with colonoscopy, if unexplained positive FOBT or iron deficiency is present

Therapy

The least expensive oral iron replacement is iron sulfate and it is as effective as any of the more expensive oral preparations. Oral iron for 6 months is the standard treatment. Parenteral iron preparations are indicated only for patients who cannot tolerate or absorb oral iron or are receiving hemodialysis. Transfusion is reserved for severely symptomatic anemia.

❖ **Test Yourself**

A 20-year-old woman with iron deficiency anemia does not respond to oral iron therapy. Review of systems is remarkable for IBS.

ANSWER: Test for celiac disease.

Hereditary Hemorrhagic Telangiectasia: Hereditary hemorrhagic telangiectasia can be associated with mucocutaneous telangiectasias that occur on the face, lips, tongue, buccal mucosa, fingertips, and dorsum of the hand, and are associated with GI bleeding in up to one third of patients.

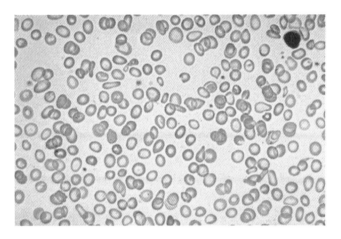

Microcytic Anemia: The erythrocytes show hypochromia, anisocytosis, and poikilocytosis. Erythrocytes in thalassemia have less variability in size and shape, and target cells are seen.

Macrocytic Anemia

Diagnosis

Macrocytic anemia is associated with an MCV of >100 fL. Macro-ovalocytes suggest megaloblastic maturation of erythrocytes. Hypersegmented neutrophils may also be present. Etiologies include:

- folate and/or cobalamin deficiencies
- drugs affecting folate metabolism and/or DNA synthesis (alcohol, zidovudine, hydroxyurea, methotrexate)
- acquired causes of megaloblastic maturation such as the MDS

Anemia associated with an MCV >115 fL is almost always due to megaloblastic disorders. Because megaloblastic causes of anemia affect trilineage hematopoiesis, leukopenia and thrombocytopenia may accompany anemia.

If serum vitamin B_{12} levels are borderline low (200-300 pg/mL), measure serum methylmalonic acid and homocysteine levels. Elevated levels confirm vitamin B_{12} deficiency; elevated homocysteine and normal methylmalonic acid levels are associated with folate deficiency.

Macrocytic anemia may be caused by nonmegaloblastic disorders.

- Large target cells (MCV 105-110 fL) and echinocytes (spur cells with multiple undulating spiny erythrocyte membrane projections) signify membrane changes associated with liver disease.
- Diminished splenic function (hyposplenism or asplenia) yields large target cells, acanthocytes (erythrocytes with only a few rather than many spiny membrane projections), Howell-Jolly bodies, and variable numbers of nucleated erythrocytes.
- Reticulocytosis (e.g., secondary to hemolysis) can also increase the MCV.

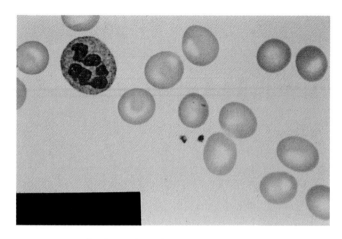

Hypersegmented Polymorphonuclear Cell: The erythrocytes are large ovalocytes, and a single PMN cell has more than 5 nuclear lobes. Consider vitamin B_{12} or folate deficiency (megaloblastic anemia).

Therapy

High-dose oral vitamin B_{12} supplementation of 1000 to 2000 µg/day is usually as effective as parenteral administration, even in patients with intrinsic factor insufficiency, and should be the initial therapy for most patients. Patients with severe anemia, neurologic dysfunction, or those not responding to oral replacement require parenteral B_{12} injections. Malabsorption syndromes always require parenteral vitamin B_{12}. Folate deficiency can be treated with oral folic acid, 1 to 5 mg daily, until complete hematologic recovery; oral therapy is effective even in malabsorption conditions.

◆ **DON'T BE TRICKED**

- Vitamin B_{12} deficiency can present with neurologic symptoms in the absence of anemia or macrocytosis.
- Folate supplementation can improve the anemia of B_{12} deficiency but not prevent the associated neurological sequelae.

Hemolytic Anemia

Diagnosis

Characteristic findings are:

- anemia
- splenomegaly
- elevated reticulocyte count
- elevated LDH and indirect bilirubin
- decreased haptoglobin
- elevated MCV is frequently elevated (due to reticulocytosis)

When laboratory tests suggest hemolytic anemia, categorize the anemia as spherocytic or nonspherocytic.

Spherocytic hemolytic anemia implicates a membrane defect, either acquired as in warm autoimmune hemolytic anemia or congenital as in hereditary spherocytosis. Nonspherocytic hemolytic anemias include bite cell hemolysis (as in oxidant stress due to G6PD deficiency) and fragmentation hemolysis (as in thrombotic microangiopathies).

Extramedullary hemolysis may be extravascular (as in hemolysis mediated by the spleen) or intravascular (as in hemolysis associated with cold agglutinin disease or thrombotic microangiopathies).

Immune-mediated hemolysis is identified by a positive direct antiglobulin (Coombs) test that detects IgG or complement on the erythrocyte surface. Hemolytic disorders "intrinsic" to the erythrocyte include membrane defects, enzymopathies, and hemoglobinopathies. In all cases, examining the peripheral blood smear is central to identifying erythrocyte morphologies that implicate certain hemolytic mechanisms.

STUDY TABLE: Peripheral Blood Smear Findings in Hemolytic Anemia

Finding	Diagnosis
Schistocytes and thrombocytopenia	TTP-HUS, DIC, HELLP
Schistocytes in a patient with a prosthetic heart valve	Valve leak
Erythrocyte agglutination	Cold agglutinin hemolysis (*Mycoplasma* infection, lymphoproliferative diseases, CLL)
Spherocytes	Autoimmune hemolytic anemia or hereditary spherocytosis
Target cells	Thalassemia, other hemoglobinopathy, or liver disease
Sickle cells	Sickle cell anemia
Bite cells	G6PD deficiency (suggested by eccentrically located hemoglobin confined to one side of the cell)

STUDY TABLE: Tests for Hemolytic Anemia

Test	Condition
Direct antiglobulin (Coombs) test	Warm-antibody autoimmune hemolytic anemia
Osmotic fragility	Hereditary spherocytosis
Cold agglutinin measurement	Cold agglutinin autoimmune hemolytic anemia
Hemoglobin electrophoresis	Thalassemia or other hemoglobinopathy
G6PD activity measurement	Test 2-3 months after event to detect deficiency (normal enzyme concentration after a hemolytic episode)
Flow cytometry for CD55 and CD59 proteins	PNH

Therapy

Warm-antibody autoimmune hemolytic anemia: initial therapy is glucocorticoids. Alternative agents are azathioprine, cyclophosphamide, cyclosporine, IV immune globulin, rituximab, or danazol for patients unresponsive to glucocorticoids or splenectomy.

Cold agglutinin autoimmune hemolytic anemia: primary therapy is cold avoidance or rituximab for persistent symptoms; glucocorticoids or splenectomy are usually ineffective.

TTP: emergent plasma exchange.

Any chronic hemolytic anemia: folic acid supplements.

Severe symptomatic anemia: select transfusion even if fully matched erythrocytes are not available.

Hereditary spherocytosis and transfusion-dependent thalassemias: splenectomy is first-line therapy.

Severe thalassemia: HSCT is standard therapy.

Severe PNH: eculizumab or HSCT.

◆ DON'T BE TRICKED

- All patients with sickle cell anemia or other hemolytic anemias need pneumococcal (both 23- and 13-valent), *Haemophilus influenzae* type B, influenza, and meningococcal vaccinations.
- A personal or family history of anemia, jaundice, splenomegaly, or gallstones suggests hereditary spherocytosis.

A previously healthy 28-year-old woman has weakness and a palpable spleen. Hemoglobin concentration is 7.2 g/dL and the reticulocyte count is 9.8%. Peripheral blood smear shows occasional spherocytes.

ANSWER: The probable diagnosis is hemolytic anemia. A Coombs test is indicated.

Sickle Cell Disease

Diagnosis

Hemoglobin S results from a single-base mutation in the β-globin chain resulting in abnormal hemoglobin. The sickle cell syndromes can be diagnosed by hemoglobin electrophoresis. Most clinical findings in sickle cell disease are related to vaso-occlusion from sickled erythrocytes. Characteristic findings include elevated reticulocyte, platelet, and leukocyte counts, and sickle cells on a peripheral blood smear. Aplastic crisis is common and may be due to coexisting infection, especially parvovirus B19 infection. Several complications of sickle cell disease mimic other diseases. Keep the following diagnostic points in mind:

ACS vs. pneumonia, fat embolism, and PE:

- ACS is usually characterized by pulmonary infiltrates, fever, chest pain, tachypnea, and hypoxemia (and is often treated empirically as pneumonia).
- Fat embolism presents with chest pain, fever, dyspnea, hypoxia, thrombocytopenia, and multiorgan failure, and may be associated with fat bodies in bronchial washings or sputum.
- Presence of lower extremity thrombophlebitis may help differentiate PE from ACS, but pulmonary CT arteriography may be needed.

Cholecystitis vs. hepatic crisis:

- Chronic hemolysis may result in gallstones and acute cholecystitis.
- Fever, RUQ pain, and elevated aminotransferase levels may also be due to ischemic hepatic crisis; abdominal ultrasonography can differentiate between the two.

Sickle cell anemia vs. aplastic crisis and hyperhemolysis:

- Anemia that decreases by ≥2 g/dL during a painful crisis could be due to aplastic crisis or hyperhemolysis.
- Aplastic crisis could be due to parvovirus B19 infection or cytotoxic drugs or be idiopathic.
- Hyperhemolysis could be due to infection (*Mycoplasma*), transfusion reaction, or coexistent G6PD deficiency.
- The reticulocyte count is decreased with aplastic crisis and increased with hyperhemolysis.
- Bilirubin, LDH, and aminotransferase levels are elevated in hyperhemolysis but normal or at baseline in aplastic crisis.

Sickle cell pain crisis vs. appendicitis:

- Abdominal pain, fever, and leukocytosis may suggest appendicitis.
- A high LDH level and normal bowel sounds support sickle cell pain syndrome.

STUDY TABLE: Long-Term Complications of Sickle Cell Disease	
If you see this...	**Think this...**
Chronic pain involving hips and shoulders	Osteonecrosis (avascular necrosis)
CVAs	Ischemic infarction in children and hemorrhage in adults
Exertional dyspnea	HF or PH
Infection with encapsulated organisms	Functional asplenia
	(Continued on next page)

STUDY TABLE: Long-Term Complications of Sickle Cell Disease (*Continued*)	
If you see this...	**Think this...**
Liver disease	Viral hepatitis, iron overload from transfusions, or ischemic-induced hepatic crisis
Impotence	Prolonged or repeated episodes of priapism
Proteinuria	CKD
Isosthenuria (inability to concentrate urine)	CKD
Decreased visual acuity	Retinopathy

Therapy

Vaccinate all patients against pneumococcus (13- and 23-valent vaccines), meningococcus, *Haemophilus influenzae* type B, hepatitis B, and influenza. All patients require folate supplementation.

The three common disease-altering strategies are HSCT, prophylactic transfusions, and hydroxyurea therapy.

- HSCT should be considered for patients with severe symptoms unresponsive to transfusions and hydroxyurea or end-organ damage if there is a HLA-matched sibling donor.
- Exchange transfusion is indicated for patients with an acute stroke, fat embolism, or ACS.
- Prophylactic exchange transfusion for patients with a history of ischemic stroke.
- Hydroxyurea for patients with more than two pain crises each year or for those with ACS.

Because of transfusion-related hyperviscosity, persons with sickle cell disease should not receive transfusion unless they have significant symptoms from their anemia or they have signs of end-organ failure (acute neurologic symptoms, acute chest syndrome, multiorgan failure). Transfusion target is hemoglobin <10 g/dL (hemoglobin A level >70%).

Simple transfusion to a hemoglobin level of 10 g/dL has been shown to be equivalent to exchange transfusions in low- to medium-risk surgeries (e.g., adenoidectomy, inguinal hernia repair, cholecystectomy, joint replacement).

Erythropoietin is used for patients with severe anemia, low reticulocyte counts, and CKD.

Vaso-occlusive crisis is managed with hydration, supplemental oxygen for hypoxemia, treatment of any precipitating event, and opioids.

Sickle Cells: Erythrocyte anisocytosis and poikilocytosis involving several sickle cells.

Iron overload due to multiple transfusions may require chelation therapy.

◆ DON'T BE TRICKED
- Hydroxyurea is contraindicated in pregnancy and kidney failure.
- Do not use meperidine to treat painful crises because the accumulation of the metabolite normeperidine can lead to seizures.
- Do not transfuse patients with simple vaso-occlusive pain.

◇ Test Yourself

A 32-year-old woman with sickle cell disease has a low-grade fever and exertional dyspnea. Hemoglobin concentration is 4.2 g/dL, and the reticulocyte count is 0.2%.

ANSWER: Diagnose aplastic crisis due to parvovirus B19 infection.

Thalassemia

Diagnosis

Hemoglobin is a tetrameric molecule. The two α-globin chains and two β-globin chains are linked to heme (iron and protoporphyrin) and reversibly bind one molecule of oxygen. The thalassemic syndromes result from defects in synthesis of α or β chains and lead to ineffective erythropoiesis and hemolysis. Patients with α-thalassemia or β-thalassemia have microcytosis and target cells on the peripheral blood smear, may have splenomegaly, and may develop pigmented gallstones.

STUDY TABLE: α-Thalassemia		
Gene Deletion	**Clinical Syndrome**	**Treatment**
(- α/$\alpha\alpha$) [single-gene deletion]	Silent carrier state that is clinically normal	None
(- -/$\alpha\alpha$; or -α/-α) [two-gene deletion]	α-Thalassemia trait; mild microcytic anemia; normal or elevated erythrocyte count; normal hemoglobin electrophoresis	None
(- -/- α) [three-gene deletion]	Hemoglobin H (β_4); severe anemia and usually early death	Intermittent transfusion
(- -/- -) [four-gene deletion]	Hemoglobin Bart's; hydrops fetalis; fetal death	In utero transfusion

β-Thalassemia is most common among persons from the Mediterranean, Southeast Asia, India, and Pakistan. β-Thalassemia results from several abnormalities in the β-gene complex. Decreased β-chain synthesis leads to impaired production of hemoglobin A ($\alpha_2\beta2$) and resultant increased synthesis of hemoglobin A_2 ($\alpha_2\delta2$) and/or hemoglobin F ($\alpha_2\gamma2$).

STUDY TABLE: β-Thalassemia		
Condition	**Characteristics**	**Treatment**
β-Thalassemia major (Cooley anemia)	No effective production or severely limited production of β-globin	Transfusion, iron chelation; consider splenectomy and HSCT
β-Thalassemia minor (β-thalassemia trait)	A single β-gene leading to reduced β-globin production with no or mild anemia	None
β-thalassemia intermedia	Intermediate severity, such as in those who are compound heterozygotes of two thalassemic variants	Intermittent transfusion, iron chelation

β-Thalassemia trait and α-thalassemia trait are most commonly confused with iron deficiency anemia.

STUDY TABLE: Iron Deficiency Anemia and β-Thalassemia Trait		
Iron Deficiency Anemia	**α-Thalassemia Trait**	**β-Thalassemia Trait**
Low serum ferritin level	Normal serum ferritin level	Normal serum ferritin level
Low erythrocyte count	Normal or high erythrocyte count	Normal or high erythrocyte count
High RDW	Normal RDW	Normal RDW
Normal hemoglobin electrophoresis	Normal hemoglobin electrophoresis	Elevated hemoglobin A_2 and fetal hemoglobin
RDW = red cell distribution width.		

◆ DON'T BE TRICKED

- β-Thalassemia can be associated with iron overload even in the absence of transfusion therapy.

Therapy

Treatment of β-thalassemia varies with the type of disease. β-Thalassemia minor requires no therapy. β-Thalassemia major requires early-onset, lifelong transfusion therapy. Iron chelation therapy may be indicated if serum ferritin concentrations exceed 1000 ng/mL. Allogeneic HSCT is indicated for severe β-thalassemia major.

❖ **Test Yourself**

An asymptomatic 18-year-old man has a hemoglobin concentration of 13.0 g/dL, an MCV of 64 fL, and a reticulocyte count of 4.0%.

ANSWER: The probable diagnosis is β-thalassemia or α-thalassemia trait. Order serum ferritin measurement and hemoglobin analysis or electrophoresis.

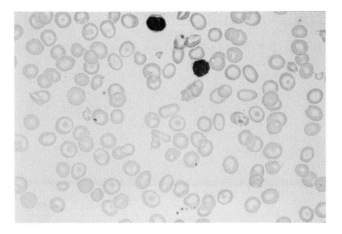

Thalassemia: Microcytosis, hypochromia, and target cells consistent with thalassemia.

Transfusion Medicine

Treatment Parameters

Erythrocytes, platelets, plasma, cryoprecipitates, and (rarely) whole blood may be used for transfusion.

Each unit of packed erythrocytes results in an increase of hemoglobin of 1 g/dL. Each unit of platelets transfused results in a 20,000 to 30,000/μL increase in platelets. Platelet transfusion refractoriness is defined as an increase in the platelet count of <10,000/μL, measured 10 to 60 minutes after transfusion on at least two separate occasions. Nonimmune causes of platelet transfusion refractoriness include sepsis, DIC, drugs, and splenic sequestration. Alloimmunization is an important cause of platelet transfusion refractoriness due to the development of antibodies to antigens expressed on platelets.

FFP is used to replace coagulation factors. FFP is not needed for treating mild coagulopathies characterized by an INR of <1.9.

Cryoprecipitates (factor VIII, fibrinogen, vWF) are an adjunct to FFP replacement therapy and are used mainly for their fibrinogen content in patients with DIC.

Inactivated 4f-PCCs contain factors II, VII, IX, and X and are indicated for the treatment of major warfarin-associated bleeding in conjunction with vitamin K.

In emergencies:

- Group O erythrocytes can be transfused to anyone.
- Group AB plasma and platelets can be transfused to anyone.
- Rh(D)-positive patients can safely receive either D-positive or D-negative blood, but Rh(D)-negative patients must receive D-negative blood and platelets.

STUDY TABLE: Threshold Values for Prophylactic Transfusion	
Condition	**Threshold to Transfuse**
Platelet transfusion; no other risk factors for bleeding	10,000/μL
Platelet transfusion for intracranial bleeding	100,000/μL
Hemoglobin for most medical and surgical patients	7.0 to 8.0 g/dL
Platelet transfusion; bleeding or planned surgery	50,000/μL

Transfusion Reactions

An acute hemolytic transfusion reaction results from ABO incompatibility. Characteristic findings are:

- fever and chills
- flank and abdominal pain
- dyspnea
- hypotension and tachycardia
- red plasma and urine
- free hemoglobin in the plasma
- A direct antiglobulin (Coombs) test is positive

Therapy for acute hemolytic transfusion reaction consists of transfusion discontinuation, IV hydration, and appropriate cardio-vascular support.

A delayed hemolytic transfusion reaction is due to delayed emergence of an alloantibody that causes rapid extravascular clearance of transfused erythrocytes 2 to 10 days after transfusion. Characteristic findings are an unexplained drop in hemoglobin concentration, elevated serum bilirubin and LDH levels, increased reticulocyte count, decreased haptoglobin concentration, and the presence of a new alloantibody.

Posttransfusion purpura is associated with thrombocytopenia that occurs ≥1 week after a transfusion. This reaction is most common in women who become sensitized to HPA-1a after pregnancy or an earlier transfusion. A subsequent transfusion may then cause immune-mediated thrombocytopenia. The diagnosis is made by an assay showing antibodies to HPA-1a. Treatment is IV immune globulin.

A febrile nonhemolytic transfusion reaction occurs at the end of or after a transfusion and is caused by donor leukocyte cytokines or recipient alloantibodies directed against donor leukocytes. The transfusion is stopped, a hemolytic transfusion reaction is ruled out, and antipyretic agents are given.

Transfusion-related acute lung injury (TRALI) is a rare, severe reaction caused by donor antileukocyte antibodies reacting with recipient leukocytes and causing leukocyte aggregation in the pulmonary capillary bed, usually occurring during or within 6 hours of transfusing erythrocytes, platelets, or FFP. Characteristic findings are hypoxemia, noncardiogenic PE, and ARDS. The transfusion is stopped, respiratory support is provided, and vasopressors are given for hypotension.

An allergic transfusion reaction occurs when donor plasma constituents react with a recipient's IgE on mast cells. Characteristic findings are rash, hives, wheezing, and mucosal edema. Treatment includes antihistamines and glucocorticoids. Patients with IgA deficiency are at high risk for allergic reaction because of the presence of anti-IgA antibodies, which may result in anaphylaxis.

Transfusion-associated graft-versus-host disease (GVHD) is a rare but fatal complication in which donor lymphocytes engraft in an immunocompromised or HLA-similar recipient and cause reactions that affect the bone marrow, skin, liver, and GI tract. Patients at risk include those undergoing chemotherapy, recipients of blood components from first-degree relatives, and premature infants.

STUDY TABLE: Cellular Transfusion Product Modifications	
Modification	**Notes**
Leukoreduction	Reduces the number of leukocytes present in the transfused product. Reduces class I HLA alloantibody production and subsequent platelet transfusion refractoriness, febrile nonhemolytic transfusion reactions, and transmission of CMV.
Irradiation	Used to prevent transfusion-associated GVHD, which is mediated by donor lymphocytes. Indicated in patients with congenital immunodeficiencies, stem cell or organ transplants, or hematologic or solid-organ cancers; in patients receiving chemotherapy; and in immunocompetent patients receiving HLA-matched platelets or transfusions from relatives.
Washing	Removes the proteins residing in the small amount of plasma of erythrocyte and platelet transfusions and is used in patients with a history of severe/recurrent allergic reactions, IgA deficiency (when IgA-deficient donors are unavailable), or complement-dependent autoimmune hemolytic anemia.

Approach to Bleeding Disorders

Diagnosis

Bleeding disorders are characterized by defects in primary and secondary hemostasis. Primary hemostasis involves the formation of a platelet plug at the site of vascular disruption. Secondary hemostasis is initiated by the exposure of tissue factor at the site of vascular damage and initiation of the coagulation cascade.

- A mucocutaneous bleeding pattern (epistaxis, gingival bleeding, easy bruising, and menorrhagia) is the hallmark of primary hemostasis failure.
- Secondary hemostasis failure is characterized by bleeding into muscles and joints as well as delayed bleeding.
- Excessive bleeding after childbirth, surgery, or trauma can occur in either category.

Remember these general rules when evaluating bleeding disorders:

- The PT and aPTT screen for factor deficiencies and factor inhibitors.
- A mixing study differentiates factor deficiency from factor inhibitor by mixing patient plasma with normal plasma and retesting the PT and aPTT.
- Bleeding time identifies platelet disorders and vessel-wall integrity; the commercially available Platelet Function Analyzer-100 (PFA-100) also assesses platelet function.
- Thrombin time tests the conversion of fibrinogen to fibrin.
- Fibrinogen, fibrinogen degradation products, and D-dimer are used to identify excessive fibrinolysis.

Common Acquired Bleeding Disorders

Diagnosis

Liver disease: Patients with liver failure will have prolonged PT and aPTT values due to decreased levels of coagulation factors. Despite this, patients are not protected against thrombosis, because protein C and S levels and antithrombin levels are low as well. Fibrinogen levels are low, and the fibrinogen may be dysfunctional. Patients experiencing bleeding may require vitamin K if deficiency is suspected or transfusion with cryoprecipitate, FFP, and platelets.

Vitamin K deficiency: Patients with liver disease and a prolonged PT require oral or subcutaneous vitamin K. Active bleeding because of vitamin K deficiency is treated with FFP. Depending on the severity of the bleeding and urgency, other options include prothrombin complex concentrate and FFP or 4f-PCC.

Factor inhibitors: Bleeding mimics hemophilia A and B. A factor inhibitor is diagnosed with a mixing study that fails to correct the coagulation abnormality. This disorder may be associated with an underlying condition such as SLE or malignancy (either lymphoproliferative or solid tumor) but is more commonly idiopathic. Bleeding is treated with activated factor concentrate, and the patient should receive immunosuppression to decrease the inhibitor levels.

DIC: Characteristic findings are thrombocytopenia, prolonged PT and aPTT, decreased plasma fibrinogen level, and elevated serum D-dimer. Schistocytes are seen on a peripheral blood smear. Treatment is of the underlying disorder.

STUDY TABLE: Management Strategy for Elevated INRs and Bleeding in Patients Taking Warfarin

INR	Bleeding	Risk Factors for Bleeding	Intervention
<5	No	N/A	Lower or omit next VKA dose(s)
			Reduce subsequent dose(s)
5-9	No	No	Omit next VKA dose(s)
			Reduce subsequent dose(s)
5-9	No	Yes	Vitamin K 1-2.5 mg PO
>9	No	N/A	Vitamin K 2.5-5 mg PO
Serious bleeding at any INR	Yes	N/A	Vitamin K 10 mg IV + 4f-PCC (or 3f-PCC + FFP or rFVIIa)

STUDY TABLE: Differential Diagnoses for Patients Experiencing Bleeding

Clotting Assay Abnormality	Differential Diagnoses
Prolonged PT, normal aPTT	Factor VII deficiency or inhibitor
	DIC
	Liver disease
	Vitamin K deficiency
	Warfarin ingestion
Normal PT, prolonged aPTT	Deficiency of factors XI or VIII
	vWD (if severe and factor VIII level is quite low)
	Heparin exposure
Prolonged PT and aPTT	Deficiency of factors V, X, II, or fibrinogen
	Severe liver disease, DIC, or vitamin K deficiency
	Heparin overdose
Normal PT and aPTT	Platelet dysfunction (acquired and congenital)
	vWD (if mild and factor VIII level is not too low)
	Scurvy
	Ehlers-Danlos syndrome
	Hereditary hemorrhagic telangiectasia
	Deficiency of factor XII

Hemophilia

Diagnosis

Factor VIII (hemophilia A) and factor IX (hemophilia B) deficiencies are X-linked disorders with clinical manifestations seen almost exclusively in men and should be considered in patients with a personal or family history of spontaneous, excessive posttraumatic, or unexpected surgical bleeding. Mild hemophilia can be missed until adulthood. Up to one third of patients with hemophilia A may develop factor VIII inhibitor antibody. The presence and quantity of inhibitor is measured with the Bethesda assay and the level of the assay determines therapy.

The PT is normal and the aPTT is prolonged in hemophilia A and B. A factor deficiency is confirmed by a mixing study using the patient's plasma and normal plasma. The results of a mixing study will normalize in a patient with a factor deficiency but will remain abnormal if an inhibitor is present.

Factor XI deficiency is rare and is most prevalent in persons of Ashkenazi Jewish descent. Affected patients typically do not have excessive bleeding; they have a prolonged aPTT but normal PT, thrombin time, and bleeding time.

Inherited factor XII deficiency is also rare and usually does not cause excessive bleeding; it is associated with a prolonged aPTT.

Therapy

Transfusions and factor VIII or factor IX replacement are indicated for patients with hemophilia A or B, respectively, and severe bleeding or hemarthrosis. Patients with mild hemophilia A should be given desmopressin for acute bleeding or before undergoing minimally invasive procedures (e.g., dental procedures). Prophylactic factor replacement has been proven to reduce the incidence of arthropathy in patients with severe hemophilia. If factor VIII inhibitor is present in low quantities (<5 Bethesda units), factor VIII replacement can overcome the inhibitor and control bleeding. Higher levels of inhibitor may require activated procoagulant concentrate to control bleeding.

❖ **Test Yourself**

A 57-year-old man has a left-sided ecchymosis. The hemoglobin concentration is 8.0 g/dL, platelet count is 220,000/μL, PT is 12 s, and aPTT is 67 s. The abnormal aPTT does not correct with a mixing study.

ANSWER: The diagnosis is acquired factor VIII inhibitor.

von Willebrand Disease

Diagnosis

The most common inherited bleeding disorder is vWD, an autosomal codominant disorder. Clinically, patients have mild to moderate bleeding evidenced by nosebleeds, heavy menstrual flow, gingival bleeding, easy bruising, and bleeding associated with surgery or trauma. vWF adheres platelets to injured vessels and acts as a carrier for factor VIII. Secondary hemostatic dysfunction can occur because of concomitantly low factor VIII levels in vWD. This distinction is important for treatment purposes.

Diagnostic testing includes a prolonged bleeding time and a normal or prolonged aPTT. Definitive diagnosis is based on the vWF antigen level, vWF activity assay, factor VIII level, and a multimer study used to diagnose subtypes of vWD.

Therapy

For mild symptoms, estrogen-containing oral contraceptives can regulate menstrual bleeding and increase vWF levels. Select DDAVP for mild to moderate bleeding or before minor invasive procedures (e.g., dental procedures). Intermediate-purity factor VIII concentrates, which contain vWF, can also be given for more severe bleeding.

◆ **DON'T BE TRICKED**

- Do not use cryoprecipitate to treat vWD because of its increased transfusion infection risk.

❖ **Test Yourself**

A 33-year-old man is evaluated for continued bleeding following a tooth extraction. His mother has easy bruising, and his sister required a transfusion following the birth of her first child. The hemoglobin concentration is 13.0 g/dL, and the platelet count is 210,000/μL.

ANSWER: The probable diagnosis is vWD. Order an aPTT and bleeding time as an initial diagnostic study.

Immune Thrombocytopenia

Diagnosis

Look for causes associated with decreased platelet production or accelerated destruction. Disorders associated with decreased bone marrow production often affect other cell lines, causing additional cytopenias. Common causes of nonimmune thrombocytopenia include:

- toxins (alcohol)
- idiosyncratic drug reactions
- metastatic cancer
- infections
- vitamin B_{12} or folic acid deficiency
- acute leukemia
- MDS
- aplastic anemia

Thrombocytopenia and the presence of schistocytes on the peripheral blood smear suggest DIC, TTP, and HUS.

Immune thrombocytopenia occurs when antibodies targeting platelet antigens mediate accelerated destruction. The characteristic finding in immune thrombocytopenic purpura (ITP) is isolated thrombocytopenia in a patient without other apparent causes for the reduced platelets. Antibodies arise in three distinct clinical settings: drug induced, disease associated, and idiopathic.

Drug-induced ITP is most often linked to heparin and certain antibiotics but any new drug, supplement, or herbal remedy could be causative. Discontinuation of the offending drug should result in platelet recovery.

Common causes of disease-associated immune thrombocytopenia include HIV, hepatitic C infection, hyperthyroidism, hypothyroidism, SLE, and lymphoproliferative malignancy (e.g., CLL or Hodgkin and non-Hodgkin lymphomas).

In immune thrombocytopenia, a peripheral blood smear shows reduced numbers of large platelets and normal erythroid and myeloid cells. A bone marrow biopsy/aspiration is usually not necessary to make the diagnosis but should be done if there are abnormalities in two cell lines, in older patients with new-onset ITP, or if the peripheral blood smear is abnormal.

◆ DON'T BE TRICKED

- Anemia does not exclude a diagnosis of ITP if the anemia can be explained by bleeding.
- Measurement of platelet-associated antibody is not helpful because the test lacks both sensitivity and specificity.

STUDY TABLE: Thrombocytopenia Associations	
If you see this...	**Think this...**
Schistocytes	DIC, TTP-HUS, HELLP
Platelet clumps	Pseudothrombocytopenia caused by EDTA-dependent agglutinins leads to falsely decreased platelet counts. Repeat count using a citrated or a heparinized tube.
Teardrop (erythrocyte) cells, disorders in two cell lines	MDS
Anemia, leukopenia, and lymphocytosis	Aplastic anemia
Pancytopenia, macrocytosis, macro-ovalocytes, hypersegmented neutrophils	Vitamin B_{12} or folate deficiencies
Thrombocytopenia following heparin administration or thrombocytopenia and thrombosis	HIT
Thrombocytopenia 5 to 10 days after blood transfusion	Posttransfusion purpura
Cirrhosis and thrombocytopenia	Splenic sequestration

Therapy

At the time of diagnosis, initiate therapy when the platelet count is <30,000/μL or with evidence of bleeding.

- Glucocorticoids are first-line therapy for ITP.
- IV immune globulin or anti-D immune globulin in persons who are Rh(D)-positive is indicated for glucocorticoid-resistant ITP or for management of severe bleeding.
- Splenectomy or rituximab is for patients who are unresponsive to drug therapy or who relapse after glucocorticoids are tapered.
- Thrombopoiesis-stimulating agents (romiplostim, eltrombopag) may be attempted in refractory cases.

Pseudothrombocytopenia: Platelet clumps on peripheral blood smear associated with pseudo-thrombocytopenia.

Thrombotic Thrombocytopenic Purpura–Hemolytic Uremic Syndrome

Diagnosis

TTP-HUS is a clinical diagnosis. Patients with TTP-HUS develop consumptive thrombocytopenia and microangiopathic hemolytic anemia from platelet thrombi that form throughout the microvasculature. Fever, kidney disease, and fluctuating neurologic abnormalities also occur but are seldom all present during earlier phases of the illness.

Laboratory studies show fragmented erythrocytes on peripheral blood smear and elevated serum bilirubin and LDH levels. Patients with TTP have been found to have unusually large multimers of vWF in their plasma and also have ADAMTS13 (vWF-cleaving protease) deficiency. TTP can also occur by other mechanisms in patients with cancer, in transplant recipients, and following administration of chemotherapeutic agents and other drugs (quinine, clopidogrel, ticlopidine, cyclosporine, gemcitabine).

TTP and HUS are difficult to differentiate and are sometimes considered as an overlap syndrome. *Escherichia coli* O157:H7 or *Shigella* infections are more common in patients with HUS. Infection leads to the development of abdominal pain and watery diarrhea 1 to 2 days after toxin exposure, followed by bloody diarrhea. As many as 20% of patients with infection-related bloody diarrhea progress to HUS microangiopathic hemolytic anemia and AKI, generally within 6 days after diarrhea onset.

◆ DON'T BE TRICKED

- Do not order ADAMTS13 activity and inhibitor level to make the diagnosis of TTP because of poor sensitivity and specificity; begin therapy without these tests.

Therapy

TTP caused by immune-mediated drug hypersensitivity requires immediate discontinuation of the causative drug. Treat TTP with plasma exchange. Treat HUS with plasma exchange; it may also require dialysis.

◆ DON'T BE TRICKED

- Do not order platelet transfusion in TTP-HUS because it can exacerbate the microvascular occlusion.
- PT, aPTT, D-dimer, and fibrinogen levels are normal in TTP-HUS and abnormal in DIC.
- Plasma exchange is superior to simple plasma infusion for TTP-HUS.

Heparin-Induced Thrombocytopenia and Thrombosis

Diagnosis

The characteristic findings of HIT and HITT are a platelet decrease of >50% in a patient taking heparin or a thromboembolic event 5 to 10 days after starting heparin. A syndrome of delayed-onset HIT may develop up to 3 weeks after discontinuing heparin. Patients with recent exposure to heparin may experience the onset of HIT more rapidly after re-exposure to heparin. A clinical score (called "the 4 T's") should be used to determine the pre-test probability of disease prior to obtaining diagnostic tests.

Diagnostic testing for HIT includes ELISA for heparin/PF4 antibodies and the functional assays, of which the serotonin release assay is the gold standard.

Therapy

Therapy is instituted before the results of diagnostic testing are returned. Heparin must be discontinued immediately. Use a nonheparin anticoagulant (e.g., argatroban, fondaparinux, bivalirudin) to stabilize the patient.

◆ DON'T BE TRICKED

- For HIT or HITT, warfarin or LMWH cannot be substituted for UFH.

❖ Test Yourself

A 75-year-old man who has been hospitalized multiple times for ischemic heart disease is admitted with increasing chest pain. The morning after admission, he has a painful, cold left lower leg. The platelet count is 30,000/μL.

ANSWER: The diagnosis is HITT. Stop heparin and begin argatroban.

Thrombophilia

Screening

Screening asymptomatic patients for thrombophilia is not recommended, even if there is a family history of thrombophilia.

Diagnosis

Testing patients with venous thromboembolism (VTE) for thrombophilic disorders is not recommended because identification of inherited abnormalities does not alter the length of recommended anticoagulation or reliably predict the risk of recurrence.

In the patient with VTE at intermediate risk for recurrence by traditional predictors, finding an inherited thrombophilia that results in higher risk for VTE is an argument used by experts for long-term anticoagulation. High risk might be defined as an increase in first or recurrent VTE by 10-fold and more than 1.6-fold compared with persons without a thrombophilia. Because of these uncertainties, examination questions on testing and treating inherited thrombophilias are unlikely.

Most examination questions will ask how to manage an identified thrombophilia in patients with VTE or in asymptomatic family members of a patient with an inherited thrombophilia. The most likely answer will be "no change in therapy."

Factor V Leiden mutation is the most common hereditary thrombophilia in white populations. The factor V Leiden mutation is screened for by testing resistance to activated protein C with a clotting assay and then confirming positive results by genetic analysis.

The second most common inherited thrombophilia is the prothrombin gene mutation. A molecular genetic test is used to diagnose the prothrombin G20210A mutation.

Heterozygosity for factor V Leiden and prothrombin mutation modestly increase the risk of first-time VTE. Recurrent VTE is only slightly increased by factor V Leiden and not increased by prothrombin gene mutation. Therefore, extended anticoagulation to prevent a recurrence of VTE is not indicated in these patients.

Protein C deficiency is a risk factor for primary VTE, recurrent VTE, and arterial thromboembolism.

If testing is performed, it should not be done in the setting of an acute thrombotic event but rather weeks or months after it has occurred and when anticoagulant therapy has been discontinued, because active thrombosis and anticoagulation may alter the level of some proteins.

Antiphospholipid syndrome can be a primary disease with no underlying comorbidity, or a secondary disorder associated with autoimmune diseases, malignancy, or drugs. The APLA is an antibody to a protein bound to an anionic phospholipid identified as β_2-GPI.

APLAs are detected and measured in numerous ways.

- Lupus anticoagulants (LACs) are APLAs that prolong clotting times (aPTT) and are not corrected with a mixing study. Confirmation is made with the Russel viper venom time or kaolin clotting time.
- Anticardiolipin antibodies react with proteins associated with cardiolipin and may be measured directly (IgM and IgG).

Any positive result should be confirmed later to rule out transient abnormalities from viral infection or even thrombosis itself. Positivity of LAC, anticardiolipin antibody, and anti–β_2-GPI antibodies are associated with the highest risk for thrombosis and pregnancy loss.

STUDY TABLE: Diagnosis of Antiphospholipid Syndrome	
Clinical Criteria	**Laboratory Criteria**
Presence of at least 1 of the following:	Presence of at least 1 of the following:
vascular thrombosis	LAC
≥1 fetal deaths before 34th week gestation	anticardiolipin antibody
≥3 spontaneous abortions before 10th week gestation	anti–β2-GPI antibody

Skin necrosis can occur in patients receiving large doses of warfarin without heparin because of rapid depletion of protein C and the development of a hypercoagulable state.

◆ DON'T BE TRICKED
- The LAC is most commonly associated with thrombosis, not bleeding.

Therapy

The treatment of patients with an inherited thrombophilia and VTE is generally the same as for those patients without an inherited thrombophilia.

For individuals with antiphospholipid syndrome and a thromboembolic event, long-term oral anticoagulant therapy is indicated.

❖ Test Yourself

A 23-year-old woman with a history of two miscarriages develops a VTE. Before beginning heparin, the aPTT is found to be prolonged.

ANSWER: The probable diagnosis is a LAC. A mixing study is indicated.

Deep Venous Thrombosis and Pulmonary Embolism

Screening

Routine extensive screening for underlying cancer in all patients with unprovoked VTE is not recommended.

Prevention

Pharmacologic prophylaxis is recommended in most hospitalized nonsurgical patients without a contraindication. Mechanical VTE prophylaxis with graduated compression stockings or intermittent pneumatic compression devices is not generally recommended. VTE prophylaxis is often only given during a patient's hospitalization with the exception of postdischarge prophylaxis (up to 5 weeks) following hip fracture, hip replacement, and major cancer surgery.

Diagnosis

Use the Wells DVT or PE scores for all patients. In patients with low pretest probability for DVT (score ≤1) or PE (score ≤4) obtain a D-dimer blood test; if negative, no further testing is needed. If the D-dimer is positive or the Wells score indicates a DVT or PE are likely (Wells DVT score >1; Wells PE score >4), obtain an imaging study. Duplex ultrasonography and CTA are the diagnostic tests of choice for DVT and PE, respectively. PEs are categorized as "low risk" if cardiac enzyme levels and echocardiography are normal.

Therapy

Hospital admission is appropriate for patients needing supplemental oxygen or IV pain medications, otherwise outpatient management can be considered.

STUDY TABLE: Duration of Anticoagulant Therapy for VTE	
Type of Thrombotic Event	**Duration of Anticoagulant Therapy**
Distal leg DVT	
• Provoked or unprovoked, mild symptoms	No anticoagulation, but monitor with serial duplex ultrasonography for 2 weeks
• Provoked or unprovoked, moderate-severe symptoms	3 months
Proximal leg DVT or PE	
• Provoked (by surgery, trauma, immobility)	3 months
• Unprovoked	Extended
• Recurrent	Duration of therapy depends on whether VTE events were provoked or unprovoked
• 2 provoked VTE events	3 months after each event
• 2nd unprovoked VTE	Extended
Upper extremity DVT, proximal	At least 3 months
Cancer-associated DVT or PE	As long as the cancer is active or being treated
	LMWH is the preferred anticoagulant
CTEPH	Extended

For PE with hypotension, systemic thrombolytic therapy is appropriate.

Anticoagulant treatment options include initial parenteral administration of LMWH, UFH, or fondaparinux followed by oral administration of warfarin, dabigatran, and edoxaban, or monotherapy (oral anticoagulant started without initial parenteral anticoagulant) with rivaroxaban or apixaban.

The only clear indication for an IVC filter is in patients with acute pelvic or proximal leg DVT who cannot be anticoagulated because of active bleeding or a very high risk for bleeding.

◆ DON'T BE TRICKED

- If DVT is diagnosed, a CTA is not needed because the treatment is the same.
- Do not select thrombolytic therapy for most patients with DVT.
- Parenteral anticoagulant administration must overlap with warfarin for at least 5 days and until the INR is >2 for 24 hours.
- Do not use a new oral anticoagulant (dabigatran, edoxaban, rivaroxaban, apixaban) if BMI >40 or GFR <30 mL/min/1.73 m².

Anemia and Thrombocytopenia in Pregnancy

Diagnosis

Pregnancy results in significant changes in fluid balance circulation which results in a normal dilutional anemia. However, hemoglobin values less than 11 g/dL in the first trimester or less than 10 g/dL in the second and third trimesters should prompt a search for other causes of anemia. Most other causes are due to iron or folate deficiency.

The most common cause of a decreased platelet count in a pregnant woman is gestational thrombocytopenia (incidental thrombocytopenia of pregnancy). HELLP syndrome, preeclampsia, and AFLP can cause thrombocytopenia and are part of a spectrum of disorders referred to as the "thrombotic microangiopathy of pregnancy." Symptoms and laboratory features for each overlap. Making the distinction between the disorders may not be critical, because the most effective therapy for each is emergent delivery of the fetus.

STUDY TABLE: Thrombocytopenia During Pregnancy	
Disorder	**Characteristic**
Gestational thrombocytopenia	Benign thrombocytopenia typically >50,000/μL; second or third trimester; no schistocytes on peripheral blood smear
	No treatment needed
Preeclampsia	Hypertension and proteinuria and thrombocytopenia developing at >20 weeks' gestation
	Treatment is delivery
HELLP syndrome	Microangiopathic hemolytic anemia; AST >70 U/L, platelet count <100,000/μL developing at >20 weeks' gestation
	Treatment is delivery
AFLP	Microangiopathic hemolytic anemia, hepatic failure, hypoglycemia, and coagulopathy >20 weeks' gestation
TTP-HUS	See TTP-HUS section; develops at >20 weeks' gestation; not affected by pregnancy termination
ITP	May present before or early in pregnancy
	Treatment same as for nonpregnant patients
DIC	In setting of obstetric emergency, elevated levels of fibrin degradation products and/or D-dimer, decreased fibrinogen level, possible prolongation of the PT and aPTT, and thrombocytopenia

Infectious Disease

Bacterial Meningitis

Diagnosis

The two most common organisms causing bacterial meningitis are *Streptococcus pneumoniae* and *Neisseria meningitidis*, accounting for >80% of cases.

Bacterial meningitis is associated with fever, nuchal rigidity, and altered mental status.

CT of the head is indicated before proceeding with LP if signs or symptoms of increased intracranial pressure are present (papilledema, focal neurologic deficits, altered mental status).

STUDY TABLE: Typical CSF Findings in Patients with Viral and Bacterial Meningitis		
CSF Parameter	**Viral Meningitis**	**Bacterial Meningitis**
Opening pressure	≤250 mm H_2O	200-500 mm H_2O
Leukocyte count	50-1000/μL	1000-5000/μL
Leukocyte differential	Lymphocytes	Neutrophils
Glucose	>45 mg/dL	<40 mg/dL
Protein	<200 mg/dL	100-500 mg/dL
Gram stain	Negative	Positive in 60%-90%
Culture	Negative	Positive in 70%-85%

CSF Gram stain and cultures are usually diagnostic for the infecting organism.

Therapy

STUDY TABLE: Empiric Antibiotic Management of Bacterial Meningitis	
Clinical Characteristics	**Empiric Antibiotic Regimen**
Immunocompetent host with community-acquired bacterial meningitis	IV ceftriaxone **or** cefotaxime **plus** IV vancomycin
Patient >50 years old or those with altered cell-mediated immunity	IV ampicillin (*Listeria* coverage) **plus** IV ceftriaxone **or** cefotaxime **plus** IV vancomycin
Allergies to β-lactams	IV moxifloxacin **instead of** cephalosporin
	IV trimethoprim-sulfamethoxazole **instead of** ampicillin
Hospital-acquired bacterial meningitis	IV vancomycin **plus either** IV ceftazidime, cefepime, or meropenem
Neurosurgical procedures	IV vancomycin **plus either** IV ceftazidime, cefepime, or meropenem

In patients with suspected or confirmed pneumococcal meningitis, adjunctive dexamethasone should be given approximately 15 minutes before administration of antimicrobial agents and continued for 4 days.

Therapy duration, which varies depending on the causative agent:

- *N. meningitidis*, *H. influenzae*, 7 days
- *S. pneumoniae*, 10 to 14 days
- staphylococcal, gram-negative, or *Listeria* meningitis, up to 21 days

Treatment of viral meningitis is symptomatic and supportive. Empiric antimicrobial agents may be initiated in viral meningitis until bacterial meningitis is excluded.

Brain Abscess

Diagnosis

Clinical presentation typically includes severe headache; fever and neck stiffness may not always be present.

CNS imaging is the cornerstone of diagnosis; MRI is more sensitive than CT, but contrast-enhanced CT can be obtained more rapidly.

Therapy

Empiric antimicrobial therapy should be started and continued for 4 to 8 weeks. Abscesses larger than 2.5 cm should be excised or drained stereotactically.

◆ DON'T BE TRICKED

- LP is contraindicated because of the potential for increased intracranial pressure and risk of herniation.

Herpes Simplex Encephalitis

Diagnosis

Infection with HSV-1 is the most common cause of endemic encephalitis in the United States. Focal neurologic deficits such as dysphasia and personality change suggest the diagnosis. CSF testing shows lymphocytic pleocytosis and, when necrosis is extensive, erythrocytes. The presence of temporal lobe abnormalities on imaging suggests HSE. Periodic lateralizing epileptiform discharges on EEG suggest HSE but is not sensitive.

HSV PCR of the CSF allows rapid diagnosis of HSE.

◆ DON'T BE TRICKED

- Do order HSV PCR on all cases of encephalitis, even if not typical for HSV encephalitis.
- Don't order CSF culture for HSV or serologic testing for HSV.

Therapy

High-dose IV acyclovir should be continued for 14 to 21 days.

West Nile Neuroinvasive Disease

Diagnosis

Mosquitoes serve as the primary vector, and most human infections occur during the summer and early fall. WNND may present with meningitis, encephalitis, or myelitis.

Severe disease may manifest as acute asymmetric flaccid paralysis and may progress to cause respiratory failure.

Diagnosis is established by detecting CSF IgM antibody to WNV.

- Don't order viral culture for WNND because it is rarely positive.

Therapy

Treatment is limited to supportive care. Monitor patients with significant muscle weakness for respiratory failure in an intensive care setting.

Autoimmune Encephalitis

Diagnosis

Anti-NMDA receptor antibody encephalitis is an increasingly common cause of encephalitis. It is associated with ovarian teratomas in >50% of patients. Clinical findings include choreoathetosis, psychiatric symptoms, seizures, and autonomic instability. Diagnosis is confirmed by detection of anti-NMDA receptor antibody in serum.

Therapy

Treatment includes removal of the teratoma and immunosuppression with glucocorticoids or IV immune globulin.

Cellulitis and Soft Tissue Infection

Diagnosis

Folliculitis is inflammation of hair follicles recognized as erythematous papules and pustules that are centered around a follicle on the face, chest, back, or buttocks. Infection is most often caused by *Staphylococcus aureus*, although pseudomonas folliculitis secondary to hot tub exposure and gram-negative folliculitis secondary to acne therapy can be seen.

A carbuncle is a superficial inflammatory mass consisting of several inflamed hair follicles and multiple sites of drainage.

A furuncle is an infection centered on a hair follicle with pus extending into the dermis forming a small abscess.

Impetigo, a streptococcal or staphylococcal infection of the epidermis, is characterized by yellow or golden-colored crusted pustules.

Erysipelas affects the superficial skin layers, including the dermis and dermal lymphatics. It classically involves the malar region. The key clinical finding is a sharply raised border and orange-peel texture. It is usually due to streptococcal infection.

Cellulitis, an infection of the dermis and deeper subcutaneous tissue, features a well-demarcated area of warmth, swelling, tenderness, and erythema.

Deep tissue infection is indicated by violaceous bullae, necrosis, rapidly increasing extent of infection, massive swelling, and pain out of proportion to apparent injury. Loss of sensation may indicate compartment syndrome (increased tissue pressure within a closed muscle compartment) secondary to deep tissue infection and may be present even if peripheral pulses are palpable.

Most diagnoses are based on clinical findings alone. Choose blood cultures in the presence of signs and symptoms of systemic toxicity.

STUDY TABLE: Skin and Soft Tissue Infection

If you see...	Think...
Honey-colored, crusted pustules	Impetigo caused by β-hemolytic *Streptococcus* or *Staphylococcus*
Sepsis, cellulitis, and hemorrhagic bullae after exposure to saltwater fish or shellfish in patient with cirrhosis	*Vibrio vulnificus* infection
Skin ulcer in a patient with neutropenia	Ecthyma gangrenosum from *Pseudomonas* infection
Chronic nodular infection of distal extremities with exposure to fish tanks	*Mycobacterium marinum*
Chronic nodular infection of distal extremities with exposure to plants/soil	*Sporotrichosis* and *Nocardia*
Sepsis following a dog bite in an asplenic patient	*Capnocytophaga canimorsus*
Swelling and erythema with pain out of proportion to physical examination findings	Necrotizing (deep) soft tissue infection (surgical emergency)
Acute, tender, well-delineated, purulent lesions	Abscess caused by *S. aureus*
Follicle-centered pustules in beard and pubic areas, axillae, and thighs	*S. aureus* folliculitis
Follicle-centered erythematous papules and pustules on the trunk, axillae, and buttocks 1-4 days after hot tub or whirlpool exposure	*Pseudomonas* folliculitis
Symmetric, pink-to-brown patches with thin scale in intertriginous areas (axillae, groin, inframammary)	Erythrasma caused by *Corynebacterium minutissimum*. Erythrasma will fluoresce to a coral red color with a Wood lamp
Malodorous superficial bacterial infection characterized by small pits primarily on the plantar aspects of feet or palms	Pitted keratolysis

Therapy

Cellulitis associated with purulent drainage or exudate should be treated empirically for MRSA pending culture results. Nonpurulent cellulitis should be treated empirically for β-hemolytic streptococci and MSSA. IV antibiotics are reserved for unsuccessful outpatient treatment or patients with signs of toxicity.

Prompt surgical debridement for deeper soft tissue infection is required for:

- toxicity, purple bullae, ecchymoses, or sloughing of skin
- necrotizing fasciitis or myonecrosis on CT or MRI
- infection following recent trauma, surgery, or childbirth
- evidence of compartment syndrome

Cellulitis: Cellulitis is characterized by well-demarcated areas of tender erythema.

STUDY TABLE: Drug Therapy for Cellulitis and Soft Tissue Infection	
Diagnosis	**Treatment**
Nonpurulent cellulitis	Dicloxacillin, cephalexin, clindamycin (all oral)
Purulent cellulitis	Clindamycin, trimethoprim-sulfamethoxazole, minocycline, doxycycline, linezolid (all oral)
Purulent cellulitis with extensive disease or signs of systemic toxicity	Vancomycin (IV) or linezolid (oral or IV)
Impetigo	Extensive disease, cephalexin (oral); limited disease, mupirocin (topical)
Erysipelas	With systemic symptoms, ceftriaxone (parenteral); if mild/asymptomatic, penicillin or amoxicillin (oral)
Folliculitis (staphylococcal and pseudomonal)	Spontaneous resolution is typical. Topical mupirocin or clindamycin lotion can be used
Human bites (clenched fist injury)	Ampicillin-sulbactam (IV)
Animal bites	Ampicillin-sulbactam (IV) or amoxicillin-clavulanate (oral)
Neutropenia	Vancomycin and cefepime
Necrotizing fasciitis	Imipenem, clindamycin, vancomycin, and debridement
Erythrasma	Topical erythromycin, clarithromycin, or clindamycin
Pitted keratolysis	Antiperspirants, topical clindamycin, and erythromycin

Treat risk factors for recurrent cellulitis, such as lymphedema, tinea pedis, and chronic venous insufficiency.

◆ DON'T BE TRICKED

- Pyoderma gangrenosum is a noninfectious skin ulceration that is associated with IBD, arthritis, or lymphoproliferative disorders.
- Skin abscesses <5 cm not associated with significant surrounding cellulitis or systemic toxicity can be treated with incision and drainage alone.

❖ Test Yourself

A 60-year-old woman has a temperature of 38.8 °C (101.8 °F). Her right thigh is swollen and extremely tender to palpation, with a 5-cm red patch in the middle of the tender area. She requires morphine for pain.

ANSWER: The diagnosis is myonecrosis. Select urgent MRI followed by surgical debridement.

A 20-year-old college football player has a fever, furuncles, and associated cellulitis.

ANSWER: Likely MRSA infection; treat with trimethoprim-sulfamethoxazole.

Vibrio vulnificus Infection: Deep tissue infection associated with hemorrhagic bullae due to *V. vulnificus* in a patient with cirrhosis.

Impetigo: Erosions with golden-yellow crusts confirm the presence of impetigo.

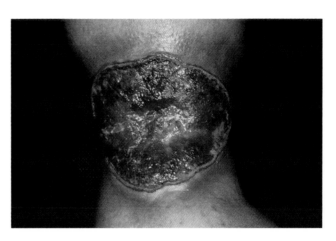

Ecthyma Gangrenosum: Ecthyma gangrenosum is characterized by single or multiple cutaneous ulcers evolving from painless nodular lesions, with surrounding erythema progressing to central hemorrhage, ulceration, and necrosis due to *Pseudomonas* infection, typically in a neutropenic patient.

Pyoderma Gangrenosum: Pyoderma gangrenosum involves a rapidly evolving, irregular, blue-red ulcer with undermined borders and a purulent, necrotic base.

Diabetic Foot Infections

Diagnosis

Mild infections are associated with at least two of the following factors:

- purulent discharge
- warmth
- pain/tenderness
- swelling/induration
- erythema

The infection does not extend deeper than the skin and subcutaneous tissues and erythema is ≤2 cm beyond the ulcer. There is no evidence of SIRS.

Moderate infections are associated with either:

- erythematous infection >2 cm around the ulcer
- infection deeper than the skin and subcutaneous tissues

The patient must not meet SIRS criteria.

Severe infections are associated with SIRS criteria and additional evidence of systemic infection (hypotension, confusion, vomiting, acidosis, severe hyperglycemia, AKI).

Assess all patients for arterial insufficiency (using ABI). Obtain foot imaging for all new diabetic foot infections.

Therapy

STUDY TABLE: Treatment of Diabetic Foot Infections	
Category of Infection	**Empiric Antibiotic Selection**
Mild (nonpurulent)	Single oral antibiotic including cephalexin, dicloxacillin, amoxicillin-clavulanate, or clindamycin
Mild (purulent and at risk for MRSA)	Clindamycin, doxycycline, or trimethoprim-sulfamethoxazole
Moderate	2-drug therapy including trimethoprim-sulfamethoxazole plus amoxicillin-clavulanate or clindamycin plus ciprofloxacin or levofloxacin or moxifloxacin
Severe	β-lactam/β-lactamase inhibitor (e.g., ampicillin-sulbactam), a carbapenem (e.g., imipenem-cilastin) and a fluoroquinolone (e.g., moxifloxacin) and surgical debridement

The use of vacuum-assisted wound closure is effective in achieving complete closure in diabetic foot ulcers.

◆ DON'T BE TRICKED

- Cultures obtained should not be from superficial swab specimens but from deep tissue specimens.

Toxic Shock Syndrome

Diagnosis

Toxic shock syndrome is characterized by fever, vomiting, diarrhea, hypotension, and rash. Exfoliation (peeling) of the skin occurs several days after the onset of the infection.

Staphylococcus aureus and group A β-hemolytic streptococci are the usual causative microorganisms. The syndrome is caused by bacterial exotoxins that act as superantigens.

Look for:

- menstruation history and tampon use
- abscess, nasal packings, and gauze-packed wounds
- fever >38.9 °C (102.0 °F) and hypotension (SBP <90 mm Hg)
- diffuse sunburn-type rash or erythema, vaginal and oropharyngeal erythema
- multisystem organ failure: kidney (elevation of serum creatinine), liver (elevated aminotransferase levels), GI tract (vomiting and diarrhea), ARDS, coagulopathy

Therapy

Remove sources of infection and toxin production and begin aggressive IV fluid resuscitation (up to 10–20 L/d). Start broad-spectrum antibiotics initially with a carbapenem or penicillin with a β-lactamase inhibitor plus clindamycin; narrow to clindamycin plus nafcillin if MRSA is identified. IV immune globulin may be helpful.

◆ DON'T BE TRICKED

- Do not select glucocorticoids to treat toxic shock syndrome.

✦ Test Yourself

A 25-year-old man has three episodes of epistaxis that are stopped by packing his nares with petrolatum-covered cotton balls. The next day, he is confused, his temperature is 39.0 °C (102.2 °F), and BP is 90/82 mm Hg. Erythema of his face, shoulders, and palms is present. The nasal packing is still in place.

ANSWER: Diagnose toxic shock syndrome, remove the nasal packing, and begin antibiotics.

Community-Acquired Pneumonia

Diagnosis

Streptococcus pneumoniae is the most common identified bacterial cause of CAP in patients of all ages. CAP due to *Moraxella* and *Haemophilus* species occurs mainly in patients with chronic pulmonary disease. Atypical microorganisms that cause CAP include *Mycoplasma pneumoniae* and *Chlamydophila pneumoniae*. Pneumonia due to atypical microorganisms is more common in persons 20 to 40 years of age.

Look for poor dentition and aspiration risk (anaerobic pneumonia) owing to GI or neurologic disease, episodes of altered consciousness (e.g., alcohol use), injection drug use (*Staphylococcus aureus* pneumonia), and antibiotic therapy during the past 3 months. Pay attention to travel and occupational history.

STUDY TABLE: Possible Microbial Causes of CAP	
Clinical Presentation	**Commonly Encountered Pathogens**
Aspiration	Gram-negative enteric pathogens, oral anaerobes
Cough >2 weeks with whoop or posttussive vomiting	*Bordetella pertussis*
Lung cavity infiltrates	Community-associated MRSA, oral anaerobes, endemic fungal pathogens, *Mycobacterium tuberculosis*, nontuberculous mycobacteria
Epidemiology or Risk Factor	**Commonly Encountered Pathogens**
Alcoholism	*S. pneumoniae*, oral anaerobes, *Klebsiella pneumoniae*, *Acinetobacter* species, *M. tuberculosis*
COPD and/or smoking	*Haemophilus influenzae*, *Pseudomonas aeruginosa*, *Legionella* species, *S. pneumoniae*, *Moraxella catarrhalis*, *C. pneumoniae*
Exposure to bat or bird droppings	*Histoplasma capsulatum*
Exposure to birds	*Chlamydophila psittaci*
Exposure to rabbits	*Francisella tularensis*
Exposure to farm animals or parturient cats	*Coxiella burnetii*
Exposure to rodent excreta	Hantavirus
HIV infection (early)	*S. pneumoniae*, *H. influenzae*, *M. tuberculosis*

Severity of illness scores such as the CURB-65 criteria (Confusion, Uremia, Respiratory rate, low BP, and age ≥65 years) may help predict a complicated course. Scoring 1 point for each positive criterion, patients with a score of 0 to 1 can be managed as outpatients, those with a score of 2 should be admitted to a hospital, and those with a score of 3 or higher often require ICU care. Also consider hospitalization for patients who do not respond to outpatient therapy or have decompensated comorbid illness, complex social needs, or require IV antibiotics or oxygenation.

Fever and a chest x-ray demonstrating one or more focal pulmonary infiltrates are diagnostic of pneumonia. Sputum cultures are indicated for inpatients and those with severe disease (ICU admission), complications (pleural effusions, cavitary lesions), underlying lung disease, active alcohol abuse, asplenia, liver disease, leukopenia, or ineffective outpatient antimicrobial therapy.

Blood cultures are not recommended for ambulatory patients but should be performed in patients with an indication for sputum culture.

Legionella and pneumococcal urinary antigen testing are also recommended when confirmation of a microbiologic diagnosis is indicated, when ICU admission is being considered, and when outpatient antimicrobial therapy fails. However, *Legionella* urinary antigen testing only detects *Legionella pneumophila* type 1 and is, therefore, not sensitive.

CRP is a marker of inflammation, and levels are increased in bacterial pneumonia. Procalcitonin is produced by cells as a response to bacterial toxins, which result in serum procalcitonin elevations in bacterial infections. In viral infections, procalcitonin levels are reduced.

◆ **DON'T BE TRICKED**

- Sputum culture does not influence outcomes relative to empiric antibiotic therapy and are not recommended.

STUDY TABLE: Risks and Pathogens for CAP	
Modifying Factor Putting Patient at Risk	**Pathogen**
Residence in a nursing home; underlying cardiopulmonary disease; multiple medical comorbidities; recent antibiotic therapy	Enteric gram-negative bacteria
Structural lung disease (bronchiectasis); glucocorticoid therapy (prednisone >10 mg/d); broad-spectrum antibiotic therapy for >7 days in the past month; malnutrition	*P. aeruginosa*
Influenza epidemic in the community	Influenza virus, *S. pneumoniae, S. aureus, H. influenzae*
COPD; smoking history	*S. pneumoniae, H. influenzae, M. catarrhalis, P. aeruginosa, Legionella* species, *C. pneumoniae*
Poor dental hygiene; aspiration; presence of a lung abscess	Oral anaerobes
Animal exposure	Farm animals (*C. burnetii*); birds (*C. psittaci, Cryptococcus, Histoplasma*); bat or bird droppings (*Histoplasma*)
Travel or residence in southwestern United States	*Coccidioides* species, *Hantavirus*
Travel or residence in Southeast and East Asia	*Burkholderia pseudomallei* (melioidosis)

◆ **DON'T BE TRICKED**

- Do not use chest CT for diagnosing CAP.

- Edentulous patients do not get anaerobic pneumonias.

- The presence of cavities with air-fluid levels suggests abscess formation (staphylococci, anaerobes, or gram-negative bacilli), whereas the presence of cavities without air-fluid levels suggests TB or fungal infection.

Therapy

STUDY TABLE: Empiric Therapy for CAP	
Patient Characteristics	**Therapy**
Outpatient, no comorbidities	Macrolide (azithromycin, clarithromycin, erythromycin, or doxycycline)
Risk factors for drug-resistant *S. pneumoniae* infection (chronic heart, lung, kidney, or liver disease; diabetes, alcoholism, cancer, asplenia, immunosuppressive conditions [or drugs], antimicrobial use within 3 months)	Oral β-lactam (amoxicillin-clavulanate [preferred], high-dose amoxicillin, cefpodoxime, cefuroxime) plus a macrolide or doxycycline; or monotherapy with a respiratory fluoroquinolone (levofloxacin or moxifloxacin)
Inpatient, general medicine ward	IV β-lactam (cefotaxime, ceftriaxone, ampicillin) plus a macrolide or doxycycline; if allergic, a respiratory fluoroquinolone plus aztreonam
	Antipneumococcal fluoroquinolone or β-lactam and a macrolide or doxycycline
	Consider risk factors for *Pseudomonas* infection, and add coverage if appropriate
ICU, no risk factors for *P. aeruginosa*	IV β-lactam plus azithromycin or a respiratory fluoroquinolone; if allergic, a respiratory fluoroquinolone plus aztreonam
ICU, risk factor(s) for *P. aeruginosa* (cardiopulmonary disease, glucocorticoid use), or gram-negative rods on sputum Gram stain	Combination therapy with an antipseudomonal β-lactam (piperacillin-tazobactam, cefepime, imipenem, or meropenem) plus ciprofloxacin or levofloxacin; or an antipseudomonal β-lactam plus aminoglycoside and azithromycin; or an antipseudomonal β-lactam plus an aminoglycoside and a respiratory fluoroquinolone
ICU with risk factors for community-associated MRSA, cavitary infiltrates, or compatible Gram stain	Add vancomycin or linezolid to IV β-lactam plus either azithromycin or a fluoroquinolone

◆ **DON'T BE TRICKED**

- For inpatients, administer antibiotic while in emergency department.
- Do not select the same class of antibiotics that patients have received in the past 3 months.

General rules for antibiotic administration:

- switch from parenteral to oral agents when 1) temperature ≤37.8 °C [100.0 °F], 2) HR ≤100/min, 3) respiration rate ≤24/min, 4) SBP ≥90 mm Hg, 5) arterial oxygen saturation ≥90% or breathing ambient air
- total duration of antimicrobial therapy in patients who respond clinically within the first 2 to 3 days of treatment is generally not longer than 7 days
- treat severe infections, empyema, lung abscess, meningitis, or documented infection with pathogens such as *P. aeruginosa* or *S. aureus* for ≥10 days
- treat bacteremic *S. aureus* pneumonia for 4 to 6 weeks and obtain TEE to rule out endocarditis
- follow-up chest x-ray is not routine; consider in adults age >50 years 2 to 3 months following antimicrobial treatment

◆ **DON'T BE TRICKED**

- Antimicrobial treatment duration for CAP is typically 5 days in outpatients.

Lyme Disease

Prevention

The risk of Lyme disease following a tick bite is low. Watchful waiting is preferred to giving a prophylactic antibiotic.

Diagnosis

Lyme disease has three stages (early, disseminated, and late) based on the time that has elapsed after exposure. The clinical presentation differs for each stage of the disease.

STUDY TABLE: Common Manifestations of Lyme Disease by Stage		
Stage	**Findings**	**Management**
Acute, localized	Within 30 days of exposure: erythema migrans, fever, fatigue, headache, arthralgia, myalgia	Treat without serologic confirmation
Acute, disseminated	Weeks to months after exposure: multiple erythema migrans lesions, heart conduction block, cranial neuropathy, radiculoneuropathy, lymphocytic meningitis, acute attacks of monoarticular or oligoarticular arthritis	Treat if ELISA is positive Obtain Western blot if ELISA is indeterminate
Late	Months to years after exposure: attacks of monoarticular or oligoarticular arthritis and/or chronic monoarthritis or oligoarthritis, peripheral neuropathy, or encephalomyelitis	Treat if ELISA is positive Obtain Western blot if ELISA is indeterminate

◆ **DON'T BE TRICKED**

- Serologic test results are often negative in acute localized Lyme disease so treat empirically.
- Do not test for Lyme disease in patients with nonspecific complaints of fatigue, myalgia, arthralgia, or fibromyalgia in the absence of exposure history or appropriate clinical findings.

Therapy

In patients with erythema migrans and early disease, begin doxycycline, amoxicillin, or cefuroxime for 28 days without laboratory confirmation of *Borrelia burgdorferi*. Manage late carditis or neurologic disease with ceftriaxone, and manage arthritis and facial nerve palsy with doxycycline.

◆ **DON'T BE TRICKED**

- Do not select the diagnosis "chronic Lyme disease" (post–Lyme disease syndrome) or treat with antibiotics.
- Do not rely on serologic test results to decide on the adequacy of treatment.
- Do not prescribe doxycycline for pregnant women.

Erythema Migrans: A large erythematous ring characterizes erythema migrans and early Lyme disease.

Babesiosis

Diagnosis

Babesiosis is a tick-borne malaria-like illness endemic to the northeast coast of the United States. Mild cases present with a febrile illness variably associated with myalgia, headache, and fatigue. Severe hemolytic anemia, jaundice, kidney failure, and death are more common in patients who are older, immuno-compromised, or have functional or anatomic asplenia. A Wright- or Giemsa-stained peripheral blood smear will show intraerythrocytic parasites in ring, or more rarely, tetrad formations (Maltese cross shaped). Consider PCR for *Babesia* DNA in cases of low parasitemia.

◆ **DON'T BE TRICKED**

- Babesia trophozoites appear as ring forms inside erythrocytes, and may be confused with malaria unless a thorough travel history is obtained.

Babesiosis: Peripheral blood smear that shows intraerythrocytic parasites arranged in tetrads, resembling a "Maltese cross."

Therapy

When *Babesia* infection is detected in an asymptomatic patient, monitoring for resolution of parasitemia without treatment is recommended. Atovaquone plus azithromycin is the treatment of choice for mild to moderate disease. In severe disease, clindamycin plus quinine is preferable.

Ehrlichiosis and Anaplasmosis

Diagnosis

Ehrlichia chaffeensis and *Anaplasma phagocytophilum* are rickettsia-like organisms that infect leukocytes. *E. chaffeensis* causes human monocytic ehrlichiosis (HME) and *A. phagocytophilum* causes human granulocytic anaplasmosis (HGA). Ehrlichiosis and anaplasmosis are spread by ticks.

The clinical syndromes of HME and HGA are very similar:

- fever, headache, and myalgia
- multiorgan failure (AKI, ARDS, meningoencephalitis)
- fever of unknown origin (symptoms can persist for months)
- elevated aminotransferases with normal alkaline phosphatase and bilirubin
- leukopenia and thrombocytopenia
- presence of morulae (clumps of organisms in the cytoplasm of the appropriate leukocyte)

Human Granulocytic Ehrlichiosis: HGE with demonstration of morulae recognized as clumps of organisms in the cytoplasm.

Whole blood PCR is the most sensitive test for diagnosis of acute infection.

◆ DON'T BE TRICKED

- HGA is transmitted by the same vector as Lyme disease and babesiosis, so double or triple infection is possible.

Treatment

IV or oral doxycycline is the treatment of choice for HME and HGA.

Rocky Mountain Spotted Fever

Diagnosis

Rocky Mountain spotted fever is a tick-borne rickettsial infection most prevalent in the southeastern and south central states. Look for a history of tick bite and recent travel to an endemic area; febrile illness in spring and summer months; and nonspecific symptoms such as nausea, myalgia, dyspnea, cough, and headache. Also look for a macular rash starting on the ankles and wrists; lesions spread centripetally and become petechial. Thrombocytopenia and elevated aminotransferase levels are characteristic. Immunohistochemistry or PCR of a skin biopsy specimen allows diagnosis at the time of acute infection.

Therapy

Select doxycycline. In patients who are pregnant, choose chloramphenicol. Failure to respond in 72 hours suggests an alternative diagnosis.

Cystitis

Prevention

Screen for and treat asymptomatic bacteriuria only in patients who are pregnant or are about to undergo an invasive urologic procedure.

Diagnosis

UTIs (either cystitis or pyelonephritis) are classified as uncomplicated or complicated.

- Acute cystitis and pyelonephritis occurring in healthy, premenopausal, nonpregnant women with no history of urinary tract abnormalities are uncomplicated.
- Complicated UTI is defined as infection occurring in a patient with comorbid conditions or anatomic abnormalities of the urinary tract, including diabetes, pregnancy, male gender, advanced age, kidney transplantation, anatomic or functional abnormalities of the urinary tract, urinary catheterization or manipulation, recent antibiotic exposure, and recent hospitalization.

Patients with complicated UTI are at risk for infection with antibiotic-resistant microorganisms.

Symptomatic cystitis is associated with dysuria, frequency, and urgency. Hematuria may be present.

Patients with uncomplicated cystitis do not require a urine culture but can be diagnosed with a urinalysis:

- urine dipsticks positive for leukocyte esterase and nitrites
- ≥10 WBCs/µL of unspun urine or 5-10 WBCs/hpf on a centrifuged specimen of urine

Obtain a culture for suspected cystitis only if:

- suspected pyelonephritis
- complicated UTI
- recurrent UTI
- suspected unusual or antimicrobial-resistant microorganism
- patient is pregnant

Therapy

For women with symptoms of uncomplicated cystitis, prescribing antibiotics over the telephone without seeing the patients or obtaining a urinalysis is acceptable.

For empiric treatment of nonpregnant women with uncomplicated cystitis, select one of the following:

- 3 days of oral trimethoprim-sulfamethoxazole
- 5 days of oral nitrofurantoin
- single 3-g oral dose of fosfomycin

In patients at high risk for complicated UTI, obtain a urine culture and initiate treatment empirically for 7 to 14 days with a fluoroquinolone.

Choose 7 days of empiric therapy for pregnant women with amoxicillin-clavulanate, nitrofurantoin, cefpodoxime, or cefixime. Obtain a urine culture after treatment.

For recurrent uncomplicated UTIs, select one or more of the following:

- postcoital antibiotic prophylaxis, particularly if UTIs are temporally associated with coitus
- continuous antibiotic prophylaxis
- self-initiated therapy for frequent recurrent episodes

◆ DON'T BE TRICKED

- Trimethoprim-sulfamethoxazole should not be used if it was taken in the preceding 3 months.
- Do not schedule a routine follow-up urinalysis or culture for nonpregnant women with uncomplicated cystitis after treatment.
- Old age is not an indicator of a complicated UTI in the absence of other indicators.

Pyelonephritis

Diagnosis

Pyelonephritis is associated with the abrupt onset of fever, chills, nausea, and flank or abdominal pain. Urinary frequency and dysuria may precede pyelonephritis. Hypotension and septic shock may occur. Look for risk factors including obstruction, kidney stones, neurogenic bladder, and indwelling catheters.

Bacteriuria and pyuria are the gold standard for the diagnosis of pyelonephritis. Gram stain of the urine sediment is particularly useful when selecting empiric antibiotic therapy. Obtain urine cultures for all patients and blood cultures for clinically ill patients. Imaging studies are indicated only for patients in whom an alternative diagnosis or a urologic complication is suspected.

Therapy

For patients with uncomplicated infection who are able to tolerate oral therapy, select an oral fluoroquinolone. Use an IV fluoroquinolone if nausea and vomiting precludes use of oral medications. Treat uncomplicated infection for 5 to 7 days and complicated infection for 14 days.

Choose broad-spectrum antibiotic coverage with an extended-spectrum β-lactam or a carbapenem in the following settings:

- suspected infection with resistant organisms
- recent antibiotic use
- urinary obstruction
- immunosuppression

Patients admitted from a long-term care facility should also receive empiric coverage for vancomycin-resistant *Enterococcus* and fluoroquinolone-resistant gram-negative rods.

Obtain ultrasonography or CT for persistent fever or continuing symptoms after 72 hours of antibiotics to evaluate for complications of pyelonephritis (e.g., perinephric abscess). CT and MRI should be considered in patients with persistent or relapsing pyelonephritis despite a negative ultrasound.

◆ DON'T BE TRICKED

- Do not use ampicillin, nitrofurantoin, trimethoprim-sulfamethoxazole, or first-generation cephalosporins to treat pyelonephritis.

Tuberculosis

Screening

The TST or IGRA is the initial screening and diagnostic study for TB infection. Low-risk persons should not be screened, with the exception of those beginning employment in a hospital setting.

◆ DON'T BE TRICKED

- Interpret a positive TST in a patient with a history of bacillus Calmette-Guérin vaccination the same as in a person without a history of this vaccination.
- Neither TST nor IGRA can distinguish latent from active infection.
- Do not obtain both a TST and IGRA.

Diagnosis

Know the different TST threshold measurements for TB infection.

STUDY TABLE: Interpretation of Tuberculin Skin Test Results		
Criteria for Tuberculin Positivity by Risk Group		
≥5 mm Induration	**≥10 mm Induration**	**≥15 mm Induration**
Persons who are HIV positive	Recent (<5 yr) arrivals from high-prevalence countries	All others with no risk factors for TB
Recent contacts of persons with active TB	Injection drug users	
Persons with fibrotic changes on chest x-ray consistent with old TB	Residents or employees of high-risk congregate settings: prisons and jails, nursing homes and other long-term facilities for older adults, hospitals and other health care facilities, residential facilities for patients with AIDS, homeless shelters	
Patients with organ transplants and other immunosuppressive conditions (receiving the equivalent of ≥15 mg/d of prednisone for >4 weeks)	Mycobacteriology laboratory personnel; persons with clinical conditions that put them at high risk for active disease; children aged <4 years or those exposed to adults in high-risk categories	

Latent TB infection is defined by a positive TST or IGRA in the absence of any systemic manifestation of active infection and a normal chest x-ray. Pulmonary TB accounts for 70% of active disease cases and is characterized by constitutional or pulmonary signs or symptoms that are often insidious and include:

- cough >3 weeks, chest pain, and hemoptysis
- fever, chills, and night sweats
- weight loss

Obtain acid-fast bacilli smears and cultures, chest x-ray, and TST (or IGRA) in patients with suspected active TB. A false-negative skin test (or IGRA) may occur in anergic patients and in up to 25% of patients with active TB. Sputum or tissue culture is the gold standard for diagnosis, but results may be delayed for weeks. Acid-fast bacillus stains are rapid, but neither sensitive nor specific. Nucleic acid amplification testing (NAAT) of sputum may be used to exclude TB in patients with false-positive sputum results (nontuberculous mycobacteria) or to confirm the disease in some patients with false-negative smears. Select drug susceptibility testing on all culture isolates.

STUDY TABLE: Chest X-ray Patterns for Pulmonary TB	
Syndrome	**Pattern**
Reactivation TB	Infiltrates in the apical-posterior segments of the upper lung and superior segments of the lower lobe
Primary progressive TB	Hilar lymphadenopathy or infiltrates in any part of the lung
Cavitary TB	Cavities without air-fluid levels; may be associated with either primary progressive or reactivation TB
Immunocompromised patients	Typical or absent radiologic findings are common
Miliary TB	Characteristic "millet seed" appearance (uniform reticulonodular infiltrate)

CT scans may identify abnormalities not yet visible on chest x-ray.

Perform thoracentesis for analysis and culture (positive in only 50% of cases). If negative, perform pleural biopsy. Pleural fluid adenosine deaminase levels are helpful in the evaluation of suspected pleural TB in patients with a negative culture and pleural biopsy.

TB meningitis is associated with CSF showing lymphocytic pleocytosis with elevated protein and decreased glucose levels. NAAT of the CSF is highly specific.

◆ DON'T BE TRICKED

- In persons not already known to be HIV positive, test for HIV infection.

Pulmonary Tuberculosis: Upper lobe infiltrates and cavitation consistent with pulmonary TB.

Miliary Tuberculosis: Chest x-ray reveals the bilateral presence of innumerable 1- to 3-mm nodules, predominantly seen within the lower lung fields, typical of miliary TB.

Therapy

Exclude active TB before starting treatment for latent TB. Select daily isoniazid daily for 9 months or daily rifampin for 4 months. These will be the options most likely to appear on the test. Many other options are available, including short-course intermittent options, but must be provided via directly observed therapy in which a health care worker observes the ingestion of medication.

The core first-line agents for active TB include isoniazid, rifampin, pyrazinamide, and ethambutol. These agents are administered for 8 weeks as part of the initiation phase, and then isoniazid and rifampin are continued for either 4 or 7 months as part of the continuation phase.

The 3 criteria that establish a patient as no longer infectious:

- adequate TB treatment >2 weeks
- improvement of symptoms
- 3 consecutive negative sputum smears

◆ DON'T BE TRICKED

- Drug susceptibility testing should be performed on the initial isolate in all patients.
- If pyrazinamide or ethambutol is used, uric acid levels or visual acuity and color vision testing are recommended, respectively.
- Never add a single drug to a failing TB regimen.

A 40-year-old asymptomatic female hospital employee has a 10-mm TST reaction following routine screening. The employee was born in India and has lived in the United States for 10 years. She was vaccinated with bacillus Calmette-Guérin as a child. Her chest x-ray is normal.

ANSWER: Diagnose latent TB and treat with isoniazid.

Mycobacterium avium Complex Infection

Diagnosis

Pulmonary disease is a classic presentation of MAC infection seen in middle-aged to older adult male smokers with underlying lung disease who clinically and radiographically resemble patients with TB. X-rays reveal nodular bronchiectatic disease. Another common presentation is in elderly, thin, otherwise healthy white women presenting as right middle lobe or left lingular lobe lung infection. These women often have scoliosis, pectus excavatum, or MVP, suggesting an underlying connective tissue defect.

Disseminated MAC infection develops in patients with HIV who have CD4 cell counts less than 50/μL and are not receiving MAC prophylaxis. The clinical presentation often consists of fever, night sweats, weight loss, and GI symptoms.

Therapy

Clarithromycin susceptibility testing is routinely recommended for all MAC isolates. Treatment for MAC infection usually consists of clarithromycin or azithromycin with ethambutol and either rifampin or rifabutin.

◆ DON'T BE TRICKED

- *Mycobacterium abscessus, Mycobacterium fortuitum,* and *Mycobacterium chelonae* are causes of localized skin and soft tissue infections, usually after trauma, surgery (often associated with implanted prosthetic material), cosmetic procedures, pedicures, tattooing, and body piercing. Contaminated, nonsterile water is the source of these infections.
- *Mycobacterium marinum* is a cause of localized skin and soft tissue infection associated with exposure to contaminated water via fish tanks or fish.

Aspergillosis

Diagnosis

STUDY TABLE: Pulmonary Aspergillosis Syndromes	
Condition	**Characteristics**
Allergic bronchopulmonary aspergillosis	Usually occurs in the setting of asthma or CF
	Other findings are a positive skin test, elevated IgE, and eosinophilia
	Presents as difficult-to-control asthma and recurrent pulmonary infiltrates
Aspergilloma (fungus ball)	Occurs in preexisting pulmonary cavities or cysts, or in areas of devitalized lung
	Symptoms are cough, hemoptysis, dyspnea, weight loss, fever, and chest pain
Invasive sinopulmonary aspergillosis	Occurs in immunocompromised hosts
	CT scan may show the "halo sign", a target lesion with surrounding ground-glass attenuation (hemorrhage)

Neutropenic patients and organ transplant recipients are at increased risk for developing *Aspergillus* infections. Blood cultures are rarely positive. The gold standard diagnostic test for *Aspergillus* infection is obtaining cultures from deep-body specimens. The serum galactomannan enzyme assay can support the diagnosis in the right clinical setting, and it can be followed serially to assess response to therapy.

Therapy

Voriconazole is first-line treatment in patients with documented or suspected invasive aspergillosis. Surgical resection is indicated for aspergilloma and hemoptysis and is considered definitive therapy. Treat allergic bronchopulmonary aspergillosis with oral glucocorticoids.

◆ DON'T BE TRICKED

- Patients with aspergilloma who are asymptomatic and have stable x-rays do not require therapy.

Aspergilloma: This enlarged image from a frontal chest x-ray shows a cavitary lesion (*arrowheads*) containing round mass (*arrow*) representing a fungus ball.

Candida Infections

Diagnosis

Mucocutaneous candidiasis may present as an erythematous intertriginous rash with satellite lesions. Oral candidiasis appears as adherent, painless white plaques on the tongue and buccal mucosa. Local invasion is most apparent in the esophagus and tends to occur in persons with reduced cell-mediated immunity or severe neutropenia.

Invasive candidiasis includes candidemia, focal organ involvement, and disseminated candidiasis, with candidemia being the most common. Candidemia occurs most frequently in the presence of an intravascular catheter.

In suspected disseminated disease, white exudates may be seen in the retina on ophthalmoscopic examination, and painless skin papules or pustules on an erythematous base may be present on the skin. Diagnosis is made by positive culture from the blood or a normally sterile body fluid or site.

Esophageal *Candida*: White mucosal plaque-like lesions consistent with *Candida* are seen on upper endoscopy.

◆ DON'T BE TRICKED

- When *Candida* is isolated from the sputum, it usually reflects contamination from the oral mucosa.
- *Candida* in a blood culture is never a contaminant.

Therapy

An echinocandin (anidulafungin, caspofungin, or micafungin) is recommended as initial therapy for most patients with candidemia.

Fluconazole is effective in preventing *Candida* infections in neutropenic oncology patients, but it has limited effectiveness for preventing other fungal infections.

◆ **DON'T BE TRICKED**

- Treatment is not indicated for *Candida* in the sputum of patients receiving mechanical ventilation.
- Do not treat asymptomatic candiduria except in neutropenic patients or those undergoing invasive urologic procedures.
- Catheter removal and antifungal therapy has been associated with a shorter duration of infection and improved patient outcomes in **nonneutropenic patients** with candidemia, but not in neutropenic patients.

Cryptococcal Infection

Diagnosis

The least-severe cryptococcal syndrome is characterized by lung involvement without dissemination. Disseminated disease may include bacteremia and meningitis. Cryptococcal meningitis is the most common form of meningitis in patients with AIDS, who typically present with symptoms such as headache, irritability, and nausea. Most patients have a CD4 cell count of less than 100/μL. The diagnosis is based on detection of cryptococcal antigen in the CSF or culture of *Cryptococcus neoformans* in the CSF. The opening CSF pressure is typically elevated.

Therapy

Choose amphotericin B plus flucytosine for induction treatment of meningitis followed by fluconazole maintenance therapy. Maintenance therapy is indicated for patients with AIDS and cryptococcal meningitis until the CD4 cell count is ≥100/μL for ≥3 months and have been receiving antifungal therapy for at least 1 year. Management of elevated intracranial pressure is by serial therapeutic LPs or extra-ventricular drain placement.

Endemic Mycosis

STUDY TABLE: Differentiation of Endemic Mycoses		
Infection	**Geographic Distribution**	**What to Look For**
Blastomycosis (*Blastomyces dermatitidis*)	Midwestern, southeastern, and south central United States (Mississippi, Missouri, and Ohio river valleys)	Symptom onset 4-6 weeks after exposure
		Consider in patients with primary skin lesion or concurrent pulmonary and skin or bone findings
		Consider in patients being evaluated for TB, malignancy
Coccidiomycosis (*Coccidioides* species)	Southern Arizona, south central California, southwestern New Mexico, west Texas	Symptom onset 1-3 weeks after exposure
		Consider in patients with pulmonary symptoms and erythema nodosum or erythema multiforme
		Consider in patients with pulmonary symptoms and prolonged constitutional symptoms (fever, fatigue)
Histoplasmosis (*Histoplasma capsulatum*)	Midwestern states in the Ohio and Mississippi valley regions	Symptom onset 2-3 weeks after exposure
		Consider in patients with complex pulmonary disease (nodular, cavitary, lymphadenopathy)
		Consider patients being evaluated for sarcoidosis, TB, or malignancy
Sporotrichosis (*Sporothrix schenckii*)	Occurs almost exclusively in persons who engage in landscaping or gardening	A papule appears days to weeks later at the inoculation site, then similar lesions occur along lymphatic channels proximal to the inoculation site

Sporotrichosis: The most common presentation of sporotrichosis is lymphocutaneous sporotrichosis. The primary lesion is located at the site of inoculation and consists of an ulcerated nodule. Similar lesions occur proximally along the lymphatics.

Chlamydia trachomatis Infection

Diagnosis

C. trachomatis is the most commonly reported STI in the United States. It may cause several clinical syndromes but also may be asymptomatic and lead to significant complications, including ectopic pregnancy, tubal infertility, and chronic pelvic pain syndromes.

NAAT is the preferred diagnostic test for chlamydia. NAAT can be performed on first-voided urine samples or urethral swabs from men and vaginal or endocervical swabs from women.

Therapy

See *Neisseria gonorrhoeae* Infection.

Neisseria gonorrhoeae Infection

Diagnosis

N. gonorrhoeae infection should be suspected in men with purulent or mucopurulent urethral discharge and in women with mucopurulent cervicitis. Gonorrhea and *Chlamydia trachomatis* infection are also common causes of epididymitis in sexually active men aged <35 years, proctitis in persons who engage in anal receptive intercourse, and pharyngitis in persons who engage in oral sex. Infection at any site, most notably infection of the pharynx and rectum, may be asymptomatic. Disseminated gonococcal infection may cause two syndromes: an arthritis-dermatitis syndrome or purulent arthritis alone without skin findings. Characteristics of the dermatitis-arthritis syndrome include:

- sparse peripheral necrotic pustules
- monoarthritis or oligoarthritis (knees, hips, and wrists)
- tendon sheath inflammation

Consider terminal component complement deficiency as a possible cause of recurrent disseminated gonococcal infection.

NAAT is the preferred diagnostic test for *N. gonorrhoeae* infections. NAAT can be performed on first-voided urine or urethral swabs from men and vaginal or endocervical swabs from women.

STUDY TABLE: Additional Diagnostic Studies for Gonorrhea	
Condition	**Best Test**
Male urethritis	Gram stain
Proctitis or pharyngitis	Culture (not Gram stain)
Arthritis	Joint fluid culture
Disseminated infection	Blood culture

◆ DON'T BE TRICKED

- Do not select gram stain to diagnose gonorrheal cervicitis.
- Do not forget to test for chlamydia, syphilis, and HIV infection in patients with gonorrhea.

Therapy

Treat presumed chlamydial infection with azithromycin or doxycycline. Because of high coinfection rates of chlamydia with gonorrheal infections, treat uncomplicated mucosal infections (cervicitis, urethritis, and proctitis) due to gonorrhea with ceftriaxone (or other suitable third-generation cephalosporins) plus azithromycin or doxycycline. In sexually active men <35 years of age, treat epididymitis with ceftriaxone and azithromycin or doxycycline for 10 days. Treat disseminated gonococcal infection with a 7- to 14-day course of ceftriaxone.

◆ DON'T BE TRICKED

- Do not select fluoroquinolones to treat gonorrhea because of antibiotic resistance.
- The recommended dose of ceftriaxone has been increased from 125 mg to 250 mg.

Gonorrhea: Several necrotic pustules and surrounding erythema on the leg associated with disseminated gonorrhea infection.

Pelvic Inflammatory Disease

Diagnosis

PID is a polymicrobial infection of the endometrium, fallopian tubes, and ovaries that is diagnosed by the presence of abdominal discomfort, uterine or adnexal tenderness, or cervical motion tenderness. Other criteria include:

- temperature >38.3 °C (100.9 °F)
- cervical or vaginal mucopurulent discharge
- leukocytes in vaginal secretions
- documentation of gonorrhea or chlamydia infection

PID most often occurs within 7 days of the onset of menses. Gonorrhea and chlamydia are the primary identifiable causes of PID. Order NAAT to diagnose *Neisseria gonorrhoeae* and *Chlamydia trachomatis*. All sexually active women should have a pregnancy test to rule out ectopic pregnancy. In patients with RUQ abdominal pain and elevated aminotransferase levels, consider gonorrhea or chlamydia perihepatitis. Complications include infertility, ectopic pregnancy, and chronic pelvic pain.

Therapy

Outpatient treatment is as effective as inpatient treatment for women with mild to moderate PID. Acceptable treatment regimens include single parenteral dose of ceftriaxone plus doxycycline with or without metronidazole for 14 days.

Choose hospitalization for the following scenarios:

- no clinical improvement after 48 to 72 hours of antibiotic treatment
- inability to tolerate oral antibiotics
- severe illness with nausea, vomiting, or high fever
- suspected pelvic abscess
- pregnancy

Inpatients are treated with parenteral cefoxitin or cefotetan and doxycycline. If the patient is nonresponsive to antibiotics in 48 to 72 hours, choose ultrasonography for evaluation of possible tubo-ovarian abscess.

◆ DON'T BE TRICKED

- Remember to screen for other STIs such as HIV.
- Because of increasing rates of *N. gonorrhoeae* fluoroquinolone resistance, do not select fluoroquinolones for empiric treatment of PID.

Syphilis

Diagnosis

The primary lesion in patients with syphilis is an ulcer (chancre) that develops approximately 3 weeks after inoculation. The ulcer has a clean appearance with heaped-up borders, is usually painless, and resolves spontaneously.

Secondary syphilis develops 2 to 8 weeks after the appearance of the primary chancre and is characterized by widespread hematogenous dissemination involving most often the skin, liver, and lymph nodes. Secondary syphilis resolves spontaneously.

To diagnose secondary syphilis, look for:

- fever and any type of rash (except vesicles), often with palmar or plantar involvement
- nontender generalized lymphadenopathy
- headache, cranial nerve abnormalities, altered mental status, or stiff neck
- mucous patches (a slightly elevated oval erosive lesion with surrounding inflammation) and condylomata lata lesions (grey to white, raised, wart-like lesions on moist intertriginous surfaces)

Latent syphilis is the presence of serologic evidence of infection in the absence of clinical signs. Latent syphilis is divided into early latent (infection ≤1 year in duration) or late latent (infection >1 year)

Manifestations of late (tertiary) syphilis may occur years after initial infection. Tertiary syphilis may cause:

- meningitis and subarachnoid arteritis (a cause of stroke in a young patient)
- aortitis
- general paresis and tabes dorsalis
- gumma in any organ

Serologic testing is the mainstay of syphilis diagnosis.

Pearls about RPR and VDRL tests:

- often negative in primary infection
- positive in high titers in secondary syphilis
- lower titers are seen in latent and tertiary infection

Confirm positive RPR or VDRL with a fluorescent treponemal antibody absorption test (FTA-ABS) or *Treponema pallidum* particle agglutination (TPPA) assay.

Nontreponemal tests should decrease in titer and may become negative after treatment (but will rise again in the setting of reinfection); the FTA-ABS and microhemagglutination assay for *T. pallidum* (MHA-TP) antibodies will remain positive indefinitely. Test all patients for HIV infection.

Perform a CSF examination for patients with primary or secondary syphilis and the presence of any neurologic sign or symptom.

Diagnose neurosyphilis when any one of the following is present:

- CSF lymphocytes >5/μL
- elevated CSF protein
- positive CSF VDRL test

Syphilis: Primary chancre of syphilis characterized by a clean-based, nonpainful genital ulcer.

STUDY TABLE: Differential Diagnosis of Genital Ulcers	
Disease	**Characteristics**
Herpes (HSV type 1 or 2)	Multiple 1- to 2-mm tender vesicles or erosions and tender lymphadenopathy
Syphilis (*T. pallidum*)	Single 0.5- to 1.0-cm painless indurated ulcers and nontender bilateral inguinal lymphadenopathy
Chancroid (*Haemophilus ducreyi*)	Ragged, purulent, painful ulcers with tender lymphadenopathy
Lymphogranuloma venereum (*Chlamydia trachomatis*)	Single 0.2- to 1.0-cm ulcer, sometimes painful, with tender unilateral lymphadenopathy, which may suppurate
Fixed drug eruptions (NSAIDs, phenobarbital, antibiotics)	Single or multiple blisters or erosions, 1-3 cm, frequently on the glans penis

Therapy

The preferred therapy for syphilis at all stages is parenteral penicillin, which is the only acceptable therapy for pregnant patients.

- Treat primary or secondary or early latent syphilis with one dose of IM benzathine penicillin.
- Treat late latent or asymptomatic syphilis of unknown duration with 3 weekly doses of benzathine penicillin.
- Treat late (tertiary) nonneurosyphilis with three weekly doses of IM benzathine penicillin.
- Treat neurosyphilis with continuous penicillin infusion (or IM benzathine penicillin every 4 hours) for 10 to 14 days.

Doxycycline and tetracycline are alternatives for penicillin-allergic nonpregnant patients. Failure of nontreponemal serologic test results to decrease fourfold in the 6 to 12 months after treatment indicates treatment failure or reacquisition.

Secondary Syphilis: Pink to reddish-brown macules and papules on the palms, characteristic of secondary syphilis.

- Pregnant patients who are allergic to penicillin must be desensitized and treated with penicillin.
- The Jarisch-Herxheimer reaction is an acute febrile illness occurring within 24 hours of treatment for any stage of syphilis and is not an allergic reaction to penicillin.

Herpes Simplex Virus Infection

Diagnosis

Inoculation of HSV at mucosal surfaces or skin sites results in the sudden appearance of multiple vesicular lesions on an inflamed, erythematous base. Primary infection may also be associated with systemic symptoms, such as fever and malaise. After primary infection resolves, the virus lives in a latent state in nerve cell bodies in ganglion neurons and can reactivate.

Several herpetic syndromes are possible in the adult.

STUDY TABLE: Selected Herpes Simplex Virus Syndromes	
Manifestation	**Description**
Oral	First-episode infections are most commonly gingivostomatitis and pharyngitis, whereas herpes labialis is the most frequent sign of reactivation disease
Herpetic whitlow	HSV infection of the finger often mistaken for bacterial infection
Genital herpes	Multiple painful vesicular or ulcerative lesions on penis or vulva
	Initial episode frequently associated with systemic symptoms and regional lymphadenopathy
	Recurrent genital herpes is usually caused by HSV-2
Keratitis	Punctate or branching epithelial keratitis
Encephalitis	Rapid onset of fever, headache, seizures, focal neurologic signs, and impaired consciousness
Hepatitis	Rare complication of either HSV-1 or HSV-2 that is most common in immunosuppressed patients (glucocorticoid use, HIV infection, cancer, MDS, pregnancy)
Associated HIV infection	Infection can occur anywhere and often presents as extensive oral or perianal ulcers (not vesicles) or as esophagitis, colitis, chorioretinitis, acute retinal necrosis, tracheobronchitis, and pneumonia
Bell palsy	HSV is implicated in Bell palsy syndrome

PCR testing of clinical specimens obtained from ulcers and mucocutaneous sites is the most sensitive diagnostic modality available.

◆ **DON'T BE TRICKED**

- A positive HSV-2 antibody test indicates only previous infection and is not a useful diagnostic test.
- Don't obtain Tzanck test to diagnose HSV infection; it is neither sensitive nor specific.
- Patients with late-stage HIV are prone to frequent recurrences of genital herpes and chronic mucocutaneous ulceration (not vesicles).
- Recurrent erythema multiforme is most commonly caused by HSV recurrences.

Therapy

For the first episode of genital herpes, treat with acyclovir, famciclovir, or valacyclovir for 7 to 10 days. Treat recurrent disease for 3 to 5 days. Treatment decreases duration of symptoms and reduces viral shedding. Suppressive therapy may be necessary to decrease the frequency of recurrences.

Treat primary episodes of oral HSV infection the same as genital lesions. Recurrent disease is generally not treated. Suppressive therapy can be considered for frequent recurrences (≥6/year), particularly in immunosuppressed patients.

Treat primary herpes keratoconjunctivitis with topical trifluorothymidine, vidarabine, or acyclovir. Ophthalmology referral is mandatory.

Use IV acyclovir to treat suspected or confirmed herpes encephalitis. Glucocorticoids may be beneficial for Bell palsy with severe facial paralysis. The role of antiviral therapy is unclear.

◆ **DON'T BE TRICKED**

- Do not treat herpetic keratitis with topical glucocorticoid drops.
- Topical acyclovir is not effective for treating genital herpes.

Herpetic Whitlow: Herpetic whitlow involving the lateral aspect of the index finger.

Perianal Herpes Simplex: Perianal herpes simplex in an immunocompromised patient (HIV/AIDS). In patients with HIV disease, herpes simplex may appear as painful, shallow ulcers rather than the classic vesicle.

Genital Warts

Diagnosis

Genital warts are most commonly caused by HPV types 6 and 11. They are typically painless, flesh colored, and exophytic. Diagnosis is generally made based on clinical appearance.

Therapy

Most infections clear spontaneously. Treatment does not prevent HPV transmission. Patient-applied agents include podophylox (podophyllotoxin), imiquimod, and sinecatechins. Physician-administered treatments include podophyllin resin, trichloroacetic acid, cryotherapy, and surgical removal.

Osteomyelitis

Diagnosis

Microorganisms can reach the bone by:

- contiguous spread from adjacent soft tissue or joints
- hematogenous seeding
- direct inoculation as a result of surgery or trauma

Staphylococcus aureus is the most commonly isolated pathogen causing hematogenous osteomyelitis. Osteomyelitis associated with contiguous foci of infection, decubitus ulcers, and vascular insufficiency is often polymicrobial.

Adults with osteomyelitis usually have pain around the involved site without systemic symptoms. A draining sinus tract may be present over the area of involved bone. Patients who have undergone total joint arthroplasty and have new or unresolved joint pain may have a prosthetic joint infection.

Clinical clues that indicate the presence of osteomyelitis in patients with diabetic foot ulcers include ulcers that are:

- present for ≥2 weeks
- size >2 cm
- grossly visible bone or the ability to probe to bone
- ESR >70 mm/h

STUDY TABLE: Categorization and Characterization of Osteomyelitis

Category	Characteristics
Acute hematogenous osteomyelitis	Infection of intervertebral disc space and two adjacent vertebrae
Contiguous osteomyelitis	Patients >50 years old with diabetes mellitus or peripheral vascular disease and a foot ulcer
Following dog or cat bite	*Pasteurella multocida* may cause contiguous-focus osteomyelitis after dog or cat bites
Following foot puncture wound	*Pseudomonas* is frequently isolated following puncture wounds through the rubber sole of a shoe
Sternal osteomyelitis	Wound healing complications, unstable sternum, and fever after thoracic surgery
Clavicular osteomyelitis	Pain, cellulitis, or drainage after subclavian vein catheterization
Sternoclavicular joint osteomyelitis	Pain and fever in an injection-drug user
Sickle cell disease	Bone infarcts and bone marrow thrombosis predispose to osteomyelitis most commonly caused by *Salmonella* species and *S. aureus*.

Bone biopsy is the definitive diagnostic study for osteomyelitis.

MRI is the imaging procedure of choice for patients with suspected osteomyelitis. Half of patients with acute hematogenous osteomyelitis will have positive blood cultures. Cultures are less likely to be positive with contiguous osteomyelitis. A positive blood culture obviates the need for a bone biopsy.

Bone biopsy is best obtained by surgical sampling or by needle aspiration under radiographic guidance. In stable chronic osteomyelitis, antimicrobial therapy is withheld until deep bone cultures have been obtained.

◆ **DON'T BE TRICKED**

- Do not obtain sinus tract and wound drainage cultures.

Therapy

The pillars of treatment include:

- administration of adequate antimicrobials for a prolonged period of time (usually 6 weeks)
- surgical debridement (if warranted)
- removal of orthopedic prosthetic devices (if feasible)

Broad-spectrum antimicrobial therapy is usually required considering the polymicrobial nature of diabetic foot infections:

- imipenem-cilastatin
- piperacillin-tazobactam
- ampicillin-sulbactam

Vancomycin, linezolid, or daptomycin is added if there is concern or proof of MRSA coinfection.

Diabetic foot osteomyelitis is treated for at least 4 to 6 weeks. Surgically remove all devitalized bone. In patients with poor arterial vascular supply, also choose revascularization.

The most common organism found in vertebral osteomyelitis is *S. aureus* (including MRSA); coagulase-negative staphylococci are also common. MRI is the most sensitive imaging modality to detect vertebral osteomyelitis. Patients with imaging studies suggestive of vertebral osteomyelitis but negative blood cultures should undergo a CT-guided percutaneous needle biopsy.

Hematogenous Osteomyelitis: MRI shows moderate destruction of the inferior L3 and superior L4 vertebral bodies compatible with osteomyelitis. Moderate narrowing of the thecal sac is seen at this level due to retropulsion of an enhancing bony fragment.

Empiric antibiotic treatment may be given if an etiologic agent is not identified to guide specific therapy. Vancomycin or daptomycin plus ceftriaxone, ceftazidime, cefepime, or a fluoroquinolone are appropriate choices. Also consider:

- removal of orthopedic hardware for most patients with orthopedic implant–associated osteomyelitis
- a prolonged course (3-6 months) of fluoroquinolone and rifampin therapy when implant removal is not possible

◆ DON'T BE TRICKED

- A positive blood culture obviates the need for bone biopsy.
- Surgery is not needed for uncomplicated hematogenous vertebral osteomyelitis.
- A positive MRI persists long after effective therapy for osteomyelitis; do not obtain follow-up MRI to verify clinical improvement.

Test Yourself

A 60-year-old previously healthy man has nonradiating pain in his lower thoracic spine that began 10 days ago. Six weeks ago, he was unable to urinate and required an indwelling urinary catheter. Temperature is 37.9 °C (100.2 °F). Point tenderness of the lower thoracic spine is present.

ANSWER: Choose probable acute hematogenous osteomyelitis of the vertebral spine with cord compression secondary to vertebral collapse or epidural abscess formation. Select empiric antibiotic therapy and urgent surgical consultation.

Fever of Unknown Origin

Diagnosis

Fever of unknown origin is characterized by a temperature >38.3 °C (100.9 °F) for at least 3 weeks that remains undiagnosed after 2 outpatient visits or 1 week of inpatient evaluation. Fever of unknown origin can be classified into classic, nosocomial, neutropenic, and HIV-associated categories.

STUDY TABLE: Categories and Common Causes of Fever of Unknown Origin	
Category	**Common Causes**
Classic	Infection (primary CMV infection, endocarditis, TB, abscesses, complicated UTI), neoplasm, connective tissue disease
Health-care associated	Drug fever, septic thrombophlebitis, PE, sinusitis, postoperative complications (occult abscesses), *Clostridium difficile* enterocolitis, device- or procedure-related endocarditis
Neutropenic	Bacterial and fungal infections (aspergillosis, candidiasis), drug fever, PE, underlying malignancy; cause not documented in 40%-60% of cases
HIV associated	Primary HIV infection, opportunistic infections (CMV, cryptococcosis, TB and nontuberculous *Mycobacteria* infection, toxoplasmosis), lymphoma, IRIS

Drug-induced fever can occur at any time but usually appears days to weeks after initiation of a new drug. Associated features may include rash, urticaria, liver or kidney dysfunction, and mucosal ulceration. Laboratory tests may show elevated serum aminotransferases, leukocytosis or leukopenia, and eosinophilia. Look especially for use of anticonvulsants (phenytoin, carbamazepine), antibiotics (β-lactams, sulfonamides, nitrofurantoin), and allopurinol.

❖ **Test Yourself**

A 22-year-old woman begins taking phenytoin after undergoing a craniotomy for a subdural hematoma. Twelve days later, she develops a temperature of 38.3 °C (100.9 °F) and a generalized erythematous rash. The leukocyte count is 12,800/μL with eosinophilia, serum AST level is 66 U/L, and ALT level is 72 U/L.

ANSWER: Select DRESS, also known as hypersensitivity syndrome, as cause of fever and rash.

Primary Immunodeficiency

Diagnosis

Consider primary immunodeficiency syndromes in patients with multiple or recurrent infections. The most common primary immunodeficiency is congenital IgA deficiency. Most patients with isolated IgA deficiency are clinically normal, but may present with recurrent respiratory infections, giardiasis, and have an increased risk for autoimmune disorders, including RA and SLE. Patients with undetectable levels of serum IgA are at high risk for transfusion reactions because of the development of anti-IgA antibodies.

CVI is the most common symptomatic primary immunodeficiency and is characterized by low levels of one or more immunoglobulin classes or subclasses. Findings include:

- hypogammaglobulinemia
- recurrent bacterial upper and lower respiratory infections (including bronchiectasis)
- predilection for infection with encapsulated bacteria (pneumococcus, *Haemophilus*, staphylococcus)
- infectious diarrhea, specifically *Giardia lamblia* infection
- chronic diarrhea/malabsorption

Some other considerations:

- autoimmune manifestations are found in one third of cases (hemolytic anemia and thrombocytopenia, SLE, RA)
- CVI increases the risk for gastric adenocarcinoma, intestinal lymphoma, and non-Hodgkin lymphoma

Measure serum IgM, IgA, IgG (all low), and IgG subclasses (variably low), and measure the ability to mount an antibody response to tetanus toxoid (protein) and pneumococcal polysaccharide vaccine (polysaccharide) antigens.

Therapy

Choose IV immune globulin as first-line therapy for CVI. Most patients with selective IgA therapy do not require treatment.

◆ **DON'T BE TRICKED**

- Standard IV immune globulin is contraindicated in isolated IgA deficiency, because these patients may have IgG or IgE antibodies directed against the transfused IgA.

❖ **Test Yourself**

A 37-year-old woman has had eight episodes of documented sinusitis annually for the past 15 years. She had a single episode of pneumonia as a child.

ANSWER: The patient has probable CVI. Choose measurement of serum immunoglobulin levels and, if low, measurement of antibody response to pneumococcal and tetanus vaccines.

Complement Deficiency

Diagnosis

Persons with deficiencies of the terminal components of the classic complement pathway (C5, C6, C7, C8, and C9) are susceptible to recurrent neisserial infections. Defects in components of the alternative complement pathway of activation and the lectin pathway may also be associated with neisserial infections.

Obtain a CH_{50} assay. If CH_{50} is low, follow up with individual component measurements. Screen all patients with repeated episodes of disseminated gonorrhea or meningococcal infection with CH_{50} assay. Measurement of the alternative (AH_{50} assay) and lectin pathway components is indicated in patients in whom complement deficiency is suspected but CH_{50} is normal. Patients with deficiencies of the early components of the complement system will have repeated bacterial infections and often SLE.

Therapy

Patients with complement deficiency respond to standard antibiotics. Patients should maintain currency of vaccinations, especially meningococcal, pneumococcal, and *Haemophilus* b conjugate vaccine.

STUDY TABLE: Pattern Recognition Diagnosis of Repeated Infections		
Presenting Pattern	**Congenital Defect**	**Test**
Invasive skin infections	Granulocyte (chronic granulomatous disease)	Nitroblue tetrazolium dye test (respiratory burst assay)
Benign or intracellular viral or fungal infections	Cell mediated	Skin test response to PPD, mumps, and *Candida* antigen, quantitative T cell assay
Repeated sinopulmonary infections with encapsulated bacteria	Immunoglobulins	Quantitative serum immunoglobulins and response to tetanus and pneumococcal polysaccharide vaccines
Sinopulmonary infections, malabsorption, infertility, family history of CF	*CFTR* gene (CF)	Sweat chloride test
Recurrent *Neisseria meningitidis* infection and disseminated gonorrhea	Terminal complement components (C5, C6, C7, C8, and C9), alternative and lectin pathways	CH_{50} assay

❖ **Test Yourself**

A 21-year-old male college student has meningococcal meningitis for the third time in 2 years.

ANSWER: The patient has probable terminal complement deficiency. Select serum CH_{50} assay.

Bioterrorism

Biologic agents most likely to be used in bioterrorist events are anthrax, smallpox, plaque, tularemia, botulism, and viral hemorrhagic fever. Clues suggesting a bioterrorism attack include:

- sudden onset of unusual number of cases
- increased severity or uncommon clinical presentation
- unusual geographic, temporal, or demographic clustering of cases

Smallpox

Diagnosis

The last reported case of smallpox worldwide occurred in 1977. It remains a concern because of the threat of bioterrorism and the need to distinguish smallpox from similar diseases.

To diagnose smallpox, look for:

- fever >38.5 °C (101.3 °F), fatigue, and headache and backaches
- rash beginning 2 to 3 days after onset of fever
- rash beginning first on buccal or pharyngeal mucosa then the face, proximal arms, and legs and then spreading to the chest and distal extremities, including the palms and soles
- rash in the same stage at any one time, in any one location of the body (all papules, all vesicles, all pustules, or all crusts)

Smallpox can be confused with varicella (chickenpox), look for:

- generally mild prodrome of fever and constitutional symptoms in children and adolescents, occurring simultaneously with rash
- rash beginning on the trunk, then spreading to the face and extremities
- rash in different stages (mix of papules, vesicles, pustules, and crusts) at any one time

◆ DON'T BE TRICKED

- **Patients with smallpox remain contagious until all scabs and crusts are shed.**

Therapy

Therapy is supportive. Postexposure vaccination with vaccinia, targeting close contacts of patients with smallpox ("ring vaccination") within 3 days after exposure is recommended to prevent spread.

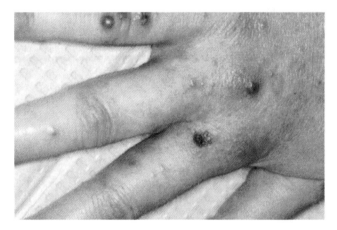

Varicella Infection: Characteristic varicella infection with rash at different stages of development (vesicles, papules, pustules, and crusts) in one region of the body.

Anthrax

Diagnosis

Three types of anthrax occur in humans: cutaneous, GI, and inhalational. Cutaneous anthrax is the most common type of anthrax in the United States. Look for anthrax risk factors, including:

- travel to the Middle East, Africa, South America, or Asia
- exposure to wool, hides, or animal hair from endemic countries
- bioterrorism

Select cutaneous anthrax if the patient has an enlarging, painless ulcer with black eschar surrounded by edema or large gram-positive bacilli on Gram stain. Look for inhalational anthrax if the patient has dyspnea, fever, chest pain, and a widened mediastinum on chest x-ray or CT scan.

Therapy

To prevent inhalational anthrax, select postexposure vaccination and ciprofloxacin for 60 days. Select oral ciprofloxacin for cutaneous anthrax and IV ciprofloxacin and two additional antibiotics (penicillin, ampicillin, imipenem, meropenem, clindamycin, linezolid, rifampin, vancomycin, clarithromycin) for inhalational anthrax, anthrax meningitis, and severe cutaneous disease (involving the head, neck). Raxibacumab, a monoclonal antibody that neutralizes *Bacillus anthracis* toxin, is approved for the treatment and prevention of inhalational anthrax.

Cutaneous Anthrax: The primary lesion of cutaneous anthrax is a painless, pruritic papule. As the lesion matures, a painless ulcer covered by the characteristic black eschar surrounded by nonpitting edema develops.

❖ Test Yourself

A 57-year-old male government clerk has 3 days of malaise, fever, cough, and headache. Temperature is 39.0 °C (102.2 °F), and lung crackles are heard bilaterally. A chest x-ray shows scattered pulmonary infiltrates and a widened mediastinum.

ANSWER: Select inhalational anthrax and IV ciprofloxacin and two other antibiotics.

Plague

Diagnosis

Yersinia pestis most often is transmitted by fleas, but may also arise from inhalation.

The forms of plague include:

- bubonic plague follows primary cutaneous exposure and is characterized by buboes (infected, swollen lymph nodes)
- septicemic plague is characterized by DIC and multiorgan system failure
- pneumonic plague most often arises secondarily through hematogenous spread from a bubo or direct inhalation

Patients with pneumonic plague present with sudden high fever, pleuritic chest discomfort, a productive cough, and hemoptysis. The chest x-ray is nonspecific. Sputum Gram stain (and possibly blood smear) may identify the classic bipolar gram-negative staining or "safety pin" shape.

Therapy

Treat with either streptomycin or gentamicin.

Tularemia

Diagnosis

Francisella tularensis is gram-negative coccobacillus that exists mainly as a zoonotic disease but can cause significant illness through inhalation.

Pneumonic tularemia is characterized by a cough, dyspnea, and substernal or pleuritic chest pain. Respiratory failure may ensue. Typical chest x-ray findings include infiltrates (at times nodular or rounded), hilar lymphadenopathy, and pleural effusion.

Therapy

Treat severe tularemia with streptomycin or gentamicin and mild or moderate infection with oral ciprofloxacin or doxycycline.

Botulism

Diagnosis

The *Clostridium botulinum* neurotoxin inhibits acetylcholine release at ganglia and neuromuscular junctions, causing bulbar palsy and symmetric flaccid paralysis beginning 12-72 hours after exposure. Remember the "Five D's" of botulism:

- Diplopia
- Dysphonia
- Dysarthria
- Dysphagia
- Descending paralysis (starting with facial muscles)

Confirmation of disease depends on identifying botulinum toxin from samples of the patient's blood, stool, gastric contents, and wound.

Therapy

Ventilatory capacity must be monitored (often in the ICU), and respiratory support may be required. In patients with wound botulism, the wounds should be débrided. A trivalent (types A, B, C) equine serum antitoxin should be administered as early as possible to prevent progression, as it cannot reverse existing paralysis.

Viral Hemorrhagic Fever

Diagnosis

Viral hemorrhagic fevers are a group of febrile illnesses caused by zoonotic RNA viruses. Ebola is the best known in this group endemic to Central Africa.

A high febrile prodrome universally occurs, accompanied by myalgia and prostration. Early signs of infection often include conjunctival injection, petechial hemorrhages, and easy bruising. As the disease advances, patients experience shock and generalized bleeding from the mucous membranes, skin, and GI tract with multiorgan failure. High titers of virus may be found in blood, urine, saliva, feces, vomit, and sweat. Isolation precautions are important to protect healthcare providers and limit the spread of infection.

Diagnostic confirmation requires RNA detection by reverse transcription PCR, the presence of viral protein antigens, development of IgM antibodies, or isolation of the virus.

Therapy

Treatment is primarily supportive.

Malaria

Prevention

Select chloroquine for travelers to areas where chloroquine-resistant *Plasmodium falciparum* has not been reported (Central America, Haiti, Dominican Republic). Otherwise, select mefloquine, atovaquone-proguanil, or doxycycline.

Diagnosis

Most infections are caused by *P. falciparum* or *Plasmodium vivax*, and most deaths are due to *P. falciparum*. Fever develops with the release of merozoites from ruptured, infected erythrocytes. Look for:

***Plasmodium falciparum* Infection:** In the center of the peripheral blood smear is a banana-shaped gametocyte diagnostic of *P. falciparum* infection.

- cyclical paroxysms of rigors
- fever, drenching sweats
- travel history and inadequate antimalarial prophylaxis
- jaundice
- splenomegaly
- coma, seizure

Select thick and thin peripheral blood smears to diagnose malaria. Parasitemia levels >2% are most consistent with *P. falciparum* infection.

◆ DON'T BE TRICKED

- Any traveler who has returned from a malaria-endemic area in the past year and has an undiagnosed febrile illness should undergo malaria evaluation.

Therapy

Use chloroquine for malaria acquired where chloroquine resistance has not been reported. Choose artemisinin derivative combinations, atovaquone-proguanil, mefloquine, and quinine-based regimens for malaria acquired where chloroquine-resistant parasites are present.

Leptospirosis

Diagnosis

Leptospirosis is a zoonosis caused by the spirochete *Leptospira interrogans*. Most clinical cases occur in the tropics (Hawaii in the United States). Patients typically become infected following exposure to animal urine or contaminated water or soil. Most patients present with the abrupt onset of fever, rigors, myalgias, and headache; kidney failure, uveitis, respiratory failure, myocarditis, and rhabdomyolysis can occur. A key physical sign is conjunctival suffusion, infrequently found in other infectious diseases. The diagnosis is usually made by serologic confirmation.

Therapy

Most cases are self-limited, but doxycycline and penicillin may be helpful in severe disease or shortening the duration of mild disease.

Infectious Gastrointestinal Syndromes

STUDY TABLE: Agents, Presentation, and Treatment of Infectious Gastrointestinal Syndromes			
Agent	**Clinical Findings**	**Diagnosis**	**Empiric Treatment**
Bacterial			
Campylobacter	Fevers, chills, diarrhea, abdominal pain Postinfectious IBD, reactive arthritis, Guillain Barré	Routine stool culture	Azithromycin or erythromycin ×3-5 days
Shigella	Dysentery Day care center or nursing home workers Rare cause of HUS	Routine stool culture	Usually self-limited Fluoroquinolone ×3 days; azithromycin ×3 days for severe symptoms or positive stool cultures to reduce transmission
Salmonella (nontyphoidal)	Fever, chills, diarrhea; bacteremia in 10%-25% of cases and may result in endothelial infection including aortitis, arteritis, mycotic aneurysm	Routine stool culture; blood cultures (with moderate to severe illness)	Do not treat mild disease – may lead to prolonged shedding of bacteria in stool If significant comorbid illness or severe illness, treat with fluoroquinolone
STEC including *Escherichia coli* O157:H7	Bloody stools in >80% of cases; fever often absent; may be associated with HUS	*E. coli* O157:H7: stool culture with specialized media followed by serology Other STEC: stool culture with specialized media followed by Shiga toxin serology or PCR	None (antibiotic treatment of STEC may increase the risk of HUS)
Enterotoxigenic *E. coli* (travelers' diarrhea)	Nonbloody, watery stools	None	Fluoroquinolone ×3 days, azithromycin ×1 dose, or rifaximin ×3 days
Yersinia	Fever, diarrhea, RLQ pain (mimics appendicitis) Postinfectious reactive arthritis	Routine stool culture	Fluoroquinolone ×3 days; trimethoprim-sulfamethoxazole ×3 days
Vibrio	Bloody stools (>25% of cases), fever, vomiting (>50% of cases) Severe infection with sepsis in patients with hepatic dysfunction or alcoholism	Stool culture with specialized media	Fluoroquinolone ×3 days; azithromycin ×3 days
Clostridium difficile	Diarrhea, fever, abdominal pain, colonic distention (including toxic megacolon in severe cases), leukocytosis, sepsis	PCR or stool EIA for toxin	Mild: metronidazole Severe: oral vancomycin
Viral			
Norovirus	Watery, noninflammatory diarrhea; vomiting in >50% of cases; highly transmissible; frequent cause of outbreaks	None	None
Parasitic			
Giardia	Watery diarrhea, abdominal cramping, steatorrhea, weight loss Prolonged infection with IgA deficiency	Microscopy or stool antigen	Metronidazole ×5-10 days or tinidazole
Cryptosporidium	Watery diarrhea HIV-infected patients at high risk	Modified acid-fast stain, stool antigen	Supportive care Nitazoxanide for symptomatic patients
Amebiasis	Dysentery	Microscopy, stool antigen	Tinidazole or metronidazole
Cyclospora	Watery diarrhea, bloating, flatulence, weight loss HIV patients have more severe illness with wasting	Modified acid-fast stain	Trimethoprim-sulfamethoxazole

STEC = Shiga toxin-producing *Escherichia coli*.

Posttransplantation Infections

Diagnosis

Within the first 4 postoperative weeks, the most common infections in transplant recipients are the same as those that develop postoperatively in patients who have undergone non–transplant-related surgery:

- bacterial wound infection
- *Clostridium difficile*–associated diarrhea
- central line–associated bloodstream infection
- CAUTI
- health care–related pneumonia

CMV frequently occurs after the first month of transplantation, occurring most often in the setting of a CMV-negative transplant recipient with an organ from a CMV-positive donor. CMV is associated with:

- an increased risk for renal graft failure
- GI perforations and significant bleeding
- CMV-related pneumonia and respiratory failure
- EBV, polyomavirus BK, polyomavirus JC, and hepatitis B and C reactivation

Polyomavirus JC infection may cause progressive multifocal leukoencephalopathy. EBV infection is found in almost all patients with posttransplantation lymphoproliferative disease.

Kidney transplant patients with polyomavirus BK infection may develop nephropathy, organ rejection, or ureteral strictures. HSCT recipients with BK infection may develop hemorrhagic cystitis.

Therapy

During neutropenia, prophylaxis usually includes an antifungal such as voriconazole. Trimethoprim-sulfamethoxazole is the preferred agent for *Pneumocystis* and *Toxoplasma* prophylaxis. Prophylaxis with valganciclovir is appropriate for transplant recipients at risk for or with known CMV infection. Patients receiving adequate anti-CMV prophylaxis have a lower incidence of polyomavirus BK and EBV reactivation. The only known effective treatment for polyomavirus JC infection is to reverse immunosuppressive therapy.

◆ DON'T BE TRICKED

- If donor and recipient are both seronegative for CMV, preventive therapy need not be given.
- Patients undergoing HSCT need revaccination with complete series after immune system reconstitution.
- Live vaccines are typically contraindicated for patients receiving immunosuppression after transplantation.

❖ Test Yourself

A 63-year-old woman is evaluated for fever and hypotension 4 days after kidney-pancreas transplantation surgery. She has erythema and tenderness around the surgical wound.

ANSWER: Select staphylococcal wound infection as the most likely cause of an early infection in a transplant patient.

Catheter-Associated UTIs

Prevention

CAUTIs can be prevented by using a urinary catheter only when indicated and removing it as soon as possible. Maintain a closed catheter system at all times, and keep the catheter bag below the level of the bladder.

Diagnosis

Typical signs and symptoms of UTI may not be present in a catheterized patient. Obtain urine cultures in patients with symptoms attributable to the urinary tract or in patients with altered mental status or fever.

Therapy

If a CAUTI is suspected, management includes catheter removal and urine culture. In general, cefotaxime, ceftriaxone, ciprofloxacin, or levofloxacin is used for suspected gram-negative infection and vancomycin for suspected staphylococcal or enterococcal infection. When culture data are available, therapy should be adjusted to the narrowest coverage spectrum possible.

◆ **DON'T BE TRICKED**

- In patients with a urinary catheter, do not obtain routine urinalysis or cultures and do not treat asymptomatic bacteriuria.
- Don't treat asymptomatic candiduria with antifungal therapy; do remove the catheter.

Hospital-Acquired and Ventilator-Associated Pneumonia

Prevention

HAP is defined as occurring ≥48 hours after admission. VAP, a subset of HAP, is defined as occurring >48 hours after endotracheal intubation.

Procedures to reduce VAP include:

- following daily weaning protocols for timely extubation
- keeping the head of the bed elevated >30 degrees
- avoiding nasal intubation and nasogastric tubes
- using chlorhexidine mouth rinse and subglottic suction catheters

Diagnosis

The diagnosis of HAP is based on a new or progressive radiographic infiltrate plus clinical signs of pneumonia (fever, purulent sputum, leukocytosis, hypoxemia).

Therapy

Antibiotic selection is based on the risk for multi–drug-resistant organisms (MDRO). Risk factors for MDRO are:

- current hospitalization ≥5 days
- admission from a health care–related facility
- recent antibiotic therapy
- immunosuppression

Choose ceftriaxone or levofloxacin for patients with no MDRO risk factors. If MDRO risk factors are present, select vancomycin plus imipenem, cefepime, or ceftazidime. Narrow the empiric therapy based on culture results.

◆ **DON'T BE TRICKED**

- Do not delay empiric antibiotic therapy to perform diagnostic studies.

❖ **Test Yourself**

A 78-year-old woman was admitted from a skilled nursing facility for treatment of a hip fracture. Two days after admission, she develops a temperature of 38.3 °C (100.9 °F) and a cough. A chest x-ray shows a new left lower lobe infiltrate.

ANSWER: Diagnose HAP and prescribe vancomycin and ceftazidime.

Clostridium difficile Antibiotic-Associated Diarrhea

Diagnosis

C. difficile antibiotic-associated colitis is produced by two toxins, A and B. The most important risk factors are antibiotic use and hospitalization, but community-acquired infection is becoming increasingly common. EIAs to detect the toxins are specific, but sensitivity using a single stool sample is 75% to 85%. PCR assays to detect the genes responsible for production of toxins A and B are more sensitive than EIAs.

Management of *C. difficile* infection is based upon disease severity. Severe disease is defined by any one of the following:

- leukocyte count >15,000/μL
- serum creatinine level ≥1.5 times baseline level
- age >60 years

Hospitalized patients with known or suspected illness should be placed under contact isolation.

Therapy

Discontinue the offending antibiotic.

Treat mild to moderate *C. difficile* infection with oral metronidazole. Treat severe infection with oral vancomycin. Severe disease associated with ileus may benefit from the addition of IV metronidazole and vancomycin enemas; select colectomy for very severe or complicated disease (e.g., toxic megacolon or severe sepsis).

A first recurrence is treated in the same way as the initial episode, based on disease severity. A second relapse is treated with oral vancomycin given as a prolonged taper or pulse therapy for >6 weeks. Fecal microbiota transplant is used for patients with multiple relapses. Fidaxomicin, a nonabsorbable macrolide, is an alternative to vancomycin.

◆ **DON'T BE TRICKED**

- Do not obtain stool cultures and cell culture cytotoxicity assays.

Catheter-Related Intravascular Infection

Prevention

Use of IV catheters should be reserved for patients with a proven need, and the catheter should be removed as soon as clinically possible.

STUDY TABLE: Prevention Strategies for Catheter-Related Intravascular Infections	
Choose...	Do not choose...
Maximum sterile barrier precautions and chlorhexidine for skin decontamination during catheter insertion	Femoral artery insertion
Antibiotic-coated catheters and dressings	Routine replacement of central venous catheters
Catheter-care teams	Routine dressing changes

Diagnosis

Consider catheter-related infection in any patient with fever and a central venous catheter. Purulence and cellulitis around the catheter site are specific, but not sensitive, for catheter-related infection. Begin the evaluation of suspected infection by removing the catheter and culturing the catheter tip.

- If the tip is culture positive and associated with fever or a positive peripheral blood culture, the diagnosis is catheter-related infection.
- A negative central blood culture has a good negative predictive value. However, a positive central or peripheral blood culture alone requires clinical interpretation to differentiate infection from colonization.

Therapy

Remove the catheter in the following situations:

- tunnel or pocket infection
- sepsis
- metastatic infection (septic thrombosis, endocarditis, or osteomyelitis)
- *Staphylococcus aureus* or gram-negative bacteremia
- fungemia

IV catheter-related *S. aureus* bacteremia that clears within 72 hours without evidence of endocarditis or metastatic infection may be treated with 10-14 days of parenteral antibiotics. Persistent *S. aureus* bacteremia >72 hours after the start of appropriate antimicrobial therapy suggests a complicated infection. Evaluate with echocardiography, preferably transesophageal. Treat complicated *S. aureus* bacteremia for 4-6 weeks.

- MSSA is treated with either nafcillin (or oxacillin) or cefazolin
- MRSA is treated with vancomycin or daptomycin

Empiric treatment for neutropenic or septic patients should cover gram-negative organisms including *Pseudomonas*. Narrow antibiotic selection based on culture and susceptibility results.

◆ DON'T BE TRICKED
- A normal TTE does not exclude endocarditis in the setting of *S. aureus* bacteremia.
- Catheter removal is not required for transient coagulase-negative staphylococcal bacteremia.

HIV Infection

Screening

Routinely screen all Americans aged 13 to 64 years for HIV infection. One-time testing is reasonable in persons at low risk, but persons engaged in high-risk behavior should be tested annually.

Screen using the following protocol:

- a fourth-generation combination immunoassay that includes an EIA for HIV antibody (HIV-1 and HIV-2) and HIV p24 antigen
- if combination immunoassay is positive, obtain immunoassay to differentiate HIV-1 from HIV-2
- detection of either HIV-1 or HIV-2 antibody confirms that diagnosis
- if differentiation immunoassay is inconclusive for either HIV-1 or HIV-2, obtain NAAT
- a positive NAAT in the setting of a negative antibody test indicates acute HIV infection

◆ DON'T BE TRICKED

- If a test is positive on the initial antigen/antibody combination immunoassay but negative on the antibody differentiation immunoassay and NAAT testing, the initial test result was a false-positive test.

Diagnosis

Diagnose primary HIV infection (initial acute HIV infection) for a febrile illness that occurs within several weeks of a potential HIV exposure. Additional symptoms may include fatigue, lymphadenopathy, pharyngitis, rash, and/or headache. During the "window period" before seroconversion, the diagnosis of primary infection is confirmed with a positive NAAT test.

Test for HIV in any patient with signs or symptoms of immunologic dysfunction, weight loss, generalized lymphadenopathy, fever and night sweats of more than 2 weeks' duration, or severe aphthous ulcers.

Certain diagnoses warrant HIV testing:

- severe or treatment-refractory HSV infection
- oral thrush or esophageal candidiasis
- *Pneumocystis jirovecii* pneumonitis
- cryptococcal meningitis
- disseminated mycobacterial infection
- CMV retinitis or GI disease
- toxoplasmosis
- severe seborrheic dermatitis or new or severe psoriasis
- recurrent herpes zoster infections

Rapid HIV tests, which give results from salivary samples in about 20 minutes, are available for clinic and home use. Positive tests must be confirmed using the same HIV testing as described above.

The HIV RNA viral load is the most reliable marker for predicting the long-term risk of progression to AIDS or death. The CD4 cell count is the most reliable marker for the current risk of opportunistic complications.

AIDS is diagnosed in an HIV-infected person if the CD4 cell count is <200/µL or if an AIDS-defining illness is present.

Therapy

Consider initiating therapy in all patients motivated to start life-long medication, regardless of CD4 cell count.

Current recommendations for initial HIV treatment, if the patient is not pregnant, include use of tenofovir and emtricitabine as the dual nucleoside reverse transcriptase inhibitor (RTI) "backbone." Options for a third agent to complete the regimen include:

- ritonavir-boosted protease inhibitors atazanavir or darunavir
- integrase inhibitors raltegravir, dolutegravir, or cobicistat-boosted elvitegravir
- nonnucleoside RTI efavirenz

Do resistance testing on all patients before starting ART. Check the viral load 4 weeks after ART is initiated or changed. Viral load should fall quickly and progressively and reach undetectable levels within a few months. Viral loads should remain undetectable while the patient is receiving ART. Persistent detectable levels of virus should be considered as treatment failure and resistance testing should be repeated.

◆ DON'T BE TRICKED

- Resistance testing should be done while the patient is still receiving the ineffective regimen.

All pregnant women should be tested for HIV infection and, if positive, treated. Preferred antiretroviral regimens combine two nucleosides (tenofovir-emtricitabine, abacavir-lamivudine, or zidovudine-lamivudine) with a protease inhibitor (either lopinavir or atazanavir, both with ritonavir boosting).

◆ DON'T BE TRICKED

- Breast feeding should be avoided in women with HIV infection.

Antiretroviral agents must be started as soon as possible after occupational (needle stick) exposure; the standard course is 3 drugs (typically tenofovir, emtricitabine, and raltegravir) for 4 weeks. Testing for HIV should be done immediately and at 6 weeks, 12 weeks, and 6 months.

Prophylaxis for nonoccupational exposures is recommended for persons presenting with an exposure within the previous 72 hours. Select preexposure prophylaxis in certain populations with ongoing high risk of infection, such as sexual partners of infected persons.

IRIS is an intense inflammatory disorder associated with paradoxical worsening of preexisting infectious processes following the initiation of ART therapy. IRIS may occur in one of two ways:

- a preexisting subclinical infection is "unmasked" by immune system recovery
- a previously treated infection may "paradoxically" recur because of the presence of persistent antigens

The most important therapy for IRIS is treatment of the underlying infection. Glucocorticoids and/or NSAIDs are sometimes added to decrease the inflammatory response.

◆ DON'T BE TRICKED

- Do not stop ART in the setting of IRIS.

STUDY TABLE: Side Effects and Precautions of Commonly Used Antiretroviral Drugs

Drug	Side Effects	Precautions
Emtricitabine	Well-tolerated, minimal toxicity	Lactic acidosis, severe hepatomegaly
	Skin discoloration or hyperpigmentation	Acute exacerbations of hepatitis B when discontinued
Tenofovir	Well-tolerated	Lactic acidosis, severe hepatomegaly
	Nausea, diarrhea, asthenia, headache	Acute exacerbations of hepatitis B when discontinued
	May cause kidney injury (Fanconi syndrome), decreased bone density	Avoid combining with didanosine
Efavirenz	CNS side effects that may diminish after 2 weeks (such as dizziness, insomnia, sleep disturbance, mood or psychiatric alterations, vivid dreams, hallucinations), rash	Avoid with pregnancy
		CYP3A4 drug interactions (including protease inhibitors)
Darunavir	Rash, diarrhea, nausea, LFT elevations, hepatotoxicity, hyperlipidemia, hyperglycemia	Substrate and inhibitor of CYP3A
		Caution with sulfonamide hypersensitivity
Atazanavir	Nausea, abdominal pain, headache, prolonged PR interval	Caution with conduction abnormalities
	Jaundice or scleral icterus due to indirect hyperbilirubinemia	CYP3A4 drug interactions

(Continued on next page)

STUDY TABLE: Side Effects and Precautions of Commonly Used Antiretroviral Drugs (*Continued*)

Drug	Side Effects	Precautions
Ritonavir	Paresthesia, nausea, vomiting, headache, diarrhea, insulin resistance, lipodystrophy, hyperlipidemia, hepatic dysfunction	Drug interactions
		Substrate and potent inhibitor of CYP3A4
	Liquid has unpleasant taste	
Raltegravir (Isentress)	Well-tolerated	
	Nausea, diarrhea, headache, elevated creatine phosphokinase	
	Rash possible (including hypersensitivity reactions, SJS, TEN)	

STUDY TABLE: Prophylaxis for Patients with HIV Infection

Preventable Condition	When	Agent
P. jirovecii pneumonitis	CD4 cell count <200/μL	Trimethoprim-sulfamethoxazole
Toxoplasmosis	CD4 cell count <100/μL and positive IgG for toxoplasmosis	Trimethoprim-sulfamethoxazole
MAC infection	CD4 cell count <50/μL	Azithromycin
Active or latent TB	TST ≥5 mm or positive IGRA	Isoniazid for 9 months
Influenza	Annual vaccination for all HIV-infected patients	Killed influenza vaccine
Pneumococcal pneumonia	Upon diagnosis	Pneumococcal conjugate vaccine (PCV-13) and pneumococcal polysaccharide vaccine (PPSV-23)
		See General Internal Medicine, Screening and Prevention
Hepatitis A and B	Completion of series	Hepatitis A and B vaccine

Discontinue *P. jirovecii*, toxoplasmosis, and *Mycobacterium avium* complex prophylaxis when ART therapy produces CD4 cell counts >200/μL and a negative viral load for at least 3 months.

◆ **DON'T BE TRICKED**

- Live vaccines are contraindicated in immunocompromised patients but the MMR and varicella vaccines can be given to HIV patients with CD4 cell counts >200/μL.

❖ **Test Yourself**

A 29-year-old man with recently diagnosed pulmonary TB is found to have late-stage HIV infection. Three-drug ART and four-drug TB therapy is initiated, and he quickly improves. Four weeks later, he develops recurrent fever and neck pain and swelling. He has bilateral tender cervical lymphadenopathy.

ANSWER: Diagnose IRIS. Continue ART and antituberculous drugs.

Protease Inhibitor Fat Dystrophy: Increase in subcutaneous fat at back of neck, creating a "buffalo hump" in a patient with HIV taking a protease inhibitor.

Pneumocystis jirovecii Pneumonia

Prevention

Select prophylaxis (usually with trimethoprim-sulfamethoxazole) for patients with HIV infection and a CD4 cell count <200/μL. In patients treated with HIV antiretroviral medications, discontinue prophylaxis in patients who maintain a CD4 cell count >200/μL for 3 months.

Diagnosis

In patients infected with HIV, *P. jirovecii* pneumonia is gradual in onset and characterized by nonproductive cough and progressive dyspnea. Other findings may include:

- fever, chills, night sweats, and weight loss
- tachypnea and crackles on lung examination
- chest x-ray that may show consolidation or diffuse infiltrates

The diagnosis is established by immunofluorescent monoclonal antibody stain or silver stain examination of induced sputum or a bronchoscopic sample showing characteristic cysts.

◆ DON'T BE TRICKED

- The most common cause of a pneumothorax in a patient with AIDS is *P. jirovecii* pneumonia.
- *P. jirovecii* pneumonia can occur in patients not infected with HIV, typically in association with immunosuppressant drug therapy.

STUDY TABLE: Classification of *P. jirovecii* Pneumonia	
ABG Findings (Ambient Air)	**Classification**
A-a <35 mm Hg and PO_2 >70 mm Hg	Mild
A-a 35-45 mm Hg and PO_2 >70 mm Hg	Moderate
A-a >45 mm Hg and PO_2 <70 mm Hg	Severe

Therapy

Select 3 weeks of therapy with:

- oral trimethoprim-sulfamethoxazole for mild to moderate pneumonia
- IV trimethoprim-sulfamethoxazole for moderate to severe pneumonia
- glucocorticoids within 72 hours for A-a ≥35 mm Hg or arterial PO_2 <70 mm Hg
- IV pentamidine or IV clindamycin plus oral primaquine for patients with sulfa allergy

❖ Test Yourself

A 45-year-old man with HIV and a CD4 cell count of 100/μL presents with 3 weeks of dry cough and progressive dyspnea on exertion, now present at rest. On examination, his temperature is 38.3 °C (100.9 °F) and PO_2 is 67 mm Hg on ambient air. His chest x-ray shows diffuse bilateral infiltrates.

ANSWER: Initiate empiric treatment with IV trimethoprim-sulfamethoxazole and glucocorticoids for presumed *P. jirovecii* pneumonia; begin diagnostic evaluation.

Toxoplasmosis

Diagnosis

Toxoplasmosis is caused by an intracellular protozoan parasite, *Toxoplasma gondii*. Immunocompetent persons with primary infection are usually asymptomatic, but latent infection can persist, and reactivation of the infection is a risk if the person becomes immunocompromised. Look for:

- encephalitis, chorioretinitis, or pneumonitis in immunocompromised patients
- any focal neurologic syndrome, acute or subacute
- mononucleosis-like syndrome

Select IgM and IgG serologic testing in patients with suspected toxoplasmosis and brain MRI or head CT for neurologic signs and symptoms. Typical findings on imaging include multiple ring-enhancing lesions.

STUDY TABLE: Differential Diagnosis of Cerebral Toxoplasmosis in Immunocompromised Patients

Diagnosis	Characteristics
Lymphoma (primary CNS, B-cell lymphoma)	Often a solitary lesion is located in the periventricular or periependymal area or in the corpus callosum
	Neither clinical nor neuroradiologic findings reliably distinguish lymphoma from toxoplasmosis
	Brain biopsy is diagnostic
Progressive multifocal leukoencephalopathy	Dementia is often the presenting symptom
	CD4 cell counts are usually <50/µL and PCR of CSF can show JCV
	Brain biopsy is diagnostic
Cryptococcus neoformans	Headache, fever, and altered mental status are present
	CD4 cell counts are usually <100/µL
	CSF culture for *Cryptococcus* or cryptococcal antigen tests on CSF and serum are diagnostic; elevated CSF opening pressure is characteristic
Mycobacterium tuberculosis	Basilar meningitis with cranial nerve abnormalities
	Culture and PCR of CSF are diagnostic
CMV	Diffuse encephalitis and fever are characteristic
	CD4 cell counts are <50/µL; CSF PCR is positive, and brain biopsy is diagnostic
Neurosyphilis	Atypical and accelerated neurosyphilis is seen in HIV infection
	Positive serum RPR or VDRL test, FTA-ABS, and MHA-TP; positive CSF VDRL

JCV = John Cunningham virus.

Therapy

Select empiric treatment with sulfadiazine, pyrimethamine, and folic acid in patients with multiple ring-enhancing lesions, positive *T. gondii* serologic test results (IgG), and immune suppression (CD4 cell count <200/µL). Treat patients with persistent immunosuppression indefinitely. Biopsy lesions that fail to respond to 2 weeks of empiric therapy.

Influenza Virus

Prevention

See General Internal Medicine, Screening and Prevention. For institutional outbreaks, vaccinate staff members and residents not already immunized and give chemoprophylaxis with zanamivir or oseltamivir for at least 2 weeks following immunization.

Intracerebral Toxoplasmosis: MRI showing a single ring-enhancing brain lesion associated with edema consistent with toxoplasmosis. Most patients with AIDS with cerebral toxoplasmosis have multiple ring-enhancing brain lesions.

◆ **DON'T BE TRICKED**

- Do not administer live attenuated influenza vaccine to persons who have close contact with immunocompromised patients.

Diagnosis

During November through April, look for acute onset of high fever, headache, fatigue, nonproductive cough, sore throat, nasal congestion, rhinorrhea, and myalgia. Use diagnostic testing (rapid antigen tests) in patients for whom results would influence management (e.g., initiating antiviral treatment, performing other diagnostic testing, or inpatient infection control measures). The most common complications of influenza are primary influenza pneumonia and secondary bacterial pneumonia (*Streptococcus pneumoniae, Staphylococcus aureus*).

Therapy

Treat all hospitalized patients with confirmed infection and outpatients at high risk for severe disease. Select zanamivir or oseltamivir, both of which are active against influenza A and B. Peramivir is available for IV administration.

Risk factors for severe disease:

- immunosuppression (highest risk)
- chronic pulmonary disease (highest risk)
- age >64 years
- pregnancy (or delivery within 2 weeks)
- diabetes
- significant cardiovascular, kidney, liver, or hematologic disease
- BMI ≥40

◆ DON'T BE TRICKED

- Do not administer amantadine or rimantadine to prevent or treat influenza virus because of the high rate of resistance.
- Zanamivir (inhaled) has been associated with bronchospasm and is contraindicated in patients with pulmonary or cardiovascular disease.

❖ Test Yourself

A 68-year-old woman with diabetes is admitted to the hospital in November with the acute onset of fever, chills, nonproductive cough, and fatigue. Her 6-year-old granddaughter has had similar symptoms for 3 days.

ANSWER: Diagnose probable influenza and start oseltamivir immediately.

Epstein-Barr Virus

Diagnosis

EBV is the primary agent of infectious mononucleosis and is associated with the development of B-cell lymphoma, T-cell lymphoma, Hodgkin lymphoma, and nasopharyngeal carcinoma. Another EBV manifestation is oral hairy leukoplakia that characteristically affects the lateral portions of the tongue as white corrugated painless plaques. Oral hairy leukoplakia is most commonly associated with underlying HIV infection.

Typical symptoms in patients with acute infectious mononucleosis include:

- severe fatigue, headache, and sore throat
- fever associated with posterior cervical lymphadenopathy
- splenomegaly
- reactive lymphocytosis

Consider EBV infection in all patients with aseptic meningitis or encephalitis, hepatitis, hemolytic anemia, and thrombocytopenia.

◆ DON'T BE TRICKED

- The morbilliform rash appearing in patients with infectious mononucleosis following the administration of ampicillin is not an allergic reaction; patients can subsequently use ampicillin without rash recurrence.

Select a Monospot test (heterophile antibody test), which is specific but not very sensitive early in disease. If the Monospot test is negative, repeat in 2 weeks or select EBV serology. Infectious mononucleosis syndrome can also be caused by CMV or HIV infection; it is often not possible to make a clinical diagnosis and serologic testing is necessary.

STUDY TABLE: Epstein-Barr Virus Serology	
Condition	**Antibody**
Acute primary infection	Elevated VCA IgM, VCA IgG, and EA IgG
	Low or undetectable EBNA-1 IgG
Past infection	Undetectable VCA IgM and EA IgG
	Elevated VCA IgG and EBNA-1 IgG

EA = early antigen; EBNA = Epstein-Barr nuclear antigen; VCA = viral capsid antigen.

Therapy

Supportive care is typically sufficient. Select glucocorticoids only if airway obstruction or other life-threatening conditions such as hemolytic anemia is present.

◆ DON'T BE TRICKED

- Do not prescribe antiviral drugs for treatment of infectious mononucleosis.

❖ Test Yourself

An 18-year-old female soccer player has malaise, anorexia, and a sore throat for 3 days. She has exudative pharyngitis, tender anterior and posterior cervical lymph nodes, and fullness in her left upper abdominal quadrant. Leukocyte count is 8500/µL with moderate atypical lymphocytes.

ANSWER: The patient has infectious mononucleosis and should avoid contact sports because of the risk of splenic rupture in the setting of splenomegaly.

Oral Hairy Leukoplakia: A patient with HIV with oral hairy leukoplakia, white corrugated painless plaques on the lateral tongue, is shown.

Nephrology

Glomerular Filtration Rate

At high levels of GFR, small changes in the serum creatinine may reflect large changes in GFR. At low levels of GFR, large changes in the serum creatinine reflect relatively smaller changes in GFR.

In patients who become functionally anephric, the serum creatinine increases 1.0 to 1.5 mg/dL per day.

Three estimation equations are commonly used: the Cockcroft-Gault equation, the Modification of Diet in Renal Disease (MDRD) study equation, and the Chronic Kidney Disease Epidemiology (CKD-EPI) Collaboration equation.

- MDRD study performs best when GFR is <60 mL/min/1.73 m^2
- CKD-EPI equation performs better at near-normal GFR values
- Cockroft-Gault is the least accurate

For drug-dosing purposes, the Cockcroft-Gault equation functions as well as the CKD-EPI and MDRD study equations.

Conditions that decrease kidney perfusion, such as dehydration or HF, are associated with increased reabsorption of BUN in the proximal tubules and a disproportionate increase in the BUN-creatinine ratio, typically to 20:1 or higher.

◆ **DON'T BE TRICKED**
- A reduction or loss of muscle mass due to advanced age, liver failure, or malnutrition may cause a disproportionately low serum creatinine concentration, which results in overestimation of the GFR.
- When the MDRD study equation is used to estimate GFR, higher levels of GFR are reported only as >60 mL/min/1.73 m^2, but this guarantees an absence of structural kidney disease.

Urinalysis

Proteinuria

Albumin is the only protein that is detected on dipstick urinalysis.

The sulfosalicylic acid (SSA) test can detect the presence of albumin and other proteins such as urine light chains or immunoglobulins but is not widely used. Protein detected by urine dipstick should always be quantified with either a 24-hour urine collection or protein or albumin to creatinine ratio on random urine samples. Levels of proteinuria are diagnostically helpful:

- >150 mg/g but <200 mg/g = tubulointerstitial disease or glomerular disease
- >3500 mg/g = glomerular disease

The albumin-creatinine ratio measures only albumin in the urine and is used to evaluate diabetic kidney disease:

- 30 to 300 mg/g, previously termed *microalbuminuria*, is now referred to as *moderately increased albuminuria*.
- >300 mg/g, previously known as *macroalbuminuria or overt proteinuria*, is now referred to as *severely increased albuminuria*.

A protein-creatinine ratio can be used to measure proteinuria (abnormal protein-creatinine ratio defined as >0.2 mg/mg).

Proteinuria is a marker of renal parenchymal and glomerular disease and an independent predictor of progressive kidney disease, cardiovascular disease, and peripheral vascular disease.

◆ **DON'T BE TRICKED**

- Dipstick urinalysis does not detect immunoglobulin light chains associated with multiple myeloma.
- Positional (orthostatic) proteinuria, a benign cause of isolated proteinuria, is diagnosed by obtaining split daytime (standing) and nighttime (supine) urine collections.

Hematuria

Hematuria is classified as glomerular and extraglomerular. Erythrocyte casts and dysmorphic erythrocytes (acanthocytes, RBCs with "Mickey Mouse" ears) in the urine indicate glomerular disease. Coexisting proteinuria supports glomerular causes of hematuria, even in the absence of casts.

Hematuria with preserved erythrocyte morphology in the urine, often without proteinuria or casts, is consistent with extraglomerular bleeding (GU cancer, kidney stones, trauma, infection, and medications) and requires additional diagnostic studies to locate the extraglomerular source. The proper evaluation is directed by findings in the history and physical examination.

Consider the following sequenced evaluation of extraglomerular bleeding:

- urinalysis or urine culture to exclude infection, and if normal . . .
- noncontrast helical CT to detect calculi and contrast CT to detect renal cell carcinoma and if normal . . .
- urine cytology, then stop evaluation if normal and patient is at low risk for malignancy (age <50 years, no other risk factors), otherwise . . .
- cystoscopy for patients with positive urine cytology, aged >50 years, or if risk factors for malignancy are present (cigarette smoking, analgesic abuse, benzene exposure, or voiding abnormalities)

◆ **DON'T BE TRICKED**

- Evaluate hematuria even in patients taking anticoagulants.

Leukocytes and Other Formed Elements

Leukocytes in the urine may be caused by glomerular or tubulointerstitial inflammation, infection, or an allergic reaction.

Remember:

- sterile pyuria (pyuria and a negative urine culture) suggests *Mycobacterium tuberculosis*, interstitial cystitis, or interstitial nephritis
- eosinophiluria suggests AIN, postinfectious GN, atheroembolic disease of the kidney, septic emboli, or small-vessel vasculitis

◆ **DON'T BE TRICKED**

- Absence of eosinophiluria does not rule out AIN, postinfectious GN, atheroembolic disease of the kidney, septic emboli, or small-vessel vasculitis.

Patients with hemolysis and rhabdomyolysis test positive for blood on dipstick urinalysis in the absence of intact erythrocytes on urine microscopy. Urine lipids and fat are almost always associated with heavy proteinuria or the nephrotic syndrome. These may appear as free lipid droplets, round or oval fat bodies, or fatty casts.

Casts are cylindrical aggregates of Tamm-Horsfall mucoproteins that trap the intraluminal contents and appear in the urine.

Different types of casts are associated with specific disorders:

- erythrocyte casts indicate glomerular disease
- leukocyte casts indicate inflammation or infection of the renal parenchyma
- muddy brown casts are associated with ATN
- broad casts are associated with CKD

Imaging

The 3 main modalities of kidney imaging are ultrasonography, CT, and MRI.

Ultrasonography indications:

- assess kidney size and cortical thickness (increased echogenicity implies parenchymal disease)
- renal cysts and tumors
- obstruction and hydronephrosis
- bladder size, postvoid residual, and the prostate in bladder outlet obstruction

CT indications:

- Noncontrast abdominal helical CT for nephrolithiasis
- Contrast abdominal CT for renal tumors and cysts
- CT urography for unexplained urologic/nonglomerular hematuria

MRI indications:

- when radiocontrast agents must be avoided
- renal masses, cysts, and renal vein thrombosis
- MRA with gadolinium contrast for renal artery stenosis (risk of nephrogenic SSc in patients with CKD)

Kidney Biopsy

Kidney biopsy should be considered in patients with:

- glomerular hematuria
- severely increased albuminuria
- acute or CKD of unclear etiology
- kidney transplant dysfunction or monitoring

Common contraindications to kidney biopsy include bleeding diatheses, severe anemia, UTI, hydronephrosis, uncontrolled hypertension, renal tumor, and atrophic kidneys.

Hyponatremia

Diagnosis

The first step in assessing low serum sodium is determining if true hyponatremia is present by measuring serum osmolality. Pseudohyponatremia is a laboratory artifact caused by severe hyperlipidemia or hyperproteinemia. In pseudohyponatremia, the measured osmolality is normal.

If true hyponatremia exists, classify it as hyperosmolar or hypo-osmolar.

Hypertonic (hyperosmolar) hyponatremia is caused by the presence of an osmotically active substance such as:

- glucose (most common)
- BUN
- alcohols

- mannitol
- sorbitol
- glycine (bladder irrigation during urological procedures)

Hypo-osmolar hyponatremia is the most common form of hyponatremia and is further classified based on the patient's volume status.

STUDY TABLE: Evaluating Hypo-osmolar Hyponatremia		
Volume Status	**Laboratory Studies**	**Differential Diagnosis**
Hypovolemia (hypotension, tachycardia)	Spot urine sodium <20 mEq/L BUN/creatinine >20:1	GI or kidney fluid losses, dehydration, mineralocorticoid insufficiency
Hypervolemia (edema, ascites)	Spot urine sodium <20 mEq/L (HF and cirrhosis in absence of diuretic therapy) Spot urine sodium >20 mEq/L (acute and chronic kidney failure)	HF, cirrhosis, kidney failure
Euvolemia (normal volume)	Spot urine sodium >20 mEq/L Urine osmolality usually >300 mOsm/L	SIADH, hypothyroidism, glucocorticoid deficiency (Addison disease)
Euvolemia (normal volume)	Spot urine sodium >20 mEq/L Urine osmolality 50-100 mOsm/L	Compulsive water drinking
SIADH = syndrome of inappropriate antidiuretic hormone secretion.		

Causes of SIADH include malignancy (SCLC), intracranial pathology, and pulmonary diseases, especially those that increase intrathoracic pressure and decreased venous return to the heart. Many medications can cause SIADH, including thiazides, SSRIs, tricyclic antidepressants, narcotics, phenothiazines, and carbamazepine.

Cerebral salt wasting syndrome causes hypo-osmolar hyponatremia and laboratory parameters exactly like that of SIADH. However, cerebral salt wasting syndrome is associated with hypovolemia, hypotension, and a neurosurgical procedure or SAH within the previous 10 days.

◆ **DON'T BE TRICKED**

- Do not miss adrenal insufficiency as a cause of hypo-osmolar hyponatremia.

Therapy

IV volume replacement with normal saline is indicated for hyponatremia due to volume depletion, including hyponatremia from thiazide diuretics and cerebral salt wasting syndrome.

Treatment of acute symptomatic hyponatremia includes 3% saline to increase serum sodium concentration by 1 to 2 mEq/L per hour to a total increase of 4 to 6 mEq/L within the first 6 hours. Should the serum sodium concentration be overcorrected, administer desmopressin and IV 5% dextrose in water. Central pontine myelinolysis (osmotic demyelination syndrome) may occur if hyponatremia is corrected too rapidly.

Fluid restriction is used initially for asymptomatic or minimally symptomatic outpatients with SIADH. Patients who do not respond to water restriction can be treated with loop diuretics combined with oral salt supplementation. Demeclocycline can also be used for outpatients who do not respond to fluid restriction. The IV V_1 and V_2 receptor antagonist conivaptan and the oral V_2 receptor antagonist tolvaptan (vaptans) are approved for treatment of euvolemic and hypervolemic hyponatremia. Oral tolvaptan should be reserved for the management of serum sodium concentration <120 mEq/L and persistent SIADH that has failed water restriction and/or oral furosemide and salt tablets. No data show the vaptans are associated with improved patient outcomes compared with conventional therapy, and the vaptans are very expensive.

◆ **DON'T BE TRICKED**

- Vaptan agents should not be used to treat hypovolemic hyponatremia, or acute symptomatic hyponatremia.

A 53-year-old man has a 3-week history of increasing weakness and anorexia. On physical examination, BP is 130/70 mm Hg, and pulse rate is 80/min without orthostatic changes. Laboratory studies: BUN, 12 mg/dL; serum creatinine, 0.8 mg/dL; serum sodium, 123 mEq/L; potassium, 3.4 mEq/L; chloride, 91 mEq/L; bicarbonate, 22 mEq/L; and urine sodium, 110 mEq/L.

ANSWER: The probable diagnosis is SIADH. Measure serum osmolality to confirm the presence of hypo-osmolality. If hypo-osmolality is present, consider SIADH (most common), thyroid disease, and adrenal insufficiency.

Hypernatremia

Diagnosis

Hypernatremia is serum sodium >145 mEq/L. Severe hypernatremia indicates a defective thirst mechanism, inadequate access to water (older patients in nursing homes), a kidney concentrating defect (DI, most commonly due to lithium), and/or impaired pituitary secretion of ADH (e.g., sarcoidosis). Most commonly, hypernatremia is due to loss of hypotonic fluids (GI, kidney, skin) with inadequate water replacement.

Therapy

Therapy is directed at sodium chloride replacement, free water replacement, and correction of the underlying problem leading to hypotonic fluid loss. The water deficit is calculated as $[(Na^+ - 140)/140] \times TBW$ where $TBW = 0.5 \times weight$ (kg) in women or $0.6 \times weight$ (kg) in men.

In volume depletion, fluid resuscitation with normal saline should precede correction of the water deficit with hypotonic fluids. Correct water deficit over 48 to 72 hours. Neurogenic (central) DI is treated with intranasal desmopressin.

Hyperkalemia

Diagnosis

The most common causes of hyperkalemia include:

- hyporeninemic hypoaldosteronism
- acute and chronic kidney failure
- low urine flow states
- medications (ACE inhibitors, ARBs, potassium-sparing diuretics, pentamidine, trimethoprim-sulfamethoxazole, and cyclosporine)
- potassium shifts (rhabdomyolysis, hemolysis, hyperosmolality, insulin deficiency, β-adrenergic blockade, and metabolic acidosis)

The earliest ECG changes of hyperkalemia are peaking of the T waves and shortening of the QT interval. As hyperkalemia progresses, there is prolongation of the PR interval, loss of P waves, and eventual widening of the QRS complexes with a "sine-wave" pattern that can precede asystole.

Pseudohyperkalemia is an in vitro phenomenon caused by the mechanical release of potassium from cells during phlebotomy or specimen processing or in the setting of marked leukocytosis and thrombocytosis. Measure the plasma potassium concentration to confirm the diagnosis of pseudohyperkalemia.

◆ **DON'T BE TRICKED**

- Significant hyperkalemia associated with a normal ECG suggests pseudohyperkalemia.

Therapy

If hyperkalemia is associated with ECG changes or arrhythmias, begin IV calcium gluconate to stabilize the myocardium and shift potassium inside the cells with insulin and glucose or inhaled β-adrenergic agonists, and by removing potassium from the body with sodium polystyrene sulfonate, loop diuretics (particularly if volume is overloaded), and dietary potassium restriction. Hemodialysis is often needed to correct life-threatening hyperkalemia but is never the "first step" because of the time delay in initiating dialysis.

◆ **DON'T BE TRICKED**

- Absolute levels of potassium cannot reliably determine if a life-threatening condition exists. Only ECG can assess the effect of hyperkalemia on the cardiac membrane.

Characteristics of Hyperkalemia: ECG showing flattened P waves; prolonged PR interval; widened QRS; and tall, peaked T waves characteristic of hyperkalemia.

Hypokalemia

Diagnosis

The most common causes of hypokalemia are vomiting and diarrhea and use of diuretics. Urine potassium loss >20 mEq/24 h, a spot urine potassium >20 mEq/L, or a spot urine potassium-creatinine ratio >20 mEq/g suggests excessive urinary losses. Conversely, urine potassium loss <20 mEq/24 h suggests cellular shift, decreased intake, or extrarenal losses of potassium.

Rare causes include:

- primary aldosteronism (hypertension, urine [Cl−] >40 mEq/L, low plasma renin activity, and elevated aldosterone level)
- Bartter syndrome (normal BP, hypokalemia, metabolic alkalosis, and elevated renin and aldosterone levels)
- Gitelman syndrome (normal BP, hypokalemia, and hypomagnesemia)
- inhaled β$_2$-agonists (may lead to hypokalemia in certain clinical settings)
- hypokalemic periodic paralysis

Hypokalemic periodic paralysis is a rare familial or acquired disorder characterized by flaccid generalized weakness from a sudden intracellular potassium shift precipitated by strenuous exercise or a high-carbohydrate meal. The acquired form occurs with thyrotoxicosis and is found in men of Asian or Mexican descent. It is resolved with treatment of hyperthyroidism.

Characteristic findings of hypokalemia include ileus, muscle cramps, rhabdomyolysis, and hypomagnesemia. ECGs may show U waves and flat or inverted T waves.

Therapy

For severe hypokalemia, IV potassium chloride is indicated. Total body potassium deficits are typically large (200-300 mEq for a serum potassium concentration of 3 mEq/L). Hypomagnesemia and metabolic alkalosis should be corrected, if present.

Hypomagnesemia

Diagnosis

The most common causes of hypomagnesemia include:

- GI losses (diarrhea, steatorrhea, intestinal bypass, pancreatitis)
- kidney losses (loop and thiazide diuretics, alcohol-induced)
- medications (cisplatin, aminoglycosides, amphotericin B, cyclosporine)
- hungry bone syndrome following parathyroidectomy

Usually the source of hypomagnesemia is obvious. If no cause is clinically apparent, GI and kidney losses can be differentiated by measuring the 24-hour urine magnesium excretion (elevated in kidney losses, low in GI losses). Hypomagnesemia is often associated with hypokalemia because of urine potassium wasting. Hypomagnesemia is also associated with hypocalcemia because of lower PTH secretion and end-organ resistance to PTH. If hypomagnesemia is suspected, look for neuromuscular irritability, hypocalcemia, and hypokalemia.

◆ DON'T BE TRICKED

- Correction of hypokalemia and hypocalcemia is difficult unless magnesium depletion is also corrected.

Therapy

Administer oral slow-release magnesium and IV magnesium sulfate to achieve a serum magnesium level >1 mg/dL.

✦ Test Yourself

A 30-year-old woman with Crohn disease has an ileostomy. For the past week, she has noted increased ostomy output, weakness, and paresthesias. Laboratory studies show serum sodium, 129 mEq/L; potassium, 2.9 mEq/L; bicarbonate, 18 mEq/L; calcium, 5.5 mg/dL; and phosphorus, 1.3 mg/dL. After treatment with isotonic saline plus potassium chloride and sodium bicarbonate, the bicarbonate concentration is 22 mEq/L. However, the serum potassium level is still 2.9 mEq/L, and the serum calcium level is 5.3 mg/dL.

ANSWER: The diagnosis is hypomagnesemia. Measure magnesium level and if low begin IV magnesium replacement.

Hypophosphatemia

Diagnosis

Phosphate is primarily excreted through the kidneys and is reabsorbed mainly in the proximal tubule. The primary hormonal factors regulating phosphorus balance are PTH (which decreases phosphorus reabsorption and promotes kidney phosphate excretion) and calcitriol (which stimulates phosphate absorption in the gut). Characteristic findings in severe hypophosphatemia are HF, muscle weakness, rhabdomyolysis, hemolytic anemia, and metabolic encephalopathy.

Common causes:

- refeeding after starvation
- insulin administration for severe hyperglycemia
- hungry bone syndrome following parathyroidectomy
- respiratory alkalosis

- chronic diarrhea
- chronic alcoholism
- hyperparathyroidism
- vitamin D deficiency

If the cause of hypophosphatemia is not evident from the history, a 24-hour urine phosphate collection or calculation of the FEPO4 from a random urine sample can help differentiate renal from extrarenal causes. The FEPO4 can be calculated as follows:

(Urine PO4 × Serum Creatinine × 100)/(Serum PO4 × Urine Creatinine)

Urine phosphate excretion >100 mg/d or an FEPO4 >5% indicates renal phosphate wasting.

Therapy

In asymptomatic patients, administer oral phosphorus replacement as a sodium or potassium salt. Parenteral therapy with either of these agents is indicated for symptomatic patients or those whose phosphorus level is <1 mg/dL.

Approach to Acid-Base Problem Solving

You must be able to diagnose double and triple acid-base disorders.

Answer these four questions when solving acid-base problems:

1. What is the primary disturbance?
2. Is compensation appropriate?
3. What is the anion gap?
4. Does the change in the anion gap equal the change in the serum bicarbonate concentration (a value called the delta-delta)?

When diagnosing a primary acid-base disorder, remember that:

- Acidemia is defined as a pH <7.38. Metabolic acidosis = [HCO_3] <24 mEq/L. Respiratory acidosis = arterial PCO_2 >40 mm Hg.

- Alkalemia is defined as a pH >7.42. Metabolic alkalosis = [HCO_3] >24 mEq/L. Respiratory alkalosis = arterial PCO_2 <40 mm Hg.

STUDY TABLE: Compensatory Response to a Primary Acid-Base Disturbance		
Condition	**Expected Compensation**	**Interpretation**
Metabolic acidosis	Acute: Δ arterial $PCO_2 = (1.5)[HCO_3^-] + 8 \pm 2$ Chronic: Δ arterial $PCO_2 = [HCO_3^-] + 15$	Failure of the arterial PCO_2 to decrease to expected value = complicating respiratory acidosis Excessive decrease of the arterial PCO_2 = complicating respiratory alkalosis
Respiratory acidosis	Acute: 1 mEq/L ↑ in [HCO_3^-] for each 10 mm Hg ↑ in arterial PCO_2 Chronic: 3.5 mEq/L ↑ in [HCO_3^-] for each 10 mm Hg ↑ in arterial PCO_2	Failure of the [HCO_3^-] to increase to the expected value = complicating metabolic acidosis Excessive increase in [HCO_3^-] = complicating metabolic alkalosis
Metabolic alkalosis	0.7 mm Hg ↑ in arterial PCO_2 for each 1 mEq/L ↑ in [HCO_3^-]	This response is limited by hypoxemia
Respiratory alkalosis	Acute: 2 mEq/L ↓ in [HCO_3^-] for each 10 mm Hg ↓ in arterial PCO_2 Chronic: 4 mEq/L ↓ in [HCO_3^-] for each 10 mm Hg ↓ in arterial PCO_2	Failure of the [HCO_3^-] to decrease to the expected value = complicating metabolic alkalosis Excessive decrease in [HCO_3^-] = complicating metabolic acidosis

Anion Gap

The normal anion gap is 10 ± 2 mEq/L; anion gap = $[Na^+] - ([Cl^-] + [HCO_3^-])$.

Always calculate the anion gap, regardless of the metabolic disturbance.

- When the primary disturbance is a metabolic acidosis, the anion gap differentiates increased anion gap from normal anion gap acidosis.
- A reduced anion gap (<4 mEq/L) suggests multiple myeloma or hypoalbuminemia.

Common causes of increased anion gap acidosis include:

- DKA
- CKD
- lactic acidosis (usually due to tissue hypoperfusion)
- aspirin toxicity
- alcoholic ketosis
- methanol and ethylene glycol poisoning (also typically associated with an osmolar gap)

Common causes of normal anion gap metabolic acidosis include:

- GI HCO_3^- loss (diarrhea)
- kidney HCO_3^- loss (ileal bladder, proximal RTA)
- reduced kidney H^+ secretion (distal RTA, type IV RTA)
- Fanconi syndrome (phosphaturia, glucosuria, uricosuria, aminoaciduria)
- carbonic anhydrase inhibitor use (acetazolamide and topiramate)

Urine Anion Gap

Increased acid excretion by the kidney is reflected as a marked increase in urine ammonium. Urine ammonium is difficult to measure, but because chloride is excreted into the urine in equal amounts with ammonium, the amount of chloride in the urine reflects the amount of ammonium present.

The ability to excrete acid in the form of ammonia is calculated with the UAG. The UAG is defined as (urine $[Na^+]$ + urine $[K^+]$) – urine $[Cl^-]$. The UAG can be helpful in these situations:

- during normal anion gap metabolic acidosis due to extrarenal bicarbonate loss (diarrhea), the kidney will excrete increased urine ammonium (and chloride), resulting in a markedly negative (-20 to -25 mEq/L) UAG
- during impaired urine acidification due to type 1 RTA (distal renal tubule), urine ammonium (and chloride) excretion is impaired, with the UAG being markedly positive (20 to 40 mEq/L)

Delta-Delta

In anion gap acidosis, the expected ratio between the change in anion gap (normal anion gap-measured anion gap) and the change in plasma $[HCO_3]$ (normal HCO_3-measured HCO_3) concentration (Δ anion gap/Δ $[HCO_3]$) is 1 to 2.

- If (Δ anion gap/Δ $[HCO_3]$) is <1, consider concurrent normal anion gap acidosis.
- If (Δ anion gap/Δ $[HCO_3]$) is >2, consider concurrent metabolic alkalosis.

Metabolic alkalosis is often caused by upper GI loss of hydrogen chloride or by kidney loss of hydrogen chloride during diuretic therapy and is maintained by extracellular fluid volume contraction, chloride depletion, hypokalemia, or elevated aldosterone activity.

You must be able to answer questions like these:

- Problem #1: pH, 7.31; arterial PCO_2, 10 mm Hg; sodium, 127 mEq/L; chloride, 99 mEq/L; bicarbonate, 5 mEq/L.
- Problem #2: pH, 7.20; arterial PCO_2, 23 mm Hg; sodium, 134 mEq/L; chloride, 80 mEq/L; bicarbonate, 8 mEq/L.

Answers:

- Mixed increased anion gap and normal anion gap metabolic acidosis and respiratory alkalosis (triple acid-base disorder)
- Mixed increased anion gap metabolic acidosis and metabolic alkalosis (double acid-base disorder)

Alcohol Poisoning

Diagnosis

Determine the presence of an osmolal gap, which is the difference between measured and calculated osmolality. The calculated plasma osmolality = $2 \times$ serum $[Na^+]$ + [BUN]/2.8 + blood [glucose]/18; sodium concentration is measured as mEq/L, and BUN and glucose concentration are measured as mg/dL.

The normal osmolal gap is 10 mOsm/kg H_2O. If a larger gap exists, consider alcohol poisoning as the source of unmeasured osmoles. Ethanol is the most common cause of alcohol poisoning.

STUDY TABLE: Clues for Ingestion of Specific Types of Alcohol	
Clues	**Alcohol Type**
Somnolence or coma and normal acid-base homeostasis	Isopropyl alcohol
Severe increased anion gap metabolic acidosis and acute visual symptoms or severe abdominal pain	Methanol (pancreatitis and retinal toxicity)
Severe increased anion gap metabolic acidosis and AKI	Ethylene glycol (metabolizes to glyoxylate and oxalic acid, which may cause calcium oxalate nephrolithiasis and AKI)
Increased anion gap metabolic acidosis and ketoacidosis that improves with IV normal saline and glucose	Ethanol

Therapy

Treat mild isopropyl alcohol poisoning with IV fluids and gastric lavage. Severe isopropyl alcohol poisoning (hypotension and shock) requires hemodialysis. Treat methanol and ethylene glycol poisoning with fomepizole and hemodialysis. Treat alcoholic ketoacidosis with IV normal saline, glucose, and thiamine.

Calcium Oxalate Crystals: Characteristic envelope-shaped calcium oxalate dihydrate crystals.

Hypertension

Diagnosis

The Joint National Committee, along with the European Society of Hypertension and the Canadian Hypertension Education Program, all currently define the treatment goal for hypertension for all nonelderly patients with or without CKD or diabetes as <140/90 mm Hg. The American Diabetes Association defines the treatment goal in patients with diabetes as <140/80 mm Hg.

The treatment goal recommended by JNC 8 for patients ≥60 years is <150/90 mm Hg.

Classification of hypertension is based on an average of two or more readings obtained at two or more visits.

STUDY TABLE: Classification of Blood Pressure			
BP Category	**Office-Based Readings (mm Hg)**	**24-Hour Ambulatory Readings (mm Hg)**	**Self-Recorded BP (mm Hg)**
Normal	SBP <120 and DBP <80	<130/80	<135/85
Prehypertension	SBP 120-139 or DBP 80-89	–	–
Hypertension, Stage 1	SBP 140-159 or DBP 90-99	≥135/85	≥135/85
Hypertension, Stage 2	SBP ≥160 or DBP ≥100	–	–
White Coat Hypertension	≥140/90	<135/85	<135/85
Masked Hypertension	<140/90	>135/85	>135/85

White coat hypertension is applied to patients with average BP readings in the office of >140/90 mm Hg and out-of-office readings <140/90 mm Hg.

Masked hypertension is defined as elevated BP detected by ambulatory BP measurement but with normal office BP measurement.

Ambulatory BP measurement is the gold standard to confirm the diagnosis of hypertension and to diagnose white coat and masked hypertension.

Most patients with established hypertension have primary (essential) hypertension. Consider secondary hypertension in patients who have atypical clinical features (early onset, absent family history, hypokalemia, evidence of kidney disease) or have resistant hypertension (not at target goal despite the use of three antihypertensive agents, including a diuretic).

Evaluation of hypertension includes collecting data on cardiovascular risk factors and symptoms or signs of a possible underlying secondary cause. Initial evaluation includes:

- laboratory testing for kidney function, fasting blood glucose, fasting lipid panel, serum potassium, and serum calcium
- ECG
- urinalysis and albumin-creatinine ratio

STUDY TABLE: Selected Secondary Causes of Hypertension	
Condition	**Notes**
Drug induced	NSAIDs, amphetamines/cocaine, sympathomimetics, oral contraceptives, glucocorticoids
CKD	Elevated BUN, serum creatinine, and potassium; most patients present at an earlier stage with minimal signs and symptoms
Renovascular disease (atherosclerotic and fibromuscular)	Onset of hypertension at young age, especially in women (fibromuscular); atherosclerotic disease often associated with cigarette smoking, flash pulmonary edema, CAD, flank bruits, advanced retinopathy, increased creatinine (usually with bilateral renovascular disease), and increased creatinine after treatment with an ACE inhibitor or ARB; notable for hypokalemia and elevated renin and aldosterone levels
Aortic coarctation	Headache, cold feet, leg pain, reduced or absent femoral pulse, delay in femoral pulse compared with radial pulse, murmur heard between scapulae, figure 3 sign and rib notching on chest x-ray

(Continued on next page)

STUDY TABLE: Selected Secondary Causes of Hypertension (*Continued*)	
Condition	**Notes**
Primary hyperaldosteronism	Muscle cramping, nocturia, thirst; physical examination normal; hypokalemia and elevated aldosterone to plasma renin activity ratio
Cushing syndrome	Weight gain, menstrual irregularity, hirsutism; truncal obesity, abdominal striae; hypokalemia, metabolic alkalosis
Pheochromocytoma	Sweating, heart racing, pounding headache; pallor; tachycardia; hypertension may be episodic with intervals of normal BP; increased urine or plasma catecholamines or metanephrine
Sleep apnea	Increased BMI >30, neck size >17, crowded oropharynx; snoring, witnessed apneic events

◆ DON'T BE TRICKED

- Do not use plasma renin activity to risk-stratify patients with hypertension or to predict response to specific drugs.

❖ Test Yourself

A 35-year-old woman is evaluated for persistent fatigue and resistant hypertension. Serum potassium is 3.3 mEq/L.

ANSWER: The diagnosis is most likely primary aldosteronism. Measure the plasma aldosterone to renin activity ratio.

Therapy

Therapeutic lifestyle changes are initiated and maintained for all patients with hypertension. Lifestyle interventions can produce reductions in BP equivalent to antihypertensive agents. Components include:

- a low sodium diet
- a diet such as DASH that emphasizes vegetables, fruits, whole grains, legumes, and low-fat dairy products and limits sweets, red meat, and saturated/total fat
- weight loss
- exercise

For patients with stage 1 hypertension, a 3- to 6-month trial of lifestyle modification alone before starting drug therapy is reasonable.

For patients with stage 2 hypertension (or end-organ disease) medications (1 or 2 drugs) and lifestyle modification are initiated simultaneously.

For initial drug therapy of stage 1 hypertension in the general nonblack population (including elderly), JNC 8 recommends monotherapy with any one of four drug classes:

- thiazide-type diuretics (thiazides)
- calcium channel blockers
- ACE inhibitors
- ARBs

From this list of preferred class of drugs, patient characteristics will influence the final choice.

STUDY TABLE: Selection of an Antihypertensive Agent		
Agent	**Potential Clinical Indications**	**Potential Clinical Contraindications**
Thiazide diuretic	Isolated systolic hypertension in elderly; hypertension in black patients; HF	Gout; hyponatremia; glucose intolerance; concomitant lithium use
ACE inhibitor/ARB	HF; post-MI; CKD; proteinuria; diabetes mellitus/metabolic syndrome	Pregnancy[a]; hyperkalemia; bilateral renal artery stenosis
Calcium channel blocker	Isolated systolic hypertension in elderly; hypertension in black patients	HF (non-dihydropyridine)
β-Blockers	Post-MI; HF; tachyarrhythmia; pregnancy; angina (NOT recommended for initial use except under these conditions)	Peripheral artery disease; COPD; glucose intolerance
[a]Absolute contraindication.		

Typically, 75% of a drug's BP-lowering effect is achieved with 50% of its maximal dose. A combination of two agents at moderate dose is often more successful at achieving BP goals than one BP agent at maximal dose.

Older adults with atherosclerotic hypertension are managed medically. Young patients with fibromuscular dysplasia can be considered for renal angioplasty and stenting.

◆ DON'T BE TRICKED

- Thiazide diuretics are not effective in patients with kidney disease (GFR <30 mL/min/1.73 m^2); select a loop diuretic.
- Do not obtain imaging studies for the diagnosis of renovascular hypertension in older adults since it is unlikely to change management.

Hypertensive Urgency

The treatment of hypertensive urgency (BP >180/120 mm Hg in the absence of symptoms or progressive target-organ damage) differs if the patient has previously treated hypertension or untreated hypertension.

In patients with preexisting treated hypertension:

- restart the medication(s) in nonadherent patients
- in adherent patients, either increase the dose of the medication(s) or add an additional agent

In patients with previously untreated hypertension:

- consider oral furosemide or small doses of clonidine or captopril and observe for several hours for a BP drop of 20-30 mm Hg (not to normal BP)
- begin a long-acting agent, discharge home with follow-up in 2 to 3 days

Hypertension in Pregnancy

Hypertension prior to the 20th week of gestation is most consistent with previously undiagnosed chronic hypertension. Treatment of hypertension less than 160/110 during pregnancy is controversial and benefits of treatment have not been demonstrated.

Antihypertensive medications absolutely contraindicated during pregnancy:

- ACE inhibitors
- ARBs
- renin inhibitors

Diuretics may induce oligohydramnios if initiated during pregnancy.

Drugs that can be used during pregnancy:

- methyldopa
- labetalol
- calcium channel blockers (e.g., long-acting nifedipine)

Gestational hypertension is hypertension that develops after 20 weeks of pregnancy without preexisting hypertension, proteinuria, or other end-organ damage. Gestational hypertension is a risk factor for preeclampsia and the development of chronic hypertension.

◆ DON'T BE TRICKED

- Treatment of gestational hypertension does not prevent the occurrence of preeclampsia or chronic hypertension.

Preeclampsia is new-onset hypertension after 20 weeks of pregnancy with proteinuria. Eclampsia is the presence of generalized, tonic-clonic seizures in a preeclamptic woman. Definitive treatment is delivery, including induction of labor in women at or near term.

Renal Tubular Acidosis

Diagnosis

Normal anion gap metabolic acidosis is associated with all three types of RTA.

STUDY TABLE: Differential Diagnosis of Renal Tubular Acidosis		
Diagnosis	**Metabolic Findings**	**Associated Findings**
Distal (classic or type 1) RTA	Normal anion gap metabolic acidosis, hypokalemia, positive UAG, urine pH >5.5 (only in the setting of systemic acidosis), serum [HCO$_3$] $\cong$ 10 mEq/L	Nephrolithiasis and nephrocalcinosis, autoimmune disorders (SLE, Sjögren syndrome), amphotericin B use, urinary obstruction
Proximal (type 2) RTA	Normal anion gap metabolic acidosis, normal or negative UAG, hypokalemia, urine pH <5.5, serum [HCO$_3$] $\cong$ 16-18 mEq/L	Glycosuria, phosphaturia, uricosuria, aminoaciduria, and tubular proteinuria (Fanconi syndrome)
Type 4 RTA	Normal anion gap metabolic acidosis, hyperkalemia, positive UAG, urine pH <5.5	Diabetes mellitus, urinary tract obstruction

Therapy

In proximal RTA, correction of acidemia in patients with bicarbonate therapy is often not possible. The addition of a thiazide diuretic may help by inducing volume depletion, lowering the GFR and thereby decreasing the filtered load of bicarbonate. The addition of a potassium-sparing diuretic may limit the degree of kidney potassium wasting.

In distal RTA, administration of bicarbonate usually corrects the metabolic acidosis. The potassium deficit should be corrected before correcting the acidemia.

In type 4 RTA, the primary goal of therapy is to correct the hyperkalemia, which will treat the acid-base disturbance. These patients may develop severe hyperkalemia following treatment with ACE inhibitors or ARBs.

❖ Test Yourself

A 31-year-old woman with IBD passes a kidney stone. Serum sodium is 142 mEq/L, potassium is 2.9 mEq/L, chloride is 112 mEq/L, and bicarbonate is 20 mEq/L. Urine pH is 6.5.

ANSWER: The diagnosis is distal RTA.

Glomerular Diseases

Glomerular disease should be suspected when proteinuria and/or hematuria are seen on urinalysis.

The most common distinction is usually made between the nephrotic syndromes and the nephritic syndromes, also referred to as GN. Some conditions may present with either or both patterns, and some may progress from one pattern to the other.

The Nephrotic Syndrome

The nephrotic syndrome is characterized by:

- urine protein excretion of >3500 mg/24 h or a urine protein-creatinine ratio of >3500 mg/g
- hypoalbuminemia, edema, and hyperlipidemia may be present

The nephrotic syndrome may be primary or secondary to systemic diseases such as diabetes, infection, or autoimmune diseases.

The 4 most common causes of nephrotic syndrome are:

- minimal change glomerulopathy
- membranous glomerulopathy
- focal segmental glomerulosclerosis
- diabetic nephropathy

◆ DON'T BE TRICKED

- Nephrotic range proteinuria in a patient with diabetes but without diabetic retinopathy is not due to diabetes.

Treatment of the consequences of the nephrotic syndrome should occur simultaneously with treatment of the specific cause:

- statins for elevated lipid levels
- anticoagulation for thrombotic complications (due to urinary loss of antithrombins)
- low salt diet and loop diuretics for edema

STUDY TABLE: Common Causes of Nephrotic Syndrome			
Condition	**Clinical Associations**	**Diagnosis**	**Treatment**
Focal segmental glomerulosclerosis	Most common cause of nephrotic syndrome in blacks "Collapsing" variety associated with HIV Associated with morbid obesity	Biopsy	Glucocorticoids or calcineurin inhibitors
Membranous glomerulopathy	Most common cause of nephropathy in whites Positive antibody against phospholipase A2 receptor Secondary causes include: infection (hepatitis B and C, malaria, syphilis); SLE; drugs (NSAIDS, gold salts); cancer (solid tumors, lymphoma) High propensity for thrombosis, especially renal vein thrombosis	Biopsy	33% spontaneously remit in 6-12 mo Glucocorticoids and cyclophosphamide or calcineurin inhibitors Treat concurrent hepatitis B
Minimal change glomerulopathy	Most common cause of primary nephrotic syndrome in children 10% of nephrotic syndrome in adults	Biopsy	Glucocorticoids
Diabetic nephropathy	Most common secondary cause of the nephrotic syndrome and the most common overall cause in adults Annual measurement of albumin-creatinine ratio measured beginning 5 years after diagnosis of type 1 diabetes and at time of diagnosis of type 2 diabetes	Clinical diagnosis	Reduce HbA_{1c} <7% and BP <140/90 mm Hg Albuminuria is treated with ACE inhibitors or ARBs

Fat Droplet: Typical "Maltese cross" appearance of a fat droplet under polarized light microscopy commonly found in the nephrotic syndrome.

The Nephritic Syndrome

The nephritic syndrome is associated with glomerular inflammation resulting in hematuria, proteinuria, and leukocytes in the urine sediment. The hallmark is the presence of dysmorphic erythrocytes. Proteinuria is variable. Systemic findings may include edema, hypertension, and kidney failure.

STUDY TABLE: Common Causes of Nephritic Syndrome	
Pathological Mechanism	**Specific Diseases**
Anti-GBM antibodies (normal complement)	Anti-GBM antibody disease
Pauci-immune GN (necrotizing GN with few immune deposits, normal complement)	Granulomatosis with polyangiitis (formerly known as Wegener granulomatosis)
	Microscopic polyangiitis
	Eosinophilic granulomatosis with polyangiitis (formerly known as Churg-Strauss syndrome)
Immune complex deposition (low complement with exception of IgA nephropathy)	IgA nephropathy
	IgA vasculitis (Henoch-Schönlein purpura)
	LN
	Infection-related GN
	Membranoproliferative GN
	Cryoglobulinemia (see Monoclonal Gammopathies and Cryoglobulinemia)

Rapidly progressive GN is a clinical syndrome characterized by evidence of GN with progression to kidney failure within weeks. It may be associated with any etiology of GN or may be idiopathic. Rapidly progressive GN is particularly common with anti-GBM antibody disease (in younger patients) and pauci-immune small-vessel vasculitis (in older patients).

Anti-Glomerular Basement Membrane Antibody Disease

- An autoimmune disease caused by antibodies directed against type IV collagen.
- If process also involves pulmonary capillaries it causes pulmonary hemorrhage (Goodpasture syndrome).
- Findings include normal complement levels and elevated levels of anti-GBM antibodies.
- Kidney biopsy shows proliferative GN with linear deposition of immunoglobulin.
- Treatment is cyclophosphamide and glucocorticoids, combined with daily plasmapheresis.

Pauci-Immune Glomerulonephritis

- Kidney manifestations range from only hematuria to rapidly progressive GN.
- Systemic symptoms may include arthritis, leukocytoclastic vasculitis (palpable purpura), and pulmonary disease (pulmonary infiltrate to pulmonary hemorrhage).
- More than 80% of patients with MPA or granulomatosis with polyangiitis are ANCA positive; granulomatosis with polyangiitis is associated with (PR3)-ANCA and MPA is associated with (MPO)-ANCA.
- Complement levels are normal.
- Kidney biopsy shows absent or minimal staining with immunoglobulin.
- Induction therapy consists of glucocorticoids and cyclophosphamide (or rituximab) with or without plasmapheresis.

IgA Nephropathy

- Most commonly presents as asymptomatic microscopic hematuria (with or without proteinuria) or episodic gross hematuria following a URI (synpharyngitic nephritis).
- Kidney biopsy shows glomerular IgA deposits on immunofluorescence.
- Complement levels are normal.
- Most patients have a benign course without treatment; patients with proteinuria and risk factors for progression may benefit from ACE inhibitors or ARBs.

IgA Vasculitis (Henoch-Schönlein Purpura)

- Kidney involvement is similar to IgA nephropathy.
- Other organ involvement may occur.
- Diagnosis is confirmed either by finding an IgA-dominant leukocytoclastic vasculitis or by kidney biopsy, which shows lesions similar to IgA nephropathy.
- Complement levels are normal.
- Heonch-Schönlein purpura is typically self-limiting without treatment.

Lupus Nephritis

- Patients typically have extrarenal symptoms of SLE at the time of diagnosis of LN.
- ANA and anti–double-stranded antibodies are positive and C3 and C4 complement levels are depressed.
- Class I and II lesions require no specific therapy directed at the kidney.
- Class III LN and class IV LN are treated with glucocorticoids with either cyclophosphamide or mycophenolate mofetil.
- Class V (membranous) LN has a course similar to idiopathic membranous glomerulopathy.

Infection-Related Glomerulonephritis

- Staphylococcal infection is as common or more common than streptococcal infection as cause of infection-related GN.
- The clinical manifestations of poststreptococcal GN typically occur after a latent period of 1 to 6 weeks (check antistreptolysin O, anti-DNase titers) but occur at the time of infection with other infectious agents.
- Diagnosis is clinical in nephritic patients who have an ongoing or preceding infection.
- Complement levels are low.
- Treatment is of the underlying infection.

Membranoproliferative Glomerulonephritis

- Membranoproliferative GN manifests in children or young adults as proteinuria or the nephrotic syndrome.
- Associated with immune complex disease (SLE), infections (hepatitis C), and monoclonal gammopathy.
- Complement levels are low.
- Treatment of the causative infection, autoimmune disease, or monoclonal gammopathy is the primary therapy.

Causes of Glomerular Diseases Associated with Low Complement Levels

- Postinfectious GN (e.g., endocarditis, Group A streptococcal infection)
- SLE
- Cryoglobulinemia
- Membranoproliferative GN
- Atheroembolic disease

Monoclonal Gammopathies and Cryoglobulinemia

Kidney manifestations of monoclonal gammopathies may include proteinuria (sometimes nephrotic range), tubular dysfunction, hypertension, and kidney failure.

Diagnosis of kidney involvement in monoclonal gammopathy usually requires biopsy.

Management of monoclonal gammopathies with kidney involvement is focused on treatment of the underlying monoclonal disorder.

STUDY TABLE: Monoclonal Gammopathies and Cryoglobulinemia-Related Kidney Diseases

Condition	Pathology	Clinical Syndrome
Amyloidosis	Deposits that stain apple green with Congo red	Proteinuria or nephrotic syndrome
Monoclonal immunoglobulin deposition disease	Congo red-negative light or heavy chain deposits	Proteinuria or nephrotic syndrome
Multiple myeloma	Accumulation of light chains in the renal tubule (cast nephropathy)	Acute kidney injury
		Acute or CKD associated with Fanconi syndrome
	Light chains absorb and crystallize in proximal tubular cells	
Cryoglobulinemia	Vasculitic syndrome with GN with membranoproliferative features	Most often associated with type II cryoglobulins (HCV infection)
		Proteinuria, hematuria, nephrotic syndrome, rapidly progressive GN
		Low C4 (sometimes C3)

◆ **DON'T BE TRICKED**

- Do not prescribe ACE inhibitors and ARBs early in the course of GN because they may worsen the GFR.

Autosomal Dominant Polycystic Kidney Disease

Diagnosis

The hallmark of ADPKD is large kidneys with multiple kidney cysts resulting from genetic mutations in *PKD1* and *PKD2*. More than 90% of the inheritance is as an autosomal dominant trait.

Kidney ultrasonography is used to diagnose ADPKD. In patients with a family history of ADPKD the number of cysts needed to diagnose ADPKD increases with age:

- ≥2 cysts (unilateral or bilateral) for ages 15-29 years
- ≥2 cysts in each kidney for ages 30-59 years
- ≥4 cysts in each kidney for ages >60 years

◆ **DON'T BE TRICKED**

- Direct mutational analysis of the *PKD1* and *PKD2* genes is reserved for equivocal cases following imaging.

Hypertension is a common presentation. More than 50% of patients develop recurrent flank or back pain from kidney stones, cyst rupture or hemorrhage, or infection.

A ruptured intracranial cerebral aneurysm is the most serious extrarenal complication of ADPKD and occurs most commonly in patients with a family history of hemorrhagic stroke or intracranial cerebral aneurysm.

Therapy

There are no specific therapies for ADPKD.

- Treat hypertension with an ACE inhibitor or an ARB.
- Treat cyst infection or pyelonephritis with fluoroquinolones or trimethoprim-sulfamethoxazole.
- Tolvaptan reduces the rate of increase in kidney size and loss of GFR but poor tolerance, hepatotoxicity, and expense limit its use.

Periodic MRA of the cerebral arteries is recommended for patients with a family history of hemorrhagic stroke or cerebral aneurysm.

Inherited Collagen Type IV-Related Nephropathies

Two important inherited collagen type IV-related nephropathies:

- hereditary nephritis
- thin GBM disease

Hereditary nephritis is a rare cause of end-stage kidney disease. When the genetic mutation is X-linked (80% of patients), the condition is termed *Alport syndrome.* Classic Alport syndrome is accompanied by sensorineural hearing loss and characteristic ocular findings such as lenticonus. Proteinuria, hypertension, and CKD usually develop over time. End-stage kidney disease occurs between the late teenage years and the fourth decade of life. There is no specific therapy for hereditary nephritis.

Thin GBM disease manifests as microscopic or macroscopic hematuria, usually first appearing in childhood. Long-term prognosis is excellent.

Acute Kidney Injury

Prevention

In patients at high risk requiring imaging with contrast, use the smallest possible dose of a low-osmolar or iso-osmolar contrast agent, and treat with isotonic saline or bicarbonate before and immediately after the procedure.

◆ DON'T BE TRICKED

- Do not prevent contrast-induced nephropathy with dialysis immediately after contrast media administration.

Diagnosis

AKI is defined as an abrupt elevation in the serum creatinine concentration or a decrease in urine output. The etiology may be secondary prerenal causes, intrinsic kidney disease, or postrenal obstruction of urine outflow. Prerenal and postrenal causes must be distinguished from intrinsic renal parenchymal disease because they are often rapidly reversible.

AKI is also divided into oliguric (≤400 mL/24 h) and nonoliguric (>400 mL/24 h) forms. The lower the urine output, the worse the prognosis.

Condition	BUN-Creatinine Ratio	Urine Osmolality (mOsm/kg H$_2$O)	Urine Sodium (mEq/L)	FE$_{Na}$	Urinalysis and Microscopy
Prerenal	>20:1	>500	<20	<1%	Specific gravity >1.020; normal or hyaline casts
ATN	10:1	~300	>40	>2%[a]	Specific gravity ~1.010; muddy brown casts and tubular epithelial cells
AIN	Variable	Variable	Variable	Variable	Mild proteinuria; leukocytes; erythrocytes; leukocyte casts; eosinophiluria
Acute GN	Variable	Variable	Variable	Variable	Proteinuria; dysmorphic erythrocytes; erythrocyte casts
Postrenal	>20:1	Variable	Variable	Variable	Variable, bland

STUDY TABLE: Diagnostic Findings in Acute Kidney Injury

[a]FE$_{Na}$ can be low in contrast nephropathy and pigment nephropathy.

FE$_{Na}$ may be >2% in prerenal patients who are on diuretics. In the setting of diuretics, the FE$_{Urea}$, calculated as $(U_{Urea} \times P_{Cr})/(U_{Cr} \times P_{Urea}) \times 100$, is more accurate in detecting volume-depleted states and prerenal AKI. A FE$_{Urea}$ of <35% is consistent with prerenal cause of AKI.

Knowing a few basic epidemiological facts can help identify the cause of AKI:

- prerenal AKI is the most common form of AKI in the outpatient setting

- a prolonged prerenal state can lead to ATN

- the most common cause of hospital-acquired AKI is ATN

- hospital-acquired ATN is most commonly caused by toxins such as radiocontrast and antibiotics (i.e., gentamicin)

- obstruction of the upper tract (ureters or renal pelvis) must be bilateral to cause AKI

Muddy Brown Granular Casts: Muddy brown granular casts consistent with kidney injury secondary to tubular necrosis.

STUDY TABLE: Differential Diagnosis of Acute Kidney Injury

When you see this...	Think of...	And select ...
Minimal proteinuria, no hematuria or pyuria; presence of muddy brown casts	ATN	FE_{Na} and/or spot urine sodium
Erythrocytes, erythrocyte casts, or dysmorphic erythrocytes	GN	As appropriate: Titers for ANA; anti-dsDNA antibodies; and antistreptolysin O antibodies; C3, C4, and CH50; hepatitis and HIV serologies and cryoglobulins; p-ANCA/c-ANCA and anti-GBM antibodies
Pyuria	Pyelonephritis, AIN	Culture urine / Examine medication list
Eosinophilia, eosinophiluria, and rash	AIN, cholesterol emboli	Examine medication list / Look for previous vascular procedure (angiography)
Livedo reticularis (violaceous reticular rash)	Cholesterol emboli / Vasculitis	Look for previous vascular procedure (angiography) / Consider cryoglobulinemia
Hypercalcemia and anemia	Multiple myeloma	Serum and urine protein electrophoresis, quantitative immunoglobulins
Nephrotic syndrome	Diabetes mellitus / Renal vein thrombosis	Plasma glucose / Renal vein Doppler study
Obstruction on kidney ultrasound	BPH, nephrolithiasis, obstructing malignant mass, retroperitoneal fibrosis	Residual bladder volume, noncontrast CT or MRI
Complete anuria	Renal cortical necrosis	Kidney ultrasonography
Large kidneys on ultrasound	Amyloidosis, diabetes (early), HIV nephropathy	SPEP, blood glucose HIV serologic studies
Kidney failure following colonoscopy	Phosphate-containing bowel prep (acute calcium phosphate crystal deposition in the kidneys)	Supportive care (fluids, stop ACE inhibitors, ARBs, NSAIDs)
Recent abdominal surgery, hemorrhage, or acute pancreatitis	Abdominal compartment syndrome	Intravesicular pressure >20 mm Hg
Peripheral blood smear schistocytes, thrombocytopenia	Thrombotic microangiopathy (HUS/TTP, DIC, scleroderma renal crisis)	As indicated CBC, coagulation parameters
Urine dipstick positive for blood, no erythrocytes on urinalysis	Hemolysis, rhabdomyolysis	Serum CK, serum haptoglobin, reticulocyte count, peripheral blood smear
AKI associated with acute leukemia or lymphoma or its treatment	Tumor lysis syndrome	Uric acid, phosphorus, potassium (all elevated)
Worsening kidney function in the setting of diuretic-resistant HF	Cardiorenal syndrome	Improving cardiac function with diuretics, ACE inhibitors or ARBs, vasodilators, and inotropes
Worsening kidney function in setting of cirrhosis and ascites	Hepatorenal syndrome	IV albumin and intravascular volume repletion. Liver transplantation (See Gastroenterology and Hepatology, Cirrhosis)

❖ **Test Yourself**

A 65-year-old man develops eosinophilia, AKI, and a net-like rash on his lower extremities following a cardiac catheterization.

ANSWER: The probable diagnosis is atheroembolic disease with cholesterol emboli to the skin and kidney.

A 35-year old with necrotizing pancreatitis and tense ascites develops AKI.

ANSWER: The probable diagnosis is abdominal compartment syndrome; measure intravesicular pressure.

Therapy

Begin IV normal saline for patients with volume depletion. Stop potential nephrotoxic drugs and look particularly for aminoglycoside antibiotics, ACE inhibitors, loop diuretics, cyclosporine, and NSAIDs.

Select dialysis for:

- refractory hyperkalemia, acidemia, or volume overload
- signs or symptoms of uremia (altered mentation, asterixis, pericardial friction rub, vomiting)
- certain drug intoxications

Generally, intermittent hemodialysis is used for stable patients with AKI, and continuous renal replacement therapy and prolonged intermittent renal replacement therapy for critically ill patients with unstable hemodynamics, multiorgan failure, or high catabolic states.

For urinary obstruction, choose a catheter to relieve bladder outlet obstruction. If the obstruction is above the bladder, select retrograde or antegrade nephrostomies.

Glomerulonephritis: Erythrocyte casts consistent with glomerulonephritis.

◆ **DON'T BE TRICKED**

- Do not withhold dialysis until BUN, creatinine, or both reach "threshold" values.

STUDY TABLE: Acute Kidney Injury Treatment Protocol	
Indication	**Treatment**
Severe acidemia (pH <7.20)	IV bicarbonate or hemodialysis
Severe hypertension	Vasodilators, β-blockers, calcium channel blockers
Rapidly progressive GN, granulomatosis with polyangiitis, and severe IgA nephropathy	Cyclophosphamide, glucocorticoids
Scleroderma renal crisis	ACE inhibitor, regardless of serum creatinine level
Hydronephrosis on ultrasound	Bladder catheter or nephrostomy tube
Abdominal compartment syndrome	Surgical decompression

◆ **DON'T BE TRICKED**

- Do not select routine loop diuretics (without evidence of volume overload), dopamine, or mannitol to treat AKI.

Nephrolithiasis

Diagnosis

Kidney stones are predominantly composed of calcium but may be formed by other substrates such as uric acid, struvite, or cystine.

Important risk factors for stone formation include:

- insufficient fluid intake
- increased dietary sodium and protein intake
- hypercalciuria, hyperuricemia, hyperoxaluria
- low urine citrate levels (citrate inhibits crystal formation)
- primary hyperparathyroidism with hypercalciuria
- metabolic syndrome and type 2 diabetes mellitus
- recurrent UTIs with urease-splitting organisms such as *Klebsiella* and *Proteus* (struvite stones)
- sarcoid (hypercalciuria/hypercalcemia)

Patients with suspected nephrolithiasis should be asked about:

- a personal or family history of stone disease
- polycystic kidney disease, medullary sponge kidney, distal RTA
- high-risk medical illness (Crohn disease, ileostomy)
- high-risk medications (indinavir, acetazolamide)
- diets with increased protein (Atkins diet)
- repeated UTIs, high urine pH, and staghorn calculi (*Proteus* infections)

The classic symptoms of nephrolithiasis are acute flank pain with radiation to the groin and hematuria. Urinalysis usually reveals blood, and the urine sediment has intact, nondysmorphic erythrocytes. Ultrasonography or noncontrast CT is the preferred imaging choice.

◆ DON'T BE TRICKED

- The absence of erythrocytes on urinalysis does not rule out nephrolithiasis.

Therapy

Therapy varies according to the specific findings. Kidney stones <5 mm in diameter typically pass spontaneously. Stones >10 mm often require invasive measures. Patients with stones 6-10 mm in size will benefit from expulsive therapy with either tamsulosin or nifedipine. These drugs induce ureteral dilatation and relaxation.

Urgent urologic consultation is indicated for patients with:

- pyelonephritis or urosepsis
- AKI
- large stones requiring surgical removal
- bilateral obstruction
- obstruction of a solitary kidney

Urologic referral is also indicated for ambulatory patients who do not pass stones with conservative management or who have stones >10 mm in diameter.

Chronic treatment:

- 2 L fluid intake per day
- For calcium composite stones, select a thiazide diuretic, allopurinol, or citrate
- Large struvite stones: percutaneous nephrostolithotomy and long-term prophylactic antibiotics

◆ DON'T BE TRICKED

- Asymptomatic kidney stones found on imaging studies do not require urgent stone removal.
- Do not select a low-calcium diet for patients with kidney stones. Calcium restriction does not prevent stones and may actually increase stone formation and contribute to bone demineralization.

❖ Test Yourself

A 35-year-old woman is evaluated in the emergency department for right flank pain and hematuria. She has a long history of Crohn disease and has had multiple operations to remove portions of her ileum and colon.

ANSWER: The probable diagnosis is calcium oxalate stones secondary to increased oxalate absorption in the GI tract and subsequent hyperoxaluria.

Chronic Kidney Disease

Diagnosis

CKD, characterized by an alteration in kidney function or structure for ≥3 months, occurs most often in patients with diabetes and hypertension. Characteristic findings of uremia are asterixis, loss of appetite, nausea, vomiting, and a pericardial rub.

Differential diagnosis of CKD:

- Diabetic kidney disease: Look for early microalbuminuria (spot albumin-creatinine ratio, 30-300 mg/g), followed by overt proteinuria, declining GFR, and a bland urine sediment. The presence of retinopathy strongly suggests coexisting diabetic nephropathy.
- Glomerular disease: Look for glomerular hematuria, proteinuria, and hypertension, often with other systemic manifestations (LN and postinfectious GN). If nephrotic syndrome is present, look for focal segmental glomerulosclerosis, membranous nephropathy, and minimal change disease. Kidney biopsy is often needed to make a specific diagnosis and guide therapy.
- Tubulointerstitial disease: Look for proteinuria, glycosuria, concentrating defect, sterile pyuria, and leukocyte casts, as well as papillary necrosis on ultrasound. Consider analgesic nephropathy (medication use, papillary necrosis), infection (TB, legionnaires disease, leptospirosis), allergic drug reaction (eosinophilia, eosinophiluria), autoimmune disorder (SLE, sarcoidosis, Sjögren syndrome), and lead nephropathy (occupational exposure).
- Vascular disease: Look for hematuria, proteinuria, and associated systemic illness. Vasculitis often presents with rapidly progressive GN and palpable purpura (leukocytoclastic vasculitis).
- After transplantation: CKD in the kidney transplant recipient may be caused by chronic allograft nephropathy, drug toxicity (cyclosporine), polyomavirus BK infection, or recurrence of disease.
- Structural disease (polycystic kidney disease): Look for hypertension, hematuria, palpable kidneys (advanced disease), and family history of CKD.

Nephrogenic Systemic Fibrosis: The patient has nephrogenic systemic fibrosis associated with an erythematous plaque, edema, and peau d'orange appearance.

◆ **DON'T BE TRICKED**

- If the kidneys are markedly scarred and small (<9 cm), do not select aggressive diagnostic or therapeutic measures.

Therapy

Avoid exposure to kidney toxins (contrast agents, NSAIDs). Avoid gadolinium-enhanced MRI, because of the risk of nephrogenic systemic fibrosis (greatest risk in patients receiving dialysis). Begin restriction of sodium, potassium, and phosphorus. Avoid significant protein restriction. Drug and alkali therapy is based on specific findings.

STUDY TABLE: Drug Therapy for CKD	
If You See This ...	**Select ...**
Hypertension	BP target <140/90 mm Hg
	Initial therapy in black patients with proteinuria is an ACE inhibitor or ARB; in black patients without proteinuria, options include a diuretic, calcium channel blocker, ACE inhibitor, or ARB
	Beneficial effect of ACE inhibitors or ARBs is limited to patients with albuminuria >300 mg/g
	Use a loop diuretic rather than a thiazide for GFR <30 mL/min/1.73m2
Hyperlipidemia	Treat patients >50 years with an eGFR of <60 mL/min/1.73 m^2 and/or albuminuria with statins
	Do not treat patients on dialysis with statins (no benefit)
Diabetes	Maintain hemoglobin A$_{1c}$ <7% for most patients
Anemia	Erythropoietin to maintain hemoglobin levels of 10-11 g/dL and iron to maintain iron stores (always check iron levels before starting erythropoietin)
Metabolic acidosis	Alkali therapy to maintain [HCO$_3$] between 23-28 mEq/L
Vitamin D deficiency	Calcitriol (or vitamin D analogues)

◆ **DON'T BE TRICKED**

- The anemia of CKD is a diagnosis of exclusion.
- Do not use ACE inhibitors, ARBs, or renin inhibitors in combination to treat CKD patients with proteinuria.

The main principle for the treatment of calcium and phosphorus disorders is to normalize the PTH:

- correct 25-hydroxy vitamin D deficiency and supplement calcium
- if PTH levels remain elevated, calcitriol or calcitriol analogues can be used to further suppress PTH
- if PTH levels remain elevated, use phosphate binders
- cinacalcet is used in patients receiving dialysis therapy who do not respond to therapy with vitamin D analogues, calcium supplements, and phosphate binders

Provide vaccinations according to guidelines with a few exceptions. All patients should be:

- vaccinated against HBV
- vaccinated with the 23- and 13-valent pneumococcal vaccines
- revaccinated with the 23-valent vaccine after a minimum of 5 years
- vaccinated annually against influenza virus (inactive vaccine)

Remember these points regarding kidney replacement therapy:

- kidney transplantation is associated with superior quality of life and improved survival and is less expensive than long-term dialysis
- all patients with end-stage kidney disease are considered candidates for kidney transplantation unless they have systemic malignancy, chronic infection, severe cardiovascular disease, or neuropsychiatric disorders
- transplantation is particularly beneficial in young patients

Remember these points about renal replacement therapy:

- clinical outcomes are equivalent for patients on peritoneal dialysis compared with hemodialysis
- peritoneal dialysis catheters are placed approximately 1 month before therapy is initiated
- patients who opt for hemodialysis should be referred for arteriovenous fistula placement before their eGFR drops below 15 mL/min/1.73 m^2 to allow sufficient time for arteriovenous fistula maturation.
- suitable candidates for kidney transplantation should be referred for evaluation once their eGFR is <20 mL/min/1.73 m^2

Patients with kidney transplants must receive immunosuppressive medications to prevent their immune system from rejecting the kidney allograft. Although immunosuppressants are usually well tolerated, they can have significant side effects.

STUDY TABLE: Common Side Effects of Immunosuppressants

Class	Medication	Common Side Effects
Calcineurin inhibitor	Cyclosporine	Hypertension; decreased GFR; dyslipidemia; hirsutism
	Tacrolimus	Diabetes; decreased GFR; hypertension
Antimetabolite	Mycophenolate	Leukopenia; anemia
	Azathioprine	Leukopenia
mTOR inhibitor	Sirolimus; everolimus	Proteinuria; dyslipidemia; diabetes; anemia; leukopenia
Glucocorticoid receptor agonist	Prednisone	Osteopenia; hypertension; edema; diabetes

Immunosuppression increases the risk for infections and cancers.

- In the first month, posttransplantation surgical wound and UTIs are most common.
- After the first month, CMV is the most important opportunistic pathogen; provide prophylactic valganciclovir and prophylaxis against *Pneumocystis jirovecii*.
- Infections with BK virus cause a rise in serum creatinine; reduce immunosuppression.
- The most common malignancy is cutaneous SCCs.
- Kaposi sarcoma is much more common in kidney transplant recipients; reduce the immunosuppression and switch to sirolimus-based immunosuppression.
- Posttransplant lymphoproliferative disease is associated with EBV infection; reduce immunosuppression and administration of rituximab in patients with CD20+ tumors.

◆ DON'T BE TRICKED

- **Do not use magnesium-containing antacids in patients with end-stage kidney disease.**

Renal osteodystrophy refers to alteration of bone morphology in patients with CKD.

STUDY TABLE: Renal Osteodystrophy

Condition	Mechanism	Characteristics
Osteitis fibrosa cystica	Secondary hyperparathyroidism	Subperiosteal resorption of bone, most prominently at the phalanges
Adynamic bone disease	Suppressed levels of PTH due to chronic illness or aggressive treatment with vitamin D analogues	Increased risk of fractures; made worse with bisphosphonate therapy
Osteomalacia	Vitamin D deficiency	Bone pain, fractures

❖ Test Yourself

A 55-year-old woman with chronic lower back pain and chronic polyuria and nocturia is found to have CKD. Urinalysis shows no protein or erythrocytes, 5-10 leukocytes/hpf, and no casts. Urine culture shows no growth. Kidney ultrasound shows only papillary necrosis.

ANSWER: The diagnosis is tubulointerstitial disease, secondary to analgesic abuse.

Neurology

Primary Headaches

More than 90% of headaches are primary headaches, including migraine, tension-type headaches, and trigeminal autonomic cephalgias.

Migraine Headache

Migraine is the most common headache in clinical practice and is frequently missed or misdiagnosed as another type of headache (tension-type or sinus headache).

Diagnosis

Approximately 30% of patients with migraine experience aura during or within the hour before the headache. An aura may manifest as visual loss, hallucinations, flashing lights, numbness, tingling, aphasia, or confusion. Migraine with brainstem aura is defined by the presence of vertigo, ataxia, dysarthria, diplopia, tinnitus, hyperacusis, or alteration in consciousness. Any aura complex that involves some degree of motor weakness is categorized as hemiplegic migraine.

STUDY TABLE: POUND Mnemonic to Diagnose Migraine
Pulsatile quality
One-day duration (between 4 and 72 hours)
Unilateral in location
Nausea or vomiting
Disabling intensity (patient goes to bed)

Four or more features are 90% predictive of migraine headache. Rule out medication overuse headache ("rebound"). Patients with this finding must be weaned off headache medications.

◆ DON'T BE TRICKED

- Ninety percent of patients with "sinus headache" have migraine headache that will respond to triptan medications.
- Neuroimaging is indicated only for atypical headache features or for headaches that do not meet the strict definition of migraine.

STUDY TABLE: Differential Diagnosis of Migraine	
Disease	**Considerations**
Tension-type headache	30 minutes to 7 days
	Typically bilateral location
	Pressure or tight quality
	Does not prohibit activity
	Not associated with nausea
	Treat acute headache with NSAIDs
	A tricyclic antidepressant may be needed for prophylaxis
Trigeminal neuralgia	Brief paroxysms of unilateral lancinating pain in the V_2 or V_3 distribution of the trigeminal nerve, often triggered by light touch of affected area
	Obtain an MRI to exclude intracranial lesions and MS
	Select carbamazepine for treatment

(Continued on next page)

STUDY TABLE: Differential Diagnosis of Migraine (*Continued*)	
Disease	**Considerations**
Medication overuse headache (rebound headache)	Chronic headache that occurs ≥15 days per month in patients using combination analgesics, ergotamine products, or triptans >10 days per month
	Must withdraw all pain medications
Chronic migraine headache	Headache occurring ≥15 days per month for >3 months
	Headache possessing the features of migraine ≥8 days per month
	Risk factors include migraine headache frequency or acute medication use >10 days per month

◆ DON'T BE TRICKED

- Avoid butalbital and opioid analgesics in headache management.
- Muscle relaxants, benzodiazepines, and botulinum toxin A have no role in the acute or preventive treatment of tension-type headache.

Therapy

Migraine treatment is categorized as acute, prophylactic, and rescue. NSAIDs or aspirin are the first-line treatment for acute mild to moderate migraine. A triptan or dihydroergotamine may be used for severe acute migraine or poor response to first-line treatment. Migraine, which is present on awakening, is associated with vomiting, or escalates rapidly, may be best treated by nasal triptans or subcutaneous sumatriptan. Metoclopramide is also effective for migraine-associated nausea and enhances the efficacy of the abortive medication.

Choose migraine prophylaxis when:

- migraines do not respond to therapy
- headache occurs ≥8 days per month
- disabling headache occurs ≥4 days per month
- use of acute migraine medications >8 days per month

Evidence-based migraine prophylaxis (in nonpregnant patients) includes topiramate, valproic acid, metoprolol, propranolol, and timolol.

◆ DON'T BE TRICKED

- Do not choose oral medications for patients with nausea and vomiting.
- Triptans are contraindicated in the presence of CAD and cerebrovascular disease, brainstem aura, and hemiplegic migraine.
- Do not use acute therapies more than 2 to 3 days per week to avoid medication overuse (rebound) headaches.
- Estrogen-containing contraceptives must be avoided in women experiencing aura with migraine because of the increased risk of stroke.

❖ Test Yourself

A 39-year-old woman has chronic headaches that occur daily and do not respond to analgesics. Medications are zolmitriptan, naproxen, acetaminophen with codeine, and amitriptyline.

ANSWER: The diagnosis is chronic daily headache from medication overuse. Taper all medications.

Trigeminal Autonomic Cephalgias

These primary headache disorders are characterized by severe unilateral pain in the first division of the trigeminal nerve (periorbital, frontal, temporal) accompanied by ipsilateral cranial autonomic symptoms. These headaches are differentiated from each other by the duration of pain and frequency of attacks.

STUDY TABLE: Trigeminal Autonomic Cephalgias	
Diagnosis	**Characteristics**
Cluster headache	Pain usually periorbital, duration 20-60 minutes, several times per day. Repeating over weeks then disappearing for months or years. Unilateral tearing and nasal congestion or rhinorrhea. Treat acute headache with a triptan (or oxygen) and verapamil for long-term prevention.
Chronic paroxysmal hemicranias	Occurs at least five times daily lasting 3 to 20 minutes. Responds completely to indomethacin.
SUNCT	Dozens to hundreds of times per day, with durations of 1 to 600 seconds. Typically resistant to treatment.
Hemicrania continua	Persistent strictly unilateral headache that responds to indomethacin.

SUNCT = Short-lasting Unilateral Neuralgiform headaches with Conjunctival injection and Tearing.

Cluster Headache: Ptosis, miosis, and increased tears in left eye in patient with cluster headache. Reprinted from Hale N, Paauw DS. Diagnosis and treatment of headache in the ambulatory care setting: a review of classic presentations and new considerations in diagnosis and management. Med Clin North Am. 2014 May; 98(3):505-27. [PMID: 24758958], with permission from Elsevier.

Selected Secondary Headache Disorders

Headaches are classified as primary, secondary, or related to a cranial neuralgia (e.g., trigeminal neuralgia). Secondary headache disorders typically display "red flags":

- first or worst headache
- abrupt-onset or thunderclap attack
- progression or fundamental change in headache pattern
- abnormal physical examination findings
- neurologic symptoms lasting >1 hour
- new headache in persons <5 years or >50 years old
- new headache in patients with cancer, immunosuppression, or pregnancy
- association with alteration in or loss of consciousness
- headache triggered by exertion, sexual activity, or Valsalva maneuver

Order as appropriate:

- MRI over CT in nonemergency situations
- CT for suspected acute ICH
- ESR or CRP for suspected giant cell arteritis
- LP for suspected infectious or neoplastic meningitis or disorders of intracranial pressure

◆ DON'T BE TRICKED

- EEG has no role in the assessment of headache disorders.

Thunderclap Headaches

An important category of secondary headaches are "thunderclap" headaches defined as reaching maximum intensity within minutes.

STUDY TABLE: Important Thunderclap Headaches		
Headache Type	**Clues**	**Therapy**
Subarachnoid hemorrhage	Sudden onset of "worst headache of my life" Many patients have warning "sentinel" headaches prior to SAH	Neurosurgery in selected cases (85% of nontraumatic cases due to ruptured aneurysm)
Carotid or vertebral dissection	Neck pain and ipsilateral headache, neurological findings in territory of involved vessel Pulsatile tinnitus	Aspirin, heparin, or oral anticoagulation
Thrombosis of cerebral vein or dural sinus	Exertional headache, papilledema, neurological findings Consider in hypercoagulable states, pregnancy, use of oral contraceptives	LMWH followed by warfarin
Reversible cerebral vasoconstriction syndrome	Premenopausal women with recurrent thunderclap headache Imaging shows strokes, hemorrhages, or cerebral edema Often triggered by exposure to adrenergic or serotonergic drugs	Normalization of BP and elimination of any triggering drug or substance

Idiopathic Intracranial Hypertension

Idiopathic intracranial hypertension, also called pseudotumor cerebri, is characterized by increased intracranial pressure without identifiable structural pathology. Patients are typically female, obese, and of child-bearing age. Papilledema is always present.

Diagnosis is confirmed by a CSF pressure >250 mm H_2O with normal fluid composition. MRI may be normal or show small ventricles.

First-line treatment is with acetazolamide.

Traumatic Brain Injury

Mild TBI presents as loss of consciousness or alteration in awareness ("dazed" after a head injury), amnesia near the time of the event, or focal neurologic deficit.

Head injury may result in epidural or subdural hematomas. Classic presentation for epidural and subdural hematomas includes headache and mental status abnormalities. Rapid neurologic decline with ipsilateral pupillary dilatation and brain herniation can occur. Some patients with epidural hematoma exhibit a brief "lucid interval" before subsequent precipitous decline. The tempo of clinical deterioration of subdural hematoma is classically slower, over days to weeks. It is often impossible to clinically distinguish between epidural and subdural hematoma.

◆ **DON'T BE TRICKED**

- Subdural hematomas can also occur in the absence of significant trauma, particularly among older persons and those taking anticoagulant drugs.

Diagnosis

Athletes who sustain a mild TBI should be immediately removed from play and undergo sideline assessment. Participation in sport is prohibited until the patient returns to cognitive baseline and is asymptomatic without taking any medication. Postconcussion syndrome describes the persistence of symptoms of mild TBI beyond a typical recovery period of several weeks.

Neuroimaging is recommended for worsening headache, repeated vomiting, drowsiness, persistent confusion, dysarthria, or focal neurologic findings.

Therapy

Management of postconcussion syndrome is supportive and rehabilitative. NSAIDs and triptans may be useful in treating posttraumatic headache. Tricyclic antidepressants, SSRIs, and SNRIs can also manage posttraumatic headache, as well as mood and anxiety disorders.

The treatment for epidural hematoma is emergent evacuation of blood to prevent death. The treatment of subdural hematoma is dependent on clinical circumstances; observation is appropriate in stable, asymptomatic patients.

Epidural Hematoma: CT scan of an epidural hematoma showing biconvex lens appearance between the skull and outer margin of the dura.

Subdural Hematoma: CT scan of a subdural hematoma showing the crescent shape of blood separating the dura from the arachnoid membrane (*arrows*).

Epilepsy

Diagnosis

Epilepsy is a collection of brain disorders characterized by two or more unprovoked seizures. Partial or localization-related seizures result from an electrical discharge that originates in a focal region of the brain. Primary generalized seizures are caused by an electrical discharge that involves all areas of the brain simultaneously. The electrical discharge in secondarily generalized seizures is focal in onset but rapidly spreads to involve the entire cerebral cortex. Clinical clues to identifying a partial seizure that progressed to a generalized seizure include:

- unilateral shaking
- head turning (versive) to one side
- aura
- postictal (temporary) weakness

STUDY TABLE: Seizure Classifications	
Seizure Type	**Characteristics**
Simple partial seizure	Normal consciousness and awareness
	Single neurologic modality (sensory, motor, olfactory, visual, gustatory) involving a single region of the body, such as the hand or arm
Complex partial seizure	Conscious but unresponsive or staring
	Automatism (lip smacking, swallowing, or manipulating objects)
	Postictal confusion
Primary generalized seizure	Loss of consciousness at onset
	No prodromal or localizing symptoms
	Whole-body stiffening (tonic) and/or jerking (clonic) seizures

Patients with complex partial seizures may recognize a typical aura before losing consciousness, but they often are unaware that they have become impaired and may have no recollection of the seizure.

STUDY TABLE: Common Epilepsy Syndromes	
Temporal lobe epilepsy	Complex partial seizures preceded by an aura. Medial temporal sclerosis is a characteristic finding on MRI.
Frontal lobe epilepsy	Nocturnal complex seizures that awaken patients from sleep. Often associated with underlying structural pathology (e.g., tumor, vascular malformations).
Idiopathic generalized epilepsy	Any combination of tonic-clonic seizures, absence seizures, and myoclonic seizures. MRI typically normal. EEG may show generalized spike-wave abnormality.
Myoclonic seizure	A generalized seizure associated with morning onset of brief, lightning-like jerks of the arms not associated with loss of consciousness (misdiagnosed as "jitteriness").

Several medical conditions can provoke seizures, such as metabolic disturbances, drug intoxication or withdrawal, or infection. Single seizures that are provoked should be addressed by correcting the underlying condition or removing the offending agent; they usually do not require treatment with an antiepileptic drug.

◆ DON'T BE TRICKED

- Consider drugs (alcohol and cocaine) as cause of first-time seizure.
- Diagnostic evaluation may not be needed for a provoked seizure if the patient has normal findings on neurologic examination.
- Seizures that occur within a week of head trauma or ICH may benefit from a short course of an AED but do not necessarily require long-term treatment.

Initial evaluation for a first unprovoked seizure:

- EEG (although a normal EEG does not rule out a seizure)
- CBC, electrolyte and glucose levels, and a toxicology screen
- brain MRI (or head CT in an emergency)
- CSF examination if the patient has fever, prolonged altered mental status after the seizure, is immunosuppressed, or has a severe headache

Psychogenic nonepileptic seizures (PNES) are a type of conversion disorder. Some of the characteristic features include:

- forced eye closure
- long duration
- hypermotor activity that starts and stops
- pelvic thrusting

Inpatient video EEG monitoring is required to make this diagnosis because of the difficulty in distinguishing between PNES and epileptic seizures. PNES is strongly associated with PTSD in military veterans.

Common comorbidities of epilepsy include mood disorders, sleep disorders, metabolic bone disease, and hyperlipidemia.

If the patient is not returning toward baseline mental status by 15 minutes after a seizure, obtain continuous EEG monitoring to rule out nonconvulsive seizures.

Convulsive status epilepticus is characterized by continuous seizure for ≥5 minutes. Complications include fever, hemodynamic instability, acidosis, rhabdomyolysis, aspiration pneumonia, and PE, and are associated with a mortality rate of approximately 20%. Thiamine and glucose can be administered if alcohol abuse is suspected or the cause of the status epilepticus is unknown. Emergent head imaging can also be useful in the absence of a known underlying cause but should not delay treatment.

◆ DON'T BE TRICKED

Avoid misdiagnosis:

- Syncope: Look for sweating and nausea, brief loss of consciousness, occasional tonic-clonic jerking, and recovery without confusion.
- Absence seizure: Do not choose this in an adult.

Therapy

For most adults who have had a first seizure, the risk for a second event is about 50% and AED therapy reduces the risk of a second seizure by only 50%. Start anticonvulsant therapy after ≥2 unprovoked seizures. Starting AED after a single unprovoked seizure can be recommended in patients with:

- age ≥65 years
- history of significant head trauma
- history of partial seizure
- history of postictal weakness or paralysis
- focal findings on neuroimaging
- focal findings on EEG

Choose single-agent therapy and increase the dosage until seizures are controlled or the patient develops adverse medication effects. If unsuccessful, discontinue the first drug, and initiate a second drug as a single agent. Although serum drug level monitoring may be helpful, targeting a clinical response is more important than achieving a specific serum level. Addition of new medications that alter the metabolism of anticonvulsants may result in loss of seizure control.

Guide to initiating AEDs:

- lamotrigine, levetiracetam, topiramate, valproic acid, and zonisamide can be used to treat both generalized and partial epilepsy syndromes
- valproic acid may be superior to other AEDs for treating generalized epilepsy
- carbamazepine is a cost-effective option for partial seizures
- levetiracetam has few drug-drug interactions and is typically well-tolerated and can be used during pregnancy

AED important side effects:

- carbamazepine: interactions with other hepatically metabolized drugs and increased risk for osteoporosis and hypercholesterolemia
- valproic acid: weight gain, hypercholesterolemia, PCOS, teratogenicity
- topiramate and zonisamide: increased risk of kidney stones
- carbamazepine and oxcarbazepine: hyponatremia
- all AEDs: drug hypersensitivity syndrome, SJS, and suicidal ideation

Patients not responding to either their first or their second AED (in sequence or combination) have refractory epilepsy and are potential candidates for epilepsy surgery. The most common surgical procedure is resection of mesial temporal lobe sclerotic lesions associated with partial seizures.

For patients with PNES, referral to appropriate psychological resources provides the best chance of a good outcome.

AEDs may be effectively withdrawn in many patients who have been seizure-free for 2 to 5 years. Predictors of relapse include:

- an abnormal EEG before or during medication withdrawal
- an abnormal neurologic examination
- mental retardation
- frequent seizures before achieving remission

◆ DON'T BE TRICKED

- Primary prophylaxis with AEDs is not indicated for a new stroke or tumor.
- Patients with juvenile myoclonic epilepsy require lifelong medication.
- Carbamazepine, oxcarbazepine, phenytoin, topiramate, clobazam, felbamate, and phenobarbital inactivate many forms of hormonal contraception.

The most common cause of convulsive status epilepticus is a low AED blood level. IV lorazepam followed by phenytoin or fos-phenytoin (valproate if phenytoin allergic) should be administered after 5 minutes of continuous seizing. All patients with convulsive status epilepticus who stop seizing but do not return to baseline within 15 minutes should be monitored with continuous EEG monitoring for nonconvulsive seizures.

AEDs raise the risk of congenital malformation. Most women will require continued drug therapy during pregnancy. The goal is to reduce the medication to the greatest extent and still maintain seizure control. Low-dose monotherapy is preferred. Lamotrigine (requires upward dose adjustment) and levetiracetam are good options. Valproic acid and topiramate should be discontinued (pregnancy risk category D drugs).

❖ Test Yourself

A 33-year-old woman has "spells" during which she is conscious but unresponsive and unaware of her environment. She has repetitive hand movements that last approximately 1 minute followed by several minutes of mild confusion.

ANSWER: The diagnosis is partial complex seizure. Begin carbamazepine.

Ischemic Stroke and Transient Ischemic Attack

Prevention

Risk factor modification is mandatory for all patients (hypertension, diabetes, hyperlipidemia, tobacco use).

Revascularization with either stenting or endarterectomy is for patients with >80% stenosis and low cardiovascular risk, as long as the operative complication rate is <3%.

Begin warfarin (or a new oral anticoagulant) in most patients with nonvalvular AF. Start aspirin therapy in patients with nonvalvular AF who are at low risk of stroke.

Surgical clipping or endovascular coiling of aneurysms are indicated for patients with aneurysms ≥7 mm in the posterior communicating and basilar arteries or ≥12 mm in the anterior circulation.

◆ DON'T BE TRICKED

- The classification of type of AF (paroxysmal, persistent, or permanent) does not affect the decision to anticoagulate.
- Warfarin is the only approved drug for AF associated with valvular heart disease.

Diagnosis

Stroke is a sudden focal neurologic deficit caused by either ischemia (85%) or hemorrhage (15%). Ischemic stroke may be further characterized by the etiologic mechanism (large-artery atherosclerosis, cardioembolic, small-vessel disease, cryptogenic). Hemorrhagic stroke is classified as either subarachnoid or intracerebral (intraparenchymal).

STUDY TABLE: Cerebrovascular Territories and Syndromes	
Artery	**Major Clinical Features**
Anterior cerebral artery	Contralateral leg weakness
Middle cerebral artery	Contralateral face and arm weakness greater than leg weakness; sensory loss, visual field cut, aphasia, or neglect (depending on side)
Posterior cerebral artery	Contralateral visual field cut
Deep/"lacunar"	Contralateral motor or sensory deficit without cortical signs (aphasia, apraxia, neglect, and loss of higher cognitive functions), clumsy hand-dysarthria syndrome, and ataxic hemiparesis
Basilar artery	Oculomotor deficits and/or ataxia with "crossed" sensory/motor deficits. Crossed signs include sensory or motor deficit on one side of the face and the opposite side of the body
Vertebral artery	Lower cranial nerve deficits (vertigo, nystagmus, dysphagia, dysarthria, tongue or palate deviation) and/or ataxia with crossed sensory deficits

TIA is a transient focal neurologic deficit resulting from ischemia rather than infarction. TIA is defined by the absence of infarction on neuroimaging, independent of symptom duration, which typically lasts 5 to 60 minutes.

All patients with stroke or TIA require:

- emergent head CT without contrast (rule out intracranial hemorrhage)
- ECG and telemetry or event monitoring (rule out AF)
- vascular studies (carotid ultrasound or carotid MRA, CTA)
- echocardiography (rule out LV thrombus)

Patients with TIA have an elevated risk of subsequent stroke, particularly in the next 48 hours. Decision to admit patients to the hospital is based upon risk stratification. The most widely used risk stratification is the ABCD² score.

Hospital admission for TIA is recommended for all patients with an ABCD^2 score of ≥3.

STUDY TABLE: ABCD^2 Scoring System	
Patient Characteristics	**Score**
Age ≥60 y	1
Blood pressure ≥140/90 mm Hg	1
Clinical Symptoms	
• Focal weakness with the TIA	2
• Speech impairment without weakness	1
Duration of TIA	
• ≥60 min	2
• 10-59 min	1
Diabetes mellitus present	1

◆ **DON'T BE TRICKED**

- Routine evaluation for thrombophilia is not indicated for patients with TIA or stroke. Patients with cryptogenic stroke should undergo prolonged cardiac rhythm monitoring to rule out AF.
- Consider vertebral-basilar stroke in elderly persons with persistent vertigo.

Therapy

Select intubation and mechanical ventilation for patients with a decreased level of consciousness.

Administer rtPA to all patients with ischemic stroke within 3 hours of stroke onset (if unknown onset, then within 3 hours of the last time the patient was seen to be well). rtPA may rarely be administered up to 4.5 hours after onset in selected patients who do not possess any of the following exclusionary criteria:

- age >80 years
- severe stroke
- diabetes mellitus with a previous infarct
- anticoagulant use

Additional exclusionary criteria for thrombolysis in general include any increased risk of bleeding or diagnosis of ICH. Specific exclusions are unlikely to be tested, but they include:

- history of ICH
- ischemic stroke or head trauma during the previous 3 months
- GI or GU bleeding during the previous 3 weeks
- major surgery or trauma during the previous 14 days
- arterial puncture at noncompressible site within 7 days
- heparin therapy within the previous 48 hours with elevated aPTT
- glucose <50 mg/dL or >400 mg/dL; INR >1.7; platelet count <100,000/μL
- SBP >185 mm Hg and DBP >110 mm Hg
- seizure at stroke onset

In patients with suspicion of a thrombolysis-induced intracranial hemorrhage manifesting as neurological deterioration, stop ongoing infusion of rtPA and evaluate with another CT.

Additional therapy in patients with stroke:

- treat temperature >38.0 °C (100.4 °F) with acetaminophen
- administer normal saline to maintain euvolemia
- allow for permissive hypertension
- give aspirin, 325 mg, unless thrombolysis is planned
- start DVT prophylaxis within 48 hours

Do not begin antihypertensive treatment unless:

- SBP is >220 mm Hg, DBP is >120 mm Hg, or MAP is >140 mm Hg
- thrombolytic therapy is planned
- ACS or aortic dissection is present

If the patient is eligible for thrombolysis, BP must be lowered and stabilized to <185 mm Hg systolic and <110 mm Hg diastolic and maintained below these levels for at least 24 hours after therapy. Preferred antihypertensive agents include IV labetalol and IV nicardipine infusion.

A swallowing assessment is recommended for patients who have experienced strokes before they start to eat or drink. Select early stroke rehabilitation to improve clinical outcomes.

STUDY TABLE: Secondary Prevention of Stroke	
Intervention	**Indication**
Antiplatelet therapy	In the acute setting begin aspirin immediately or within 24 hours after giving thrombolytic agents. In patients with ABCD^2 score ≥4 or minor ischemic stroke, a 21-day course of combination aspirin and clopidogrel, followed by clopidogrel monotherapy for a total of 90 days, reduces the risk of subsequent stroke.
	In the chronic setting, aspirin plus dipyridamole is superior to aspirin alone. Clopidogrel is equivalent to aspirin and dipyridamole.
Anticoagulation therapy	After 48 hours, treat high-risk cardioembolic etiologies of stroke and TIA with warfarin (or a new oral anticoagulant), including in patients with AF, left atrial appendage thrombus, LV thrombus, and dilated cardiomyopathy with reduced EF.
Endarterectomy	Revascularization (endarterectomy or stenting) is recommended within 2 weeks after a nondisabling stroke or TIA if ipsilateral carotid stenosis is between 70% and 99% provided the patient is likely to live 5 years.
	For ipsilateral moderate (50%-69%) carotid artery stenosis, carotid endarterectomy is also usually recommended, depending on patient-specific factors (such as age, sex, comorbidities, and severity of initial symptoms).
Statins	Begin statin therapy for all patients regardless of cholesterol level.
Hypertension	Maintain BP <140/90 mm Hg after recovery from the acute event.
Hemicraniectomy	For patients with a middle cerebral artery infarction involving >50% of the arterial territory.
Multidisciplinary stroke unit	Improves recovery and mitigates poststroke complications.
Depression	Prevalent in the acute and chronic setting and identification and treatment improve recovery.

◆ DON'T BE TRICKED

- If the patient is unable to report the time of onset and there are no witnesses to the onset, rtPA treatment is contraindicated.
- Do not select endovascular stroke therapy in lieu of, or after, thrombolytic therapy.
- Do not select heparin for most patients with ischemic stroke.
- Do not select anticonvulsant medications after stroke unless the patient has had a seizure.
- Do not combine aspirin and clopidogrel for the secondary prevention of stroke in the chronic setting.
- Do not close a PFO for secondary stroke prevention.
- Do not select carotid endarterectomy for carotid artery stenosis <50% or at 100%
- Do not select intracranial stenting.

Ischemic Stroke: CT scan of the brain without contrast shows a large wedge-shaped hypodensity with mass effect 24 hours after onset of symptoms.

Subarachnoid Hemorrhage

Prevention

Patients with small (<7 mm) unruptured aneurysms can be followed with MRI; those with larger aneurysms should consider surgery. The risk of rupture increases with size and location of the aneurysm in the posterior circulation.

Diagnosis

The most common symptom associated with SAH is altered consciousness. Spontaneous SAH most commonly results from the rupture of saccular ("berry") aneurysms of the circle of Willis. SAH less commonly results from rupture of an AVM, arterial dissection, coagulopathy, or cocaine abuse. Most patients present to the emergency department with sudden onset of the "worst headache of my life" or "thunderclap headache" (reaches maximal intensity in 30 minutes). However, up to 40% of patients with SAH experience a "sentinel hemorrhage" characterized as severe headache during the previous 2 to 3 weeks. Subhyaloid hemorrhage may be seen on funduscopy. Focal neurologic deficits occur from aneurysms that compress a cranial nerve (third nerve palsy and dilated pupil), bleed into brain parenchyma, or cause focal ischemia due to vasospasm.

Noncontrast CT establishes the diagnosis of SAH in >90% of patients. Blood in the subarachnoid space is very dense and looks white. Early conventional cerebral angiography identifies the aneurysm and determines management. Other causes of abrupt severe headache include arterial dissection and venous sinus thrombosis, both of which may be detected with vascular imaging, pituitary apoplexy, hypertensive emergency, and ICH.

◆ DON'T BE TRICKED

- If the CT scan is normal, always select CSF examination to look for erythrocytes or xanthochromia.
- If angiography is negative, order a repeat study 4 to 6 weeks later.

Therapy

The three main neurologic complications for a patient with a SAH are rebleeding, delayed brain ischemia from vasospasm, and hydrocephalus. To manage these complications, do the following:

- treat ruptured aneurysms with surgical clipping or endovascular coiling within 48 to 72 hours
- maintain BP <140/80 mm Hg to prevent rebleeding
- use vasopressors to augment the BP to treat vasospasm
- select oral nimodipine for 21 days to improve neurological outcomes

Any change in mental status should prompt emergency CT to evaluate for repeat bleeding and for signs of hydrocephalus, which is treated with ventricular drainage. Screening transcranial ultrasonography or CTA is used to detect cerebral vasospasm.

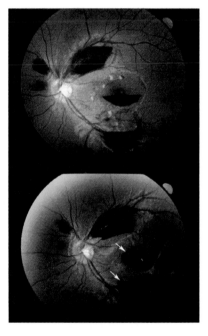

Subhyaloid Hemorrhage: Bleeding under the vitreous membrane (subhyaloid hemorrhage) is a finding associated with SAH.

✥ Test Yourself

A 44-year-old woman comes to the emergency department reporting "the worst headache of my life." She has meningism but no focal neurologic findings. CT scan is normal.

ANSWER: The diagnosis is SAH. Select CSF examination.

Intracerebral Hemorrhage

Diagnosis

The most common risk factor for ICH is hypertension (common in patients with hemorrhage in the basal ganglia, thalamus, pons, and cerebellum). Other risk factors include amyloid angiopathy (primarily in older adult patients with lobar hemorrhage), vascular malformations, coagulopathy, and use of cocaine or alcohol.

ICH, with symptoms similar to those of ischemic stroke, cannot be reliably distinguished by clinical criteria alone. CT without contrast establishes the diagnosis. Cerebral angiography is indicated for patients <45 years of age with ICH related to cocaine use (which is associated with a high incidence of vascular anomalies).

Therapy

Identify and reverse anticoagulation. Mannitol, barbiturate coma, and hyperventilation may be used to reduce intracranial pressure. IV nicardipine, or labetalol, is indicated to maintain SBP between 140 and 160 mm Hg (MAP between 70 and 130 mm Hg). Intraventricular hemorrhage requires prompt ventricular drainage to reduce intracranial pressure. Cerebellar hemorrhages require surgical posterior fossa decompression.

For warfarin-associated ICH, FFP or prothrombin complex concentrates are recommended, as is administration of IV vitamin K.

Intracerebral Hemorrhage: CT scan of the brain shows a brightly enhancing hemorrhage in the left basal ganglia.

◆ DON'T BE TRICKED

- Treatment with rfVIIa limits early enlargement of hemorrhage volume but does not improve function or survival.
- Do not select nitrates to lower BP because they can increase intracerebral pressure.
- Glucocorticoids are not recommended for intracranial hemorrhage.

Dementia

Diagnosis

Dementia is an acquired chronic impairment of memory and other aspects of intellect that impedes daily functioning.

Mild cognitive impairment (MCI) describes cognitive decline greater than expected for age but without interference with daily functioning.

The rate of progression of MCI to dementia is 10% to 15% per year compared to 1% to 2% in patients without MCI.

◆ DON'T BE TRICKED

- No test can predict the likelihood that an individual patient with MCI will develop dementia.
- No treatments delay the onset of Alzheimer disease in patients with MCI.

Alzheimer disease is the most prevalent dementia, accounting for 60% to 80% of cases.

Characteristic findings of Alzheimer disease are memory loss; getting lost; difficulty finding words; and difficulty with dressing, grooming, and doing housework.

A score <24 on the Mini–Mental State Examination is compatible with dementia. Other diagnostic tools include the Montreal Cognitive Assessment and "Mini-Cog" test.

Usual but unproved laboratory studies include a CBC, a comprehensive metabolic profile, TSH and vitamin B$_{12}$ levels, and screening tests for syphilis and HIV infection in high-risk individuals. Routinely obtain brain imaging with CT or MRI to detect nondegenerative causes that would alter management, such as cerebrovascular disease, neoplasm, subdural hematoma, or hydrocephalus. Screen all patients for depression. Consider LP and CSF examination in the following situations:

- rapidly progressive dementia
- age of onset <60 years
- history of malignancy or paraneoplastic disorders
- suspicion for acute or subacute infection; immunosuppressed or immunodeficiency state
- positive syphilis or Lyme serology
- systemic autoimmune disease; suspected CNS inflammatory disorder

Creutzfeldt-Jacob disease is the most common cause of rapidly progressive dementia. Early-onset or rapidly-progressive dementia requires early brain MRI, CSF analysis, and EEG.

Abrupt cognitive, behavioral, and neurological deterioration in patients with dementia commonly results from infection (UTI, pneumonia) or medication errors.

STUDY TABLE: Differential Diagnosis of Dementia	
When you see this...	Choose this...
Acute onset, fluctuating course, inattention, disorganized thinking, and altered consciousness	Delirium
Evidence of objective memory impairment in the absence of other cognitive deficits and intact activities of daily living	MCI
Gradual memory loss, aphasia, apraxia, agnosia, inattention, delusional thinking, decrease in executive function, and left-right confusion	Alzheimer disease
Imaging or history positive for stroke responsible for impairment of at least one cognitive domain	Vascular neurocognitive disorder
Common findings include focal neurologic findings, depression, pseudobulbar palsy, gait abnormalities, and urinary difficulties	
Mild parkinsonism characterized by postural instability and gait difficulty, fluctuating cognition, delusions, and visual hallucinations	Dementia with Lewy bodies
Early and prominent personality changes, behavioral disturbances including disinhibition and impulsivity, diminished frontal and/or temporal lobes on MRI, onset before age 60 years	Frontotemporal dementia, behavioral variant
Prominent and early changes in language function	Frontotemporal dementia, primary progressive aphasia
Dementia, shuffling gait, urinary incontinence, and ventriculomegaly in the absence of past history of meningitis, SAH, or trauma	Normal-pressure hydrocephalus
Choreoathetosis and dementia, autosomal dominant pattern of inheritance	Huntington disease
Prominent myoclonus, characteristic EEG pattern of triphasic sharp waves, CSF protein 14-3-3, rapidly progressive onset at early age	Creutzfeldt-Jakob disease
Early postural instability and falls, axial parkinsonism poorly responsive to levodopa, vertical gaze palsy, slurred speech, apathy, slow processing speed, and impaired executive dysfunction	Progressive supranuclear palsy
History of head injury followed by delayed development (10 years) of impaired concentration, short-term memory, executive dysfunction, and judgment; depression, irritability, aggression, violent behaviors, and suicidality; and parkinsonism, unsteady gait, shuffling gait, and slurred speech	Chronic traumatic encephalopathy

◆ DON'T BE TRICKED

- Do not order apolipoprotein E genotyping in patients with suspected Alzheimer disease.
- Relative sparing of memory and visuospatial function (not getting lost) are characteristic of early frontal temporal dementia, differentiating it from Alzheimer disease.
- Vascular neurocognitive disorder can mimic normal-pressure hydrocephalus but is suggested by the presence of ischemic infarctions, hypertension, ischemic heart disease, diabetes mellitus, and dyslipidemia.

Therapy

Choose cholinesterase inhibitors (donepezil, rivastigmine, and galantamine) to slow intellectual decline in patients with mild to moderate Alzheimer disease. Cholinesterase inhibitors can have prominent cholinergic side effects, including diarrhea, nausea and vomiting, bradycardia, syncope, and heart block. Memantine delays cognitive decline in patients with moderate to advanced Alzheimer disease (Mini–Mental State Examination score of 3 to 14).

Also choose:

- cholinesterase inhibitors for dementia with Lewy bodies
- risk factor modification for vascular neurocognitive disorder
- large-volume LP with symptom assessment before and after to evaluate response to shunting for normal-pressure hydrocephalus

Nonpharmacologic interventions are first-line treatment for the behavioral symptoms. Atypical antipsychotics can treat agitation, aggression, delusions, and hallucinations but have a black box warning due to increased cerebrovascular events and mortality; they are used when patient safety is jeopardized.

Treat depression with SSRIs.

◆ DON'T BE TRICKED

- Combination therapy with a cholinesterase inhibitor and memantine is no more effective than a cholinesterase inhibitor alone.
- No drug is beneficial for frontotemporal dementia.
- Benzodiazepines are not recommended for the treatment of behavioral symptoms in patients with dementia.
- Do not select tricyclic antidepressants like amitriptyline or imipramine for depression, because they can exacerbate confusion.

Delirium

Diagnosis

Diagnosis of delirium is based on the Confusion Assessment Method diagnostic algorithm, which provides greater accuracy than laboratory tests, imaging studies, or other tests. Diagnose delirium if the first two points and either point 3 or 4 are present:

1. Acute onset and fluctuating course
2. Inattention
3. Disorganized thinking
4. Altered level of consciousness

Look for triggers of delirium, particularly medications known to cause delirium and polypharmacy. Pay particular attention to sedative-hypnotics, barbiturates, alcohol, antidepressants, anticholinergics, opioid analgesics, antipsychotics, anticonvulsants, antihistamines, fluoroquinolones, and antiparkinsonian agents. Also consider fluid and electrolyte abnormalities, uncontrolled pain, hypoxemia, anemia, infections, immobility, visual and hearing impairment, sleep cycle disruption, and catheters and other "tethers" (IV lines, ECG leads, and restraints).

◆ DON'T BE TRICKED

- Two or more underlying causes are present in as many as 50% of older patients.
- Brain imaging is usually not helpful in diagnosing delirium unless there is a history of falls or evidence of focal neurologic impairment.

Therapy

Treat or eliminate precipitating factors. Achieve behavior control with environmental or social measures rather than pharmacologic or physical restraints. Choose haloperidol or risperidone for agitated delirium only in life-threatening circumstances (such as in the ICU) or when behavioral measures are ineffective.

◆ **DON'T BE TRICKED**

- Always select behavioral interventions first and order a "sitter" instead of using restraints or drugs.
- All atypical antipsychotics (aripiprazole, clozapine, olanzapine, quetiapine, risperidone, and ziprasidone) and older antipsychotics (haloperidol) are associated with an increased risk of mortality in patients with dementia and psychosis or behavioral disturbances.
- Benzodiazepines can worsen delirium and are not recommended, except in the management of alcohol withdrawal.

Parkinson Disease

Diagnosis

Parkinsonism is a generic term referring to any cause of parkinsonian symptoms and signs. Parkinson disease, a distinct clinicopathologic entity caused by the degeneration of dopaminergic neurons in the substantia nigra of the midbrain, is characterized by at least two of the following conditions:

- bradykinesia (slowed movement and decreased amplitude of repetitive movement)
- rigidity (cogwheel type)
- resting tremor (or with movement)
- postural reflex abnormality (falling)

Patients with parkinsonism are at increased fall risk and may present for evaluation of frequent falls.

Neurologic signs and symptoms are asymmetric at onset. Diminished sense of smell, constipation, and acting out dreams may precede onset of motor symptoms by years. Early dementia within the first year of the appearance of motor parkinsonism symptoms is a hallmark of dementia with Lewy bodies.

In advanced disease, look for evidence of autonomic dysfunction, such as orthostatic hypotension, urinary frequency and urgency, constipation, and diarrhea. Seborrheic dermatitis is a well-recognized Parkinson disease cutaneous association.

Clinical improvement usually occurs after administration of levodopa and/or a dopamine agonist.

Parkinson disease is a clinical diagnosis. Brain imaging may be obtained to exclude other disease processes such as vascular disease, hydrocephalus, and other degenerative diseases that may mimic Parkinson disease.

◆ **DON'T BE TRICKED**

- Early symmetric symptoms or signs, early falls, rapid progression, poor or waning response to levodopa, dementia, early autonomic failure, and ataxia suggest a diagnosis other than Parkinson disease.

STUDY TABLE: Differential Diagnosis of Parkinson Disease	
Disease	**Considerations**
Multiple system atrophy (Shy-Drager syndrome)	Severe orthostatic hypotension and ataxia
	MRI showing "necrosis" of the putamen and cerebellar atrophy
Progressive supranuclear palsy	Unexplained falls (typically backward), inability to move eyes vertically, and parkinsonian features

(Continued on next page)

STUDY TABLE: Differential Diagnosis of Parkinson Disease (*Continued*)	
Disease	**Considerations**
Corticobasal degeneration	Markedly asymmetric parkinsonism and dystonia, myoclonus, cortical sensory deficits, and cognitive deficits
Dementia with Lewy bodies	Early dementia, parkinsonism, and hallucinations
Medication-induced parkinsonism	Antiemetics (prochlorperazine, metoclopramide), antipsychotics (haloperidol), reserpine, lithium, and methyldopa

◆ **DON'T BE TRICKED**

- Drug-induced parkinsonism is distinguished from Parkinson disease by the symmetry of symptoms and the absence of typical nonmotor features.

Therapy

Levodopa is the most effective medication used in the treatment of Parkinson disease but is associated with motor fluctuations, such as dyskinesia and a "wearing-off" effect, which refers to enhanced parkinsonian symptoms due to ineffective dopamine therapy. These motor fluctuations develop at a rate of 10% annually in patients older than 60 years but seem to develop more rapidly and are more severe in younger patients. Therefore, most clinicians will initiate therapy with a dopamine agonist (pramipexole, ropinirole) in patients younger than 65 years to avoid the early appearance of these side effects. At some point, however, all patients will require the addition of levodopa therapy. Levodopa is the drug of choice in older patients. Levodopa is administered in combination with carbidopa, which prevents the peripheral conversion of levodopa to dopamine.

Side effects of dopamine agonists include sedation and increase in compulsive behaviors such as gambling, shopping, and hypersexuality.

Increasing the dose or frequency of levodopa or using a sustained release formulation is indicated to treat the symptoms of wearing off.

Deep brain stimulation is indicated for patients who have sustained motor benefit from levodopa but are limited by disabling medication-related adverse effects that are refractory to medical management.

◆ **DON'T BE TRICKED**

- Begin drug therapy when symptoms begin to interfere with function.
- Avoid cabergoline and bromocriptine, because they are associated with valvular heart disease.
- Failure to respond to dopamine therapy is the most important red flag indicating atypical parkinsonism.

✦ **Test Yourself**

A 68-year-old woman has a 2-year history of falls and imbalance. She has a staring facial expression and impaired upward gaze.

ANSWER: The diagnosis is supranuclear palsy.

Hyperkinetic Movement Disorders

Diagnosis

Hyperkinetic movement disorders include:

- tremors (rhythmic oscillation)
- dystonia (sustained contraction of opposing muscles, resulting in repetitive movements or abnormal posture)
- myoclonus (abrupt jerking movements of the extremities)
- tics (stereotyped, brief, rapid movements)
- chorea (random, nonrepetitive, flowing dance-like movements)

STUDY TABLE: Hyperkinetic Movement Disorders

Condition	Key Manifestations	Therapy
Essential tremor	Typically slowly progressive or stable over time. Bilateral postural tremor, as when the hands are outstretched, or kinetic, as during writing; improves with alcohol. Family history positive in 50%	Propranolol or primidone
Huntington disease	Most common neurodegenerative cause of generalized chorea. Also progressive dementia and psychiatric manifestations Autosomal dominant	Symptomatic only
Drug-induced dystonia	Tardive dyskinesia is associated with choreiform and dystonic craniofacial movements. Can be caused by neuroleptics, antiemetics, and serotoninergic medications	Stop the offending drug Clonazepam, tetrabenazine, anticholinergic agents, and clozapine
Cervical dystonia (torticollis)	Cervical muscle contractions resulting in abnormal posture of the head and neck	Botulinum toxin (first line) or anticholinergic medications
Restless legs syndrome	Restlessness or unpleasant sensations in the legs that are caused by rest and relieved by walking or stretching	Treat iron deficiency anemia Choose ropinirole or pramipexole, and the rotigotine patch
Periodic limb movement disorder	Repetitive triple flexion movements primarily involving the legs and occurring with sleep. Diagnosed with polysomnography Highly associated with restless legs syndrome	As above
Tourette syndrome	Childhood onset, persistence of multiple complex motor tics for at least 1 year, and presence of vocal tics (e.g., echolalia)	Reassurance or cognitive behavioral therapy
REM sleep behavior disorder	Absent muscle paralysis during the REM phase of sleep results in physically acting out dreams (e.g., shouting, kicking, punching)	Clonazepam and melatonin
Neuroleptic malignant syndrome	Exposure to therapeutic doses of dopamine-blocking agents. Hyperthermia, rhabdomyolysis, altered mental status, and rigidity and dystonia	Stop offending drug Dantrolene and bromocriptine
Myoclonus	Rapid, shock-like, jerky movements of isolated body parts. Underlying metabolic disorder, serotonin syndrome, postanoxic, Creutzfeldt-Jakob disease, corticobasal degeneration	Treat underlying metabolic disorder (uremia, hepatic failure, electrolyte imbalance)

◆ **DON'T BE TRICKED**

- Rigidity and resting tremor are not features of essential tremor.
- Screen patients <40 years with "essential tremor" or dystonia for Wilson disease with serum ceruloplasmin and 24-hour urine copper measurements.
- A neuroleptic malignant syndrome can occur with rapid withdrawal from chronic dopaminergic treatment, as in hospitalized Parkinson disease patients.

Multiple Sclerosis

Diagnosis

MS is characterized by episodes of dysfunction due to demyelinating lesions (plaques) in different areas of the CNS (brain, brain stem including optic nerve, or spinal cord) at different times.

Clinical course follows one of three patterns: relapsing-remitting (85% of cases), secondary progressive, or primary progressive disease. Relapsing-remitting MS is characterized by clinical episodes of neurologic dysfunction, typically lasting weeks before improving, that may in some patients lead to the accumulation of disability. About 50% of patients with relapsing-remitting disease develop secondary progressive disease, characterized by the disappearance of evidence of clinical relapses and by progressive disability. Primary progressive disease is characterized by progressive disability accumulation from the time of disease onset. Those who do not meet the full diagnostic criteria for MS after a first event are said to have had a clinically isolated syndrome. The 10-year risk of MS associated with a clinically isolated syndrome and lesions on MRI is 90%.

STUDY TABLE: Common Symptoms/Findings Associated with MS

Finding or Anatomical Involvement	Description
Optic neuritis	Subacute visual deficit in one eye along with pain with eye movement with reduction in visual acuity, visual field deficit, and color desaturation
Afferent pupil	Paradoxical dilation of the pupil when light is rapidly shifted from the unaffected to the affected eye
Papillitis	Inflammatory changes in the retina causing a flared appearance of the optic disc
Myelitis	Focal inflammation within the spinal cord manifesting as sensory or motor symptoms below the affected spinal level
Lhermitte sign	A shock-like sensation radiating down the spine or limbs induced by neck movements
Bladder	Urinary frequency, urgency, or retention
Cerebellum	Ataxia and vertigo
Brainstem (internuclear ophthalmoplegia)	Inability to adduct one eye and nystagmus in the abducting eye
Uhthoff phenomenon	Transient worsening of baseline neurologic symptoms with elevations of body temperature

Diagnosis requires evidence of CNS demyelination disseminated in both space and time as demonstrated through a combination of documented clinical relapses, signs on physical examination, and the distribution of lesions on an MRI. Typical lesions are contrast enhancing found in these areas:

- periventricular
- juxtacortical
- brainstem
- cerebellum
- spinal cord

CSF may contain oligoclonal IgG bands or an elevated IgG index. CSF analysis is not necessary but can be helpful when the diagnosis remains questionable.

◆ **DON'T BE TRICKED**
- MS generally is not associated with cortical syndromes, such as aphasia and neglect.
- Any patient with suspected relapse should be screened for intercurrent infection to exclude Uhthoff phenomenon before initiating MS-specific therapy.
- Migraine, microvascular ischemic disease, and head trauma can also cause white matter lesions on MRI.

Therapy

IV methylprednisolone followed by oral glucocorticoids speeds recovery from acute exacerbations, most effectively in acute optic neuritis. Treat fever and look for underlying infection before beginning glucocorticoids, because fever worsens symptoms of MS (pseudorelapse) and treatment of the underlying trigger will improve symptoms.

After the first attack of a clinically isolated syndrome (optic neuritis, spinal cord syndrome, or brain stem–cerebellar syndrome), prescribe interferon-β or glatiramer acetate if imaging suggests MS.

Prescribe interferon-β or glatiramer acetate for confirmed relapsing-remitting MS. Natalizumab is used for interferon- and glatiramer-refractory disease but has potential for serious side effects (risk of progressive multifocal leukoencephalopathy [JC virus infection]).

Other agents include mitoxantrone (cardiac toxicity and secondary leukemia), fingolimod (first-dose bradycardia effect), teriflunomide, and dimethyl fumarate.

MS relapses that have no or minimal impact on function may simply be observed. If functional status (vision, strength, balance, or coordination) is impaired, IV methylprednisolone or oral prednisone will speed recovery but will not alter the ultimate degree of recovery.

Vitamin D added to interferon-β reduces the accumulation of MRI lesions; vitamin D supplementation is recommended for all patients with MS. All patients should receive annual influenza vaccination and maintain their regular immunization schedule. Steroid-unresponsive acute exacerbations may respond to plasmapheresis.

STUDY TABLE: Symptomatic Management in Multiple Sclerosis

Symptom	Nonpharmacologic Management	Pharmacologic Management
Spasticity	Physical therapy, stretching, massage therapy	Baclofen (oral or intrathecal pump), tizanidine, cyclobenzaprine, gabapentin, benzodiazepines, carisoprodol, botulinum toxin
Neuropathic pain	None	Gabapentin, pregabalin, duloxetine, tricyclic antidepressants, tramadol, carbamazepine, topiramate, capsaicin patch
Fatigue	Proper sleep hygiene, regular exercise	Modafinil, armodafinil, amantadine, amphetamine stimulants
Depression	Individual or group counseling	Antidepressants (such as SSRIs, SNRIs, tricyclic antidepressants, antipsychotic agents)
Cognitive dysfunction	Cognitive rehabilitation and accommodation strategies	No proven therapy
Mobility	Physical and occupational therapy; use of braces, canes, rolling walkers, or electrostimulatory walk-assist devices	Dalfampridine
Urinary urgency/frequency	Timed voids, avoidance of caffeine	Oxybutynin, tolterodine
Urinary retention	Manual pelvic pressure, intermittent catheterization	None
Pseudobulbar affect	None	Dextromethorphan-quinidine
Limb tremor	Occupational therapy	Botulinum toxin

Encourage smoking cessation because of the threefold increase in the risk of secondary progression associated with cigarette smoking.

◆ DON'T BE TRICKED

- Interferon agents are contraindicated in patients with liver disease or depression.
- Pregnancy does not cause additional permanent disability in women with MS.
- Combining glatiramer acetate with interferon-β provides no added benefit to either drug alone.
- Do not prescribe natalizumab to patients with positive JC virus antibody testing.

❖ Test Yourself

A 25-year-old woman has a 2-week episode of new-onset gait ataxia, nystagmus, and dysarthria. Two years ago, she had optic neuritis. An MRI of the brain now shows brain lesions consistent with MS.

ANSWER: The diagnosis is relapsing-remitting MS. Choose IV methylprednisolone and interferon-β.

Multiple Sclerosis Lesions: Fluid-attenuated inversion recovery MRI shows MS lesions in the paraventricular white matter bilaterally.

Myelopathy

Diagnosis

Spinal cord dysfunction, or myelopathy, can occur because of a lesion arising within the spinal cord (intramedullary) or extrinsic compression of the spinal cord.

When injury to the corticospinal tracts occurs, spastic paresis or paralysis is possible, manifesting as weakness, hyperreflexia, muscle spasms, and extensor plantar responses.

Involvement of the distal cord and lower roots (cauda equina syndrome) can involve weakness of the lower motoneuron type, with decreased muscle tone and areflexia.

Causes of noncompressive myelopathy include inflammatory or demyelinating lesions, spinal cord infarction, and vitamin B_{12} or copper deficiency.

STUDY TABLE: Selected Causes of Intramedullary Myelopathy	
Cause	**Features**
MS	See Multiple Sclerosis
Neuromyelitis optica (Devic disease)	Recurrent episodes of myelitis and optic neuritis without the brain lesions typical of MS; NMO-IgG autoantibody may be present
Idiopathic transverse myelitis	Subacute onset of weakness, sensory changes, and bowel/bladder dysfunction, typically after a viral infection
	Idiopathic transverse myelitis is distinguished from MS by presence of complete (not partial) myelitis, no oligoclonal bands or elevated IgG index in the CSF, and no lesions on brain MRI
Vitamin B_{12} deficiency	Paresthesia, lower-extremity weakness, and gait instability. Findings may include paraparesis, vibration and position sense loss, and sensory ataxia. Anemia may be absent
Copper deficiency	Mimics vitamin B_{12} deficiency. May develop secondary to malabsorption after bariatric surgery or from excessive zinc ingestion
Infarction of the spinal cord	Acute onset, findings correspond to the territory of the anterior spinal artery. Flaccid paralysis or weakness and pinprick sensation loss below the level of the infarction but sparing vibration and position sense. Potential causes include emboli, hypotension during cardiovascular/aortic surgery, and AV malformations

Spinal cord compression most commonly presents with neck or back pain, followed by weakness, sensory changes, and bowel and bladder dysfunction associated with upper motoneuron signs (weakness, spasticity, hyperreflexia, extensor plantar responses) and occasionally lower motoneuron signs (atrophy, hyporeflexia).

Clues to the etiology of compression myelopathy:

- fever—epidural abscess
- anticoagulation—epidural hematoma
- cancer—metastases
- trauma—vertebral fracture
- elderly with chronic back/leg pain—spinal stenosis

Select MRI of the spine to exclude spinal cord compression in all patients with clinical suspicion of spinal cord disorder. LP may be beneficial in patients with suspected inflammatory or demyelinating spinal cord lesions.

◆ DON'T BE TRICKED

- Check methylmalonic acid and homocysteine measurements for patients with borderline B_{12} values.

Therapy

Treat traumatic spinal cord injury with high-dose IV glucocorticoids within the first 8 hours.

Treat spinal cord compression due to metastatic disease emergently with high-dose glucocorticoids and subsequent surgical decompression followed by radiation for most tumor types.

There is no treatment for spinal cord infarction.

For treatment of demyelinating diseases, see Multiple Sclerosis.

Treat vitamin B_{12} and copper deficiencies with supplementation.

Direct treatment of inflammatory and infectious myelopathy at the underlying disorder.

Treat transverse myelitis with IV methylprednisolone, and consider plasmapheresis or cyclophosphamide if transverse myelitis is refractory.

◆ DON'T BE TRICKED

- Spinal cord compression due to leukemia, lymphoma, myeloma, and germ cell tumors may be treated urgently with radiation therapy rather than surgery.
- Do not use glucocorticoids to treat spinal cord compression caused by infection or hematoma.

Amyotrophic Lateral Sclerosis

Diagnosis

Motoneuron diseases consist of an acquired group of degenerative disorders involving cortical motoneurons in the frontal lobe (primary lateral sclerosis), anterior horn cells in the spinal cord (progressive muscular atrophy), and cortical motoneurons and anterior horn cells (ALS). The defining characteristic is the combination of upper motoneuron signs (e.g., hyperreflexia, spasticity, and extensor plantar response) coexistent with lower motoneuron findings (e.g., atrophy and fasciculation). Sensory deficits are characteristically absent.

Muscle weakness in patients with ALS usually begins distally and asymmetrically, although 20% of patients have bulbar-onset ALS with difficulty speaking and swallowing. All patients with suspected ALS should undergo EMG to test for muscle degeneration and MRI of the appropriate anatomic areas to diagnose treatable neurologic disorders that may mimic ALS. Pulmonary function tests and overnight pulse oximetry studies can establish the presence of respiratory insufficiency. Patients with bulbar signs or symptoms require evaluation of swallowing function.

◆ DON'T BE TRICKED

- Findings not typical for ALS include predominant sensory symptoms or pain, early cognitive impairment, and ocular muscle weakness.
- Fasciculations in the absence of associated muscle atrophy or weakness are not due to ALS.
- Weakness in the absence of fasciculations is not due to ALS.

Therapy

Riluzole may increase survival by about 3 months. Begin noninvasive ventilatory support for patients with respiratory insufficiency. Placement of a percutaneous endoscopic gastrostomy tube is indicated when weight loss or swallowing difficulty occurs.

Myasthenia Gravis

Diagnosis

MG is an autoimmune disease caused by antibodies directed against the acetylcholine receptor, which results in impaired neuromuscular transmission. Characteristic findings of MG include:

- ptosis or diplopia
- muscle weakness, including dysphagia and dyspnea
- positive anti–acetylcholine receptor antibody titer (negative titer does not rule out MG)
- normal deep tendon reflexes and sensation

Patients may experience myasthenic crisis (rapidly progressive respiratory failure). Myasthenic crisis can occur as part of the natural history of myasthenia or be triggered by infection, surgery, or medications. Look for aminoglycosides, quinolones, magnesium, β-blockers, or calcium channel blockers as precipitants of myasthenic crisis.

Symptoms are worsened by fatigue, exertion, increased body temperature, stress, and intercurrent infections. Single-fiber EMG can also establish the diagnosis. Look for a history of hypothyroidism or elevated serum TSH levels because of the association of MG with autoimmune thyroid disorders. Perform CT of the chest to detect thymoma.

Include botulism and Eaton-Lambert myasthenic syndrome in the differential diagnosis. Botulism starts with cranial nerve involvement, including diplopia, dysphagia, and sluggish or nonreactive pupils, whereas the pupils are normal in MG.

Eaton-Lambert myasthenic syndrome involves progressive proximal weakness and diminished tendon reflexes that improve with repetitive movement of affected muscles. Diagnosis is confirmed by detection of serum anti–voltage-gated calcium channel antibodies and the EMG finding of facilitation of motor response to rapid repetitive stimulation. Fifty to sixty percent of patients with this syndrome have an undetected malignancy, typically SCLC.

Therapy

Pyridostigmine is the initial therapy. Reduce the dosage if increased salivation, respiratory secretions, sweating, or bradycardia develops. Patients with more severe symptoms may benefit from immunosuppressive therapy with agents such as prednisone, cyclosporine, azathioprine, and mycophenolate mofetil. If vital capacity decreases to <15 mL/kg, intubate the patient and begin plasmapheresis. Thymectomy is indicated if a thymoma is found on CT or MRI.

Myasthenic crisis and refractory disease should be treated with plasmapheresis or IV immune globulin.

◆ DON'T BE TRICKED

- Pyridostigmine monotherapy should be avoided in those with myasthenic crisis because the drug increases respiratory secretions.

Peripheral Neuropathy

Diagnosis

Patients with neuropathy may present with pain, paresthesia, weakness, or autonomic dysfunction. Neuropathies can be classified by:

- distribution of sensorimotor deficits (symmetric vs. asymmetric, distal vs. proximal, focal vs. generalized)
- pathology (demyelinating vs. axonal)
- size of nerve fibers involved (large vs. small fibers)
- family history
- autonomic involvement

Mononeuropathies, isolated disorders affecting a single peripheral nerve, are most frequently caused by nerve entrapment or compression (carpal tunnel syndrome).

Mononeuropathy multiplex involves multiple noncontiguous peripheral nerves, either simultaneously or sequentially. This is often the result of a systemic disease (vasculitis).

Polyneuropathy refers to a diffuse, generalized, and usually symmetric peripheral neuropathy. Polyneuropathy is often a manifestation of systemic disease (e.g., diabetes, B_{12} deficiency) or exposure to a toxin (e.g., alcohol) or medication (e.g., chemotherapy).

In all neuropathies, EMG can be helpful to characterize the type (axonal or demyelinating), severity, and distribution of the disease. Other routine tests include vitamin B_{12} level, SPEP, UPEP, ESR, and blood glucose level.

STUDY TABLE: Diagnosing and Managing Peripheral Neuropathy		
If you see this...	**Think this...**	**And choose this...**
Isolated anterolateral thigh numbness without weakness	Meralgia paresthetica (a compressive neuropathy of the lateral femoral cutaneous nerve)	Locate and relieve pressure (binding clothes, excessive weight)
Sensory loss over palmar surface of first three digits and weakness with thumb abduction and opposition	Median neuropathy (carpal tunnel syndrome)	Wrist splints or glucocorticoid injections for mild disease; surgical release if severe
Numbness of the fourth and fifth fingers and weakness of interosseous muscles	Ulnar neuropathy	Elbow splinting or elbow pads; surgical release if severe
Pain, tingling, and numbness in great toe and along medial foot	Tarsal tunnel syndrome	Local glucocorticoid injection; decompression surgery if severe
Upper and lower face weakness	Bell palsy. Assess for diabetes mellitus, vasculitis, Lyme disease, sarcoidosis, HIV infection, and compressive or infiltrative malignancies only if additional suggestive features are present	Prednisone if within 72 hours of onset
Multiple, noncontiguous nerve deficits (mononeuritis multiplex)	Consider vasculitis (especially if painful), lymphoma, amyloidosis, sarcoidosis, Lyme disease, HIV, leprosy, and diabetes	Treat underlying disorder
Distal and symmetric (stocking-glove) sensory or sensorimotor deficit	Axonal polyneuropathies; diabetes and alcohol are the most common etiologies; small fiber neuropathy will present with pain only	Treat underlying disorder; treat pain and dysesthesia symptomatically
Severe unilateral leg pain, numbness, proximal weakness, atrophy, and weight loss	Diabetic lumbosacral radiculoplexus neuropathy (diabetic amyotrophy)	Treat diabetes
Acute, ascending, areflexic paralysis and paresthesia often preceded by GI illness (usually *Campylobacter* infection); CSF shows elevated protein and a normal cell count (albuminocytologic dissociation)	Guillain-Barré syndrome	Plasma exchange and IV immune globulin
Progressive proximal motor and sensory neuropathy that evolves over months. Initial EMG and CSF findings similar to Guillain-Barré syndrome	Chronic inflammatory demyelinating polyneuropathy	Prednisone, plasma exchange, and IV immune globulin
Failure to wean from mechanical ventilation. Flaccid paralysis and distal sensory loss, cranial nerves spared; associated with long ICU stays, sepsis, organ failure, prolonged mechanical ventilation, and use of neuromuscular blocking agents	Critical illness polyneuropathy	Supportive
Progressive proximal weakness and diminished tendon reflexes that improve with repetitive movement of affected muscles	Eaton-Lambert syndrome	Search for and treat underlying malignancy
Symmetric distal sensory neuropathy in the setting of MGUS, multiple myeloma, amyloidosis, cryoglobulinemia, and other hematologic malignancies	Paraproteinemic neuropathy	Treat underlying disorder

Therapy

Carpal tunnel should be treated with surgery in the presence of refractory pain, weakness, or EMG evidence of active denervation.

Only pregabalin, duloxetine, and tapentadol (extended release) are FDA approved for the treatment of painful neuropathy.

Axonal polyneuropathies are treated by removal of the toxic agent (alcohol) or improvement of the underlying metabolic condition (diabetes, vitamin B_{12} deficiency).

All patients with Guillain-Barré syndrome are hospitalized for respiratory and cardiovascular monitoring.

◆ DON'T BE TRICKED

- When the presentation of Bell palsy is classic and without any additional neurologic deficits, brain imaging and routine laboratory testing are not necessary.
- Do not treat Bell palsy with antiviral drugs.
- If symptoms of Bell palsy do not improve by 2 months, obtain brain MRI and additional testing for secondary causes.
- Screening for glucose intolerance should be performed in all nondiabetic patients who have distal sensory neuropathy.
- Glucocorticoids are not beneficial in Guillain-Barré syndrome and may even slow the recovery.

✦ Test Yourself

A 37-year-old woman has difficulty going up stairs. She had diarrhea and low-grade fever 2 weeks ago. Physical examination shows weakness of both lower extremities and diminished deep tendon reflexes.

ANSWER: The diagnosis is Guillain-Barré syndrome. Begin plasma exchange and IV immune globulin.

Myopathy

Myopathies typically present with symmetric weakness of the proximal muscles.

- Normal sensory and reflex examination differentiates myopathy from neuropathy.
- Serum CK level is elevated and falls in response to treatment.
- EMG confirms the presence of myopathic changes (such as low amplitude, short duration, and polyphasic motor unit potentials).

See Rheumatology chapter for more detailed information on the inflammatory myopathies (polymyositis, dermatomyositis, inclusion body myositis).

STUDY TABLE: Myopathy Diagnostic Features	
Condition	**Diagnostic Clues**
Hypothyroid myopathy	Diffuse myalgia, proximal muscle weakness, and elevation of CK
	Myoedema (transient development of an edematous lump in a muscle in response to external percussion)
Hyperthyroidism	Myopathy, brisk reflexes, fasciculation, and ophthalmoplegia
Vitamin D deficiency	Proximal muscle weakness, myalgia, fatigue, and osteomalacia-related bone pain
Glucocorticoid myopathy	Proximal weakness and myalgia, normal CK levels, and normal EMG findings
Critical illness	Profound painless generalized weakness with elevated CK level
Statin myopathy	Subacute toxic myopathy associated with rhabdomyolysis
Myotonic dystrophies	Myotonia (manifested as delayed hand-grip release) and distal weakness

Primary Central Nervous System Lymphoma

Diagnosis

PCNSL is a non-Hodgkin lymphoma that commonly presents as a focal supratentorial lesion. Visual symptoms are common because of frequent tumor involvement of the optic radiations. PCNSL most commonly affects immunocompromised patients but can occur in patients with intact immune systems. A brain biopsy specimen is required to make a diagnosis. Ocular involvement in the vitreous or retina may be seen in 10% to 20% of patients and can be detected with a slit lamp examination and confirmed by vitreal biopsy.

Therapy

In patients with PCNSL and HIV infection, start ART; for those who have undergone organ transplantation, immunosuppressive therapy should be stopped. PCNSL is sensitive to both whole brain radiation and chemotherapy.

◆ **DON'T BE TRICKED**
- Resection of PCNSL is not indicated and can worsen patient outcomes.

Meningioma

Diagnosis

Meningiomas are usually benign in histology and behavior. These tumors are also typically asymptomatic and small and may be discovered incidentally during neuroimaging for unrelated symptoms. Symptomatic patients typically have progressive headache and focal neurologic lesions. CT scan of the head will show a partially calcified, homogeneously enhancing extra-axial mass adherent to the dura and an enhancing dural "tail."

Therapy

Surgical resection is the treatment of choice for symptomatic meningiomas or enlarging meningiomas. Observation is appropriate for small, asymptomatic meningiomas.

◆ **DON'T BE TRICKED**
- Chemotherapy has no established role in patients with meningioma.

Meningioma: Coronal MRI with contrast shows meningioma with the enhancing dural "tail" inferior to the tumor's dural attachment.

Metastatic Brain Tumors

Diagnosis

Parenchymal metastases usually present as multiple, ring-enhancing, centrally necrotic lesions. These lesions have a proclivity for the junction between the gray and white matter and are typically associated with significant surrounding edema and mass effect. If a metastatic brain tumor is the first indication of malignancy, evaluate the patient for lung cancer, breast cancer, and melanoma.

Lymphoma and leukemia cause leptomeningeal metastases and may present with headache or spinal pain, cranial nerve or spinal radicular pain, weakness, and mental status changes. Communicating hydrocephalus may be present. Leptomeningeal tumors are characterized on MRI by a diffuse or patchy enhancement of the surface of the brain and spinal cord or roots. When a leptomeningeal tumor is suspected in a patient with a negative MRI, obtain CSF examination to look for elevated protein and reduced glucose levels and positive cytologic findings.

◆ DON'T BE TRICKED

- MRI is required for all patients with systemic cancer and new neurologic findings.
- In patients with active, biopsy-proven systemic malignancy and multiple enhancing brain lesions, brain biopsy is not indicated.

Therapy

Glucocorticoids are a first-line treatment for parenchymal and leptomeningeal tumors. Chemotherapy (methotrexate and cytarabine) is the initial therapy for patients with leptomeningeal metastases from leukemia and lymphoma. Palliative whole-brain radiation therapy is indicated for multiple parenchymal metastases from a known primary solid tumor. Resection is an option for solitary, accessible brain metastases and controlled extracranial disease.

Parietal Lobe Metastatic Nodule: Axial postcontrast T1-weighted MRI showing an enhancing metastatic nodule in the left parietal lobe with surrounding edema and mass effect.

◆ DON'T BE TRICKED

- Chemotherapy is not indicated for parenchymal brain metastases from most solid tumors.

❖ Test Yourself

A 60-year-old woman with a history of adenocarcinoma of the lung has a 3-week history of diplopia, dysphagia, and foot drop. CT scan of the head shows only enlargement of the entire ventricular system.

ANSWER: The diagnosis is probable leptomeningeal metastases.

Coma

Diagnosis

Coma is a state of unarousable unresponsiveness. It can be caused by diffuse insults to the cerebral hemispheres, damage to the reticular activating system, or a combination of hemispheric and brain stem dysfunction. Unilateral hemispheric lesions do not result in coma unless edema and mass effect cause compression of the reticular activating system. Coma can be caused by a variety of structural lesions and toxic, metabolic, and infectious causes.

Patients in a vegetative state are unaware of self and the environment and show no purposeful responses to stimuli. They continue to have sleep-wake cycles and brain stem function.

The three cardinal findings of brain death are coma, absence of brain stem reflexes, and apnea.

STUDY TABLE: Key Points in the Evaluation of Coma	
Finding	**Consider**
Coma without focal signs, fever, or meningism	Hypoxia or a metabolic cause, toxic reaction, drug-induced state, infection, or postictal state
Coma without focal signs but with meningism	Meningitis, meningoencephalitis, or SAH
Coma with focal signs	Stroke, hemorrhage, tumor, or abscess
Quadriplegic, mute, but preserved vertical eye movements	"Locked-in" state caused by a pontine infarction or hemorrhage

Focal findings or any unexplained coma is an indication for emergent imaging of the brain to exclude hemorrhage or mass lesion. A CT scan can typically be obtained more rapidly than MRI and is the appropriate test in emergency situations. LP is indicated when meningitis or SAH is suspected but neuroimaging is normal. Emergent EEG can exclude nonconvulsive status epilepticus.

◆ DON'T BE TRICKED

- Respiratory drive and motor posturing signs are incompatible with a diagnosis of brain death.

Therapy

Attend to airway, breathing, and circulation first. All patients with unexplained coma should be urgently treated with thiamine and glucose (unless rapid finger stick rules out hypoglycemia). Give naloxone if an opiate overdose is suspected and flumazenil if a benzodiazepine overdose is being considered.

Oncology

Breast Cancer

Prevention and Screening

See General Internal Medicine, Breast Cancer Prevention and Screening.

Diagnosis

Characteristic findings include:

- a breast mass
- asymmetry of the breast
- nipple inversion
- edema and thickening of the skin (peau d'orange)
- an axillary or supraclavicular mass

Schedule mammography (and ultrasonography as needed) in women with any new breast symptoms or abnormal findings on physical examination. In premenopausal women, following the abnormality through one menstrual cycle instead of scheduling immediate imaging is reasonable. Schedule biopsy for suspicious lesions noted during physical examination or screening mammography. Any fluid discharge from the nipple requires a cytopathologic examination. If histopathologic studies confirm invasive breast cancer, determine estrogen/progesterone receptor and *HER2/neu* status. The two factors that are most prognostic are tumor size and axillary lymph node status.

◆ **DON'T BE TRICKED**

- A normal mammogram or ultrasonogram does not rule out breast cancer.
- A breast lump should always be biopsied, even if a mammogram is normal.
- Bone scan, CT scan, or tumor marker tests are not routine studies for diagnosing DCIS (stage 0) or early stage (I and II) breast cancer.

Therapy

DCIS can be treated with breast-conserving therapy, which consists of wide excision (lumpectomy) followed by breast radiation. In patients with estrogen-positive DCIS, tamoxifen decreases the risk of local recurrence but not survival.

Mastectomy and lumpectomy followed by radiation therapy are equivalent options with comparable survival in most women with invasive breast cancer.

Mastectomy is recommended for tumors involving the skin, chest wall, or more than one quadrant of the breast and for inflammatory breast cancer or if there are contraindications to radiation therapy (previous irradiation). Bilateral mastectomy is an option for women with familial breast cancer syndromes.

Axillary lymph node dissection is performed if sentinel lymph node biopsy is positive or axillary lymph nodes are clinically involved.

Chest wall radiation therapy after mastectomy is recommended in patients with tumors >5 cm, positive surgical margins, skin or chest wall involvement, inflammatory breast cancer, and for most patients with any positive axillary nodes.

Adjuvant systemic therapy is used to prevent or delay systemic recurrence for stages I to III breast cancer, stages in which the cancer is not metastatic and is potentially curable.

Most patients with hormone receptor–positive breast cancer receive adjuvant antiestrogen therapy. In premenopausal women, a 10-year course of adjuvant tamoxifen is standard of care. Premenopausal women who previously completed 5 years of tamoxifen benefit from taking an aromatase inhibitor for 5 years once they become postmenopausal.

Postmenopausal women are treated with 5 years of an aromatase inhibitor (anastrozole, letrozole, exemestane). Patients taking aromatase inhibitors should undergo DEXA scans periodically (every 1 to 2 years) and receive bisphosphonate therapy if T scores are less than -2.5.

Adjuvant chemotherapy is indicated for patients with hormone receptor–negative tumors, *HER2*-positive tumors, high-grade tumors, extensive lymphovascular invasion, and (typically) positive lymph nodes.

Molecular prognostic profiles such as the 21-gene recurrence score help determine the benefit of adjuvant chemotherapy. Patients with high-risk recurrence scores will benefit when adjuvant chemotherapy is given followed by antiestrogen therapy, whereas those with low-risk scores do not.

For patients with *HER2*-positive breast cancer, a monoclonal antibody (e.g., trastuzumab), is used as adjuvant therapy along with chemotherapy. Patients should undergo evaluation of LV function before trastuzumab treatment.

Inflammatory breast cancer is an aggressive and rapidly progressive type of cancer characterized by erythema and edema of the skin of the breast ("peau d'orange"). Inflammatory breast cancer is treated with neoadjuvant chemotherapy, followed by surgery, and then radiation.

Patients with early-stage breast cancer should receive follow-up monitoring which includes annual mammography. MRI of the breast is reserved for patients who have an especially high risk for subsequent breast cancer from *BRCA1/2* mutations or strong family history of breast cancer. Surveillance blood tests and other imaging studies are not recommended.

Hormone receptor–positive metastatic disease can be treated with antiestrogen therapy. Patients who are hormone receptor–negative or who fail to respond to antiestrogen therapy are treated with single-agent chemotherapy. Lytic bone metastases are treated with bisphosphonates to decrease bone pain and skeletal-related events. The monoclonal antibody denosumab is an alternate option. Painful skeletal disease is treated with radiation therapy.

◆ DON'T BE TRICKED

- Aromatase inhibitors are contraindicated in premenopausal women.
- Ovarian ablation or suppression can be used for premenopausal women with contraindications to tamoxifen.
- Do not select mastectomy in patients with metastatic disease unless required for local cancer control.
- Pregnancy following breast cancer treatment does not increase the risk of breast cancer recurrence.

STUDY TABLE: Breast Cancer Treatment Side-Effects	
Drug	**Side-Effect**
Aromatase inhibitors (anastrazole, letrozole, exemestane)	Arthralgia, bone pain, osteoporosis, hyperlipidemia
Tamoxifen	Endometrial cancer, VTE disease
Anthracyclines (doxorubicin, epirubicin)	Cardiomyopathy, acute leukemia
Trastuzumab	Cardiomyopathy especially if used with an anthracycline
Bisphosphonates	Osteonecrosis of the jaw, particularly in patients with dental disease
Denosumab	Hypocalcemia and osteonecrosis of the jaw, particularly in patients with dental disease

◆ DON'T BE TRICKED

- Biopsy new metastatic lesions; primary tumor and metastatic tumor estrogen receptor and *HER2* status differs in up to 15% of patients.

A 50-year-old premenopausal woman has a 1.5-cm moderately differentiated breast cancer. The lesion is completely excised (lumpectomy), and the surgical margins are negative. Three axillary lymph nodes are positive. The tumor is negative for estrogen/progesterone receptors and is highly positive for *HER2/neu*.

ANSWER: Select postoperative radiation therapy, chemotherapy, and trastuzumab, but not tamoxifen or aromatase inhibitors.

Lung Cancer

Screening and Prevention

Smoking cessation is the most effective preventive measure for lung cancer; 90% of lung cancers are smoking-related. Asbestos exposure is another risk factor.

Annual low-dose CT screening in patients with a 30-pack-year history of smoking, including those who quit smoking in the preceding 15 years, has been associated with a decrease in lung cancer and all-cause mortality.

◆ **DON'T BE TRICKED**
- Do not screen for lung cancer with chest x-ray and/or sputum cytology.
- Do not prescribe vitamin A derivatives (β-carotene and retinol) or vitamin E (α-tocopherol) to prevent lung cancer.

Diagnosis

Common symptoms include hemoptysis, pulmonary infections, dyspnea, cough, chest pain or paraneoplastic syndromes (hyponatremia, Cushing syndrome, hypercalcemia), mechanical effects of tumor (SVC syndrome), or Horner syndrome (ipsilateral ptosis, miosis, enophthalmos, and anhidrosis).

The most characteristic finding is a mass lesion on chest x-ray. Histologic confirmation is necessary for diagnosis and can be obtained by percutaneous lung biopsy, peripheral lymph node biopsy, pleural fluid cytology, or transbronchial biopsy. Whenever possible, select the biopsy site that will simultaneously diagnose and stage the disease (peripheral lymph node, mediastinal node). Treatment and prognosis vary based on whether the patient has NSCLC (adenocarcinoma, SCC, large cell carcinoma) or SCLC.

Small Cell Lung Cancer

SCLC is generally viewed as a systemic (metastatic) disease at the time of diagnosis; most patients have obvious extensive disease. Limited-stage disease is confined to one hemithorax, with hilar and mediastinal lymphadenopathy that can be encompassed within one tolerable radiotherapy portal. Extensive-stage disease consists of any disease that exceeds those boundaries, including malignant pleural effusion. Typically performed staging studies include CT of the chest, abdomen, and pelvis; whole-body bone scintigraphy; and MRI of the brain.

SCLC characteristically produces peptide hormones, which can cause endocrine syndromes, such as hyponatremia from the SIADH and hypercortisolism through secretion of ACTH. Neurologic symptoms, such as the Lambert-Eaton syndrome, cortical cerebellar degeneration, limbic encephalitis, and peripheral neuropathy, may also occur in patients with lung cancer, but they are relatively rare.

Non-Small Cell Lung Cancer

In staging NSCLC, the task is to identify metastatic disease, which eliminates surgery as a therapeutic option. Perform a staging evaluation with chest and upper abdominal CT plus a PET scan to assess for lymphadenopathy.

Measurement of the CBC and serum calcium, alkaline phosphatase, and aminotransferase levels can detect more advanced disease. A bone scan is indicated only if bone pain or elevated serum calcium or alkaline phosphatase levels are present. A brain MRI is indicated only in the presence of neurologic signs or symptoms.

◆ **DON'T BE TRICKED**

- Do not order routine bone scans or CT of the head in patients without bone or neurologic symptoms.
- If a patient has a lung mass and hypercalcemia, choose SCC as the likely cause.

Therapy

STUDY TABLE: Treatment of Small Cell Lung Cancer	
If you see this ...	**Select this ...**
Limited-stage disease	Concurrent chemotherapy and radiation therapy
Extensive-stage disease	Chemotherapy
Complete or partial response to therapy (both limited and extensive stages)	Add prophylactic cranial irradiation
Symptomatic brain metastases	Whole-brain radiation therapy

STUDY TABLE: Treatment of Non-Small Cell Lung Cancer	
If you see this ...	**Select this ...**
Stage I disease (solitary tumor 3-5 cm with no lymphadenopathy or metastases) or stage II disease (solitary tumor ≥5 cm, regional lymphadenopathy, pleura or chest wall involvement, tumors located near carina)	Surgical resection for cure followed by adjuvant chemotherapy
Stage III disease (involving mediastinum or contralateral mediastinal lymph nodes)	Chemoradiation
Stage IV disease (metastatic cancer, including malignant pleural or pericardial effusion)	Chemotherapy only if good performance status
Solitary brain metastasis	Surgical excision and postoperative whole-brain radiation therapy

Patients with EGFR mutations should receive erlotinib (or crizotinib, afatinib), whereas those with *ALK* translocations and *ROS1* mutations benefit from crizotinib. Maintenance chemotherapy is typically given until the patient experiences disease progression or an unacceptable level of toxicity.

Use glucocorticoids and radiation therapy for patients with multiple brain metastases. Select thoracic irradiation for pulmonary airway obstruction, SVC syndrome, and spinal cord metastases (following surgical decompression). Radiation therapy relieves pain, particularly bone pain, visceral pain secondary to capsular distention, or pain due to nerve compression. Treat symptomatic pleural effusions with thoracentesis and indwelling pleural catheter or pleurodesis if necessary.

Following curative-intent treatment for NSCLC, patients should undergo follow-up monitoring with periodic history, physical examination, and CT of the chest.

◆ **DON'T BE TRICKED**

- Large cell neuroendocrine carcinoma is a form of lung cancer that is distinct from SCC histologically but behaves and is treated similarly to SCLC.
- Do not treat patients who have NSCLC with poor performance status (extreme fatigue or weakness, weight loss >10%, severe symptoms) with chemotherapy, regardless of stage.
- Patients with extensive-stage SCLC and poor performance status because of tumor burden should be offered chemotherapy because it can significantly improve symptoms and increase survival.

❖ **Test Yourself**

A 51-year-old man presents with facial plethora, neck vein distention, shortness of breath, and a hilar mass.

ANSWER: The diagnosis is SVC syndrome. Establish the diagnosis with appropriate imaging and tissue diagnosis.

Gastric Cancer

Diagnosis

Because the signs and symptoms of gastric cancer are often vague and nonspecific, most patients have locally advanced or metastatic disease at diagnosis. The most common symptoms are weight loss, abdominal pain, nausea, anorexia, bleeding, and dysphagia. Findings may include any of the following:

- ascites
- periumbilical nodule (Sister Mary Joseph node)
- left supraclavicular lymphadenopathy (Virchow node)
- enlarged ovary (Krukenberg tumor)
- mass in the cul-de-sac on rectal examination (Blumer shelf)
- paraneoplastic acanthosis nigricans
- explosive onset of seborrheic keratosis (sign of Leser-Trélat)

The initial diagnostic procedure is upper endoscopy. CT scans are used to identify the presence of regional and metastatic disease. Endoscopic ultrasonography is superior to CT in the evaluation of depth of tumor invasion and lymph node involvement and aids in preoperative evaluation.

◆ DON'T BE TRICKED

- Always obtain upper endoscopy and biopsy in a patient with "achalasia" to rule out gastric cancer.

Therapy

For patients with localized tumors, standard therapy includes neoadjuvant chemotherapy (or chemoradiation therapy) followed by surgery.

Combination cisplatin-based regimens are used for metastatic cancer. Up to 20% of gastric cancers overexpress the *HER2* growth factor receptor. In these patients add the anti-*HER2* monoclonal antibody trastuzumab to the chemotherapy regimen.

Use antibiotic and PPI therapy for early-stage MALT lymphoma of the stomach and evidence of *Helicobacter pylori* infection.

Colorectal Cancer

Screening

Colorectal cancer screening is recommended for men and women beginning at age 50 years. The USPSTF does not recommend routine screening in patients 75 to 85 years of age, although considerations in individual patients may support screening. The USPSTF does not recommend screening in patients older than age 85 years. The risk for colorectal cancer is elevated in the presence of chronic colorectal inflammation from ulcerative colitis and Crohn disease of the colon. This increased risk is dependent on the proximal extent of mucosal involvement; patients with pancolitis are at highest risk, whereas risk is negligible in patients with proctitis. Risk is also increased with longer duration of disease, greater severity of inflammation, and the presence of coexistent PSC.

Acceptable USPSTF screening strategies for persons at average risk for colon cancer include:

- yearly FOBT
- sigmoidoscopy every 5 years combined with FOBT every 3 years
- colonoscopy every 10 years

More intense screening is recommended for patients at higher risk for colon cancer.

Early screening is recommended for patients with familial syndromes. The following is a partial list of hereditary syndromes that commonly appear on tests:

- familial adenomatous polyposis, which is an autosomal dominant disorder that requires prophylactic colectomy; duodenal and periampullary cancers are the second leading cause of cancer death in this group
- Gardner syndrome, which is a type of familial adenomatous polyposis with extraintestinal manifestations, including osteomas, duodenal ampullary tumors, thyroid cancers, and medulloblastomas
- HNPCC (Lynch syndrome), which is an autosomal dominant disorder

Hereditary nonpolyposis colon cancer (HNPCC) diagnostic criteria include:

- ≥3 relatives with colorectal cancer
- one relative a first-degree relative of the other two
- ≥2 successive generations affected
- one cancer diagnosed before age 50 years

Lynch syndrome is diagnosed if a patient meets the criteria for HNPCC and also has an identified germline mutation in one of the four mismatch repair genes or the epithelial cell adhesion molecule (*EPCAM*). Lynch syndrome is also associated with an increased risk for extracolonic tumors, most commonly endometrial. If an inherited colon cancer syndrome is suspected, the patient and family members should be referred for genetic testing.

Screening recommendations and frequency of screening are based on consensus opinion.

STUDY TABLE: Colon Cancer Screening

Risk Profile	When to Initiate Colonoscopy Screening
Average risk	Age 50 years – every 10 years to age 75 years (other screening modalities are available)
First-degree relative diagnosed with colon cancer at age ≤60 years	Age 50 years – every 10 years to age 75 years (other screening modalities are available)
First-degree relative diagnosed with an adenomatous polyp or colon cancer at age ≤60 years	Age 40 years, or 10 years younger than the earliest diagnosis in the family – every 5 years
Two second-degree relatives with adenomatous polyp or colon cancer at any age	Age 40 years or 10 years younger than the earliest diagnosis in the family – every 5 years
Two first-degree relatives with colon cancer	Age 40 years, or 10 years younger than the earliest diagnosis in the family – every 3-5 years
HNPCC risk	Every 1-2 years starting at age 20 or 25 years, or 10 years earlier than the age of youngest person in family diagnosed with colon cancer
Familial adenomatous polyposis risk	Age 10-15 years (annual sigmoidoscopy)
Pancolitis (ulcerative colitis or Crohn disease)	8-10 years after initial diagnosis – every 1-2 years

◆ **DON'T BE TRICKED**

- A single positive FOBT finding constitutes a positive screening test and requires follow-up colonoscopy.

Adenomatous polyps are premalignant lesions defined by their glandular architecture: tubular, villous, or a combination of both. Different levels of follow-up are recommended for patients discovered to have a colonic polyp on screening colonoscopy.

STUDY TABLE: Postpolypectomy Surveillance

Adenomatous Polyps	Interval to Next Colonoscopy
1-2 <10 mm tubular adenomas	5-10 years
3-10 adenomas, ≥10 mm, villous histology, or high-grade dysplasia	3 years
≥10 adenomas on single examination	<3 years; a genetic cause of disease should be investigated

◆ **DON'T BE TRICKED**

- Patients with a few, small (<10 mm) distal hyperplastic polyps should be screened according to average risk guidelines (i.e., every 10 years).

Diagnosis

Characteristic findings are rectal bleeding or change in bowel habits. Other findings include pelvic pain or tenesmus, weight loss, rectal or abdominal mass, hepatomegaly, and iron deficiency anemia. Patients with obstruction have hypogastric abdominal pain, abdominal distention, nausea, and vomiting. Colonoscopy is the diagnostic procedure of choice. Patients with colorectal cancer should undergo molecular testing of their tumor to determine if it has evidence of defective mismatch repair gene.

Staging generally consists of a complete colonoscopy; contrast-enhanced CT scans of chest, abdomen, and pelvis; and serum CEA level.

◆ **DON'T BE TRICKED**

- Do not obtain a serum CEA level to screen for or diagnose colon cancer.
- Do not obtain a PET scan to stage colorectal cancer.

Therapy

General rules for colorectal cancer therapy:

- confined to colon (stage I) or local invasion (stage II) → resection for cure
- metastatic to regional lymph nodes (stage III) → resection and adjuvant chemotherapy
- distant metastases (stage IV) → resection of primary lesion for palliation (if needed) and chemotherapy
- stage II-III rectal cancer → radiation therapy and chemotherapy before or after surgery

Adjuvant chemotherapy with FOLFOX or CAPOX is associated with improvement in disease-free survival for patients with stage III colon cancer.

Patients with stage II and stage III rectal cancer are treated with preoperative (neoadjuvant) radiation therapy and chemotherapy and postoperative (adjuvant) chemotherapy.

Patients with a single metastatic lesion to a single organ may be cured with surgical removal of the primary tumor and the metastasis. Patients with ≤3 liver metastases with surgical resection of the primary tumor and metastases can result in cure in about 25% of cases.

The FOLFOX regimen and FOLFIRI regimen are equally efficacious for metastatic colon cancer. The addition of bevacizumab, a monoclonal antibody against VEGF, further increases the efficacy of chemotherapy. The anti-EGFR monoclonal antibody cetuximab or panitumumab may be useful, alone or combined with other chemotherapies. These agents are inactive in nearly half of patients with the K-*ras* and N-*ras* mutations and should not be used in these patients.

Recommended follow-up includes:

- CEA measurement every 3 to 6 months for the first 2 years and then every 6 months for the subsequent 3 years
- colonoscopy 1 year following resection, 3 years later, and then every 5 years
- CT of the chest, abdomen, and pelvis annually for 3-5 years

◆ **DON'T BE TRICKED**

- In patients with metastatic colon cancer who are not eligible for curative resection, surgery is indicated only for control of bleeding or relief of obstruction.
- Do not treat asymptomatic, widely metastatic disease because treatment is not associated with improved outcomes and has significant treatment toxicity.

- Do not follow patients for recurrent colorectal cancer with PET scans.
- Anti-VEGF and anti-EGFR monoclonal antibodies should not be used together. Do not institute therapy for metastatic disease based on CEA elevation alone.

❖ **Test Yourself**

A 63-year-old man has a 4-month history of increasing fatigue and a nonobstructing colon cancer metastatic to the liver and lungs. His hemoglobin is 12.5 g/dL.

ANSWER: Begin multiagent chemotherapy. Surgery is not indicated.

Anal Cancer

Prevention

Most anal cancers are associated with HPV infection. HPV vaccine prevents anal HPV infection and anal intraepithelial neoplasia, precursors of anal cancer.

Diagnosis

Most patients present with a perianal lesion or mass associated with rectal bleeding or anal discomfort. Biopsy is essential to establish the diagnosis. Digital rectal examination; anoscopy; inguinal lymph node palpation (with biopsy or fine-needle aspiration if enlarged); and CT scan of the pelvis, abdomen, and chest are done for staging.

Therapy

Anal cancer is treated with radiation therapy and concurrent mitomycin plus 5-FU. Anal tumors may continue to regress for at least 6 months up to 1 year after completion of chemoradiation therapy.

Hepatocellular Carcinoma

Prevention

The most important preventive measure for HCC is hepatitis B vaccination.

Screening

Patients with cirrhosis and some patients with chronic hepatitis B (patients from America who are black and patients from Asia or Africa) without cirrhosis should be screened with abdominal ultrasonography every 6 months.

◆ **DON'T BE TRICKED**

- Serum AFP measurement is not recommended for HCC screening or surveillance.

Diagnosis

Order a contrast-enhanced CT or MRI of the liver when the abdominal ultrasonogram is abnormal. Because the radiographic findings of HCC are fairly characteristic (arterial phase enhancement), biopsy for confirmation is usually not necessary.

STUDY TABLE: Other Hepatic Tumors and Cysts	
Type	**Characteristics**
Cavernous hemangioma	Early peripheral nodular enhancement on contrast CT or MRI, followed by delayed fill-in toward the center of the lesion. No therapy is required.
Hepatic adenoma	Early arterial enhancement with rapid loss of enhancement and return to isointensity with the surrounding liver. Adenomas are typically heterogeneous in appearance because of regions of hemorrhage or necrosis. Patients may have a history of using oral contraceptives. Treat with resection.
Focal nodular hyperplasia	Early arterial enhancement with rapid loss of enhancement in the portal venous phase with return to isointensity with the surrounding liver. Many larger focal nodular hyperplasias have a central stellate scar. No therapy is required.
Metastatic tumors	Single or multiple hypoechoic lesions on ultrasonography that are hypovascular on contrast-enhanced CT scans. Isolated lesions may be amenable to resection.

Therapy

Surgical resection or liver transplantation is first-line therapy. Small single lesions in patients with cirrhosis but without portal hypertension and hyperbilirubinemia are managed with surgical resection. Patients with cirrhosis and 2-3 tumors ≤3 cm or 1 tumor ≤5 cm without vascular invasion or extrahepatic spread are treated with liver transplantation. Percutaneous ethanol injection or radiofrequency ablation is used for patients who cannot undergo surgery or liver transplantation. Chemotherapy is used for patients with advanced HCC who are not candidates for surgical resection, liver transplantation, or ablative therapy. Sorafenib improves overall survival in patients with advanced/metastatic HCC.

◈ Test Yourself

A 60-year-old man with chronic hepatitis C and cirrhosis is found to have a 4-cm liver mass on screening ultrasonography. A CT scan showed the mass enhances on arterial phase.

ANSWER: Select liver transplant.

Cholangiocarcinoma

Diagnosis

The most important established risk factor is the presence of PSC. Symptoms may include RUQ pain or jaundice. Diagnosis of extrahepatic bile duct cancers usually requires ERCP in combination with MRCP or contrast-enhanced CT. Surgical resection is the treatment of choice. Chemotherapy is reserved for nonresectable cholangiocarcinoma. Liver transplantation is an option for nonresectable, perihilar cholangiocarcinoma without extrahepatic spread.

◈ DON'T BE TRICKED

- CA-19 measurement is not able to confirm or exclude the diagnosis of cholangiocarcinoma.
- Percutaneous biopsy of a perihilar cholangiocarcinoma is an exclusion criterion for liver transplantation owing to the risk of tumor seeding.

Pancreatic Cancer

Diagnosis

Approximately 95% of the primary tumors are located in the exocrine pancreas, of which more than 50% occur in the head and 20% in the body or tail. Diffuse involvement of the pancreas is found in the remaining cases. Symptoms are influenced by tumor site and extent and may include:

- upper abdominal discomfort and lumbar back pain
- anorexia and weight loss
- obstructive jaundice
- marked weight loss
- vascular thromboses (Trousseau syndrome)

Physical examination findings may include a palpable gallbladder and jaundice. Contrast-enhanced multidetector CT has 90% sensitivity for detecting pancreatic cancer. Endoscopic ultrasound does not affect staging but is more sensitive in detecting small cancers (<2 cm) and allows tissue diagnosis by fine-needle aspiration when needed.

Look for the following characteristics:

- Stage I → tumor limited to the pancreas
- Stage II → tumor extending into the duodenum, bile duct, or peripancreatic tissues
- Stage III → regional lymph node involvement
- Stage IV → tumor extending directly into the stomach, spleen, colon, or adjacent large vessels or the presence of metastatic disease

◆ DON'T BE TRICKED
- Serum tumor markers are not used to diagnose pancreatic cancer.
- AIP can be mistaken for pancreatic cancer; look for elevated serum levels of IgG4 and biopsy the pancreas.

Therapy

Surgical resection is appropriate for patients with resectable pancreatic cancer. For patients with locally advanced but unresectable disease (tumor involvement of the superior mesenteric artery or the celiac trunk), treatment is controversial. Choices include:

- radiation therapy alone
- 5-FU plus radiation therapy (commonly used)
- single-agent chemotherapy (usually gemcitabine)

Gemcitabine alone is typically recommended for metastatic cancer. FOLFIRINOX has been shown to provide better outcomes but with substantially more toxicity.

Palliative measures to alleviate pain in patients with unresectable or metastatic disease include optimization of analgesic medications, radiation therapy, chemical splanchnicectomy, or celiac nerve blocks. Palliation of biliary obstruction may be achieved with:

- surgical biliary bypass
- percutaneous radiologic biliary stent placement
- endoscopic biliary stent placement

Neuroendocrine Tumors

Diagnosis

NETs arising from the endocrine cells of the pancreas are called pancreatic NETs, whereas those arising from all other neuroendocrine tissues of the aerodigestive tract are called carcinoid tumors.

Most NETs are hormonally nonfunctioning, but about 25% manifest a hormone. Carcinoid tumors can produce serotonin, which can cause diarrhea and facial flushing.

Pancreatic NETs may produce insulin, gastrin, glucagon, somatostatin, or vasoactive intestinal peptide, with resulting hormonal syndromes based on the type of hormone elaborated. This tumor may be part of the multiple endocrine neoplasia type 1 (MEN1) syndrome (primary hyperparathyroidism, pituitary tumors, enteropancreatic tumors).

Nonfunctioning tumors may be asymptomatic and develop metastatic disease many years before diagnosis. The liver is the most common site and the incidental finding of hepatomegaly is the most common presentation.

Triple-phase contrast-enhanced CT scanning or MRI with gadolinium are the preferred imaging modalities. Indium 111 pentetreotide scanning can be used to establish the presence of somatostatin receptors.

Therapy

Most NETs are indolent and can be followed until symptomatic. Surgery can be used to remove localized tumors. Hormonally active tumors with somatostatin receptors may be treated with the somatostatin analogues octreotide or lanreotide.

In pancreatic NETs, sunitinib (an anti-VEGF agent) and everolimus (an mTOR inhibitor) and chemotherapy are effective treatments.

Chemotherapy is minimally effective in carcinoid tumors.

Cervical Cancer

Prevention and Screening

See General Internal Medicine, Cervical Cancer Screening.

Diagnosis

Abnormal vaginal bleeding is the most common clinical presentation (postmenopausal, postcoital, and intermenstrual). Associated pain and abnormal discharge are usually signs of advanced disease.

Punch biopsy of obvious lesions or colposcopy-directed biopsy is usually required for diagnosis.

Therapy

Early (stage I) cancers may be treated with loop electrosurgical excision procedure or cervical conization to preserve childbearing; patients who have finished childbearing may undergo hysterectomy without lymph node dissection. Radiation therapy and cisplatin chemotherapy are used for patients with stage II, III, or IV disease. Treat metastatic disease with local radiation (for local control) or chemotherapy.

Ovarian Cancer

Prevention

Oophorectomy after childbearing or at age 35 years can be offered to women with *BRCA1/2* genetic mutations or ≥2 first-degree relatives with ovarian cancer.

Screening

Screening women at average risk for ovarian cancer is not indicated. Screening with serum CA-125, pelvic examination, and transvaginal ultrasonography is a reasonable but unproven strategy for women at high risk (e.g., ovarian cancer in a first- or second-degree family member, family member with ovarian cancer at age <50 years).

Diagnosis

Patients may have a family history of breast, ovarian, or colon cancer. Characteristic findings are abdominal swelling, ascites, and pain as well as abnormal vaginal bleeding and dyspareunia. A pelvic mass or nodularity may be present in the cul-de-sac. If ovarian cancer is suspected, CT or MRI of the abdomen and pelvis and chest imaging are done to assess disease extent. In patients with an adnexal mass without ascites, surgical removal of the mass without biopsy is associated with a survival benefit. In patients with advanced disease, diagnosis may be made by cytological examination of ascites or pleural effusion or biopsy of peritoneal masses.

◆ DON'T BE TRICKED

- Do not use CA-125 antigen to diagnose ovarian cancer.
- Women with peritoneal CUP have ovarian cancer until proven otherwise.

Therapy

Surgery is indicated to remove the ovaries and any evidence of grossly visible disease within the abdomen. Most patients with stage IA and IB disease with grade 1 (well-differentiated) histology do not receive adjuvant chemotherapy. Patients with stage IC to IV disease are treated with adjuvant platinum-based chemotherapy. Intraperitoneal chemotherapy shows a survival benefit in patients with small amounts of residual disease confined to the peritoneal cavity following surgery. Selected patients with good performance status and local recurrence of ovarian cancer may experience enhanced survival if they undergo comprehensive secondary surgical cytoreduction.

◆ DON'T BE TRICKED

- Do not opt for "second-look surgery" following completion of chemotherapy.
- All women with ovarian cancer are candidates for *BRCA1/2* testing

Limit follow-up to physical examination with pelvic examination and serum CA-125 measurement (if initially elevated).

❖ Test Yourself

A 60-year-old woman has a 3-month history of increasing abdominal girth, pain, and constipation. Physical examination is normal except for ascites. Pelvic ultrasonography is normal. Laparoscopy shows diffuse peritoneal carcinomatosis.

ANSWER: The diagnosis is adenocarcinoma of unknown primary site. Treat for ovarian cancer.

Endometrial Cancer

Diagnosis

Characteristic findings include irregular vaginal bleeding after age 40 years or in perimenopausal women, persistent pink or brown vaginal discharge, postmenopausal bleeding, and a Pap smear revealing atypical glandular cells of undetermined significance or containing endometrial cells. The diagnosis is made by endometrial biopsy.

Therapy

Surgical resection of the uterus, cervix, and adnexa is first-line treatment, and radiation therapy and/or chemotherapy may be added for higher-risk disease. Radiation therapy alone is an alternative for high-risk surgical patients.

Imaging is not more effective than a physical examination for diagnosing recurrent endometrial cancer.

◆ DON'T BE TRICKED

- Do not screen for endometrial cancer; screening does not reduce mortality.
- Women taking tamoxifen are at increased risk for endometrial cancer.

Prostate Cancer

Prevention

Finasteride reduces the incidence of prostate cancer but not cancer mortality rates and is not recommended for prevention.

Diagnosis

Most patients with prostate cancer are asymptomatic at the time of diagnosis. Characteristic findings include:

- a rapidly rising serum PSA level
- a nodule or firmness on rectal examination
- obstructive symptoms, although these are more likely associated with BPH

Obtain transrectal ultrasonography–guided prostate biopsy for a significantly elevated or rapidly rising PSA level or a nodule or firmness on digital rectal examination.

Tumors are classified according to their histology using the Gleason score. In the Gleason scoring system, tumors are graded from 1 to 5 based on the degree of glandular differentiation and structural architecture. The composite Gleason score is derived by adding together the two most prevalent differentiation patterns (a primary and a secondary grade). Patients with a Gleason score >7, serum PSA >15 ng/mL, large tumors, or the presence of bone pain require a bone scan and CT of the abdomen and pelvis to evaluate for metastatic disease.

◆ DON'T BE TRICKED

- Acute urinary retention significantly increases the PSA level regardless of the cause of obstruction.

Therapy

The NCCN has developed guidelines for the initial treatment of men with prostate cancer based on their risk score and general life expectancy. The three major treatment strategies for localized prostate cancer are surgery, radiation therapy, and active surveillance. Active surveillance is the postponement of definitive local therapy coupled with surveillance using serum PSA measurement, digital rectal examination, and repeat prostate biopsy. Men undergoing active surveillance receive referral for definitive local therapy if there is any evidence of disease progression.

General rules for treating prostate cancer:

- active surveillance is indicated for men with very low–risk cancer and a life expectancy ≥10 years
- options for local therapy include external-beam radiotherapy, brachytherapy, and radical prostatectomy
- after local therapy, high-risk disease is treated with adjuvant ADT with a GnRH agonist (e.g., leuprolide, goserelin) for 2 to 3 years
- hormonal therapy is also used for patients with a rising serum PSA level after initial definitive therapy for prostate cancer
- hormonal therapy is as effective as bilateral orchiectomy (surgical castration) in treating patients with metastatic disease

Prostate cancer that progresses despite ADT is "castrate resistant." Men who were previously treated with only a GnRH agonist may respond to the addition of an anti-androgen (e.g., flutamide). Castrate-resistant disease may also respond to ketoconazole, megestrol, glucocorticoids, and estrogens. The new anti-androgens abiraterone and enzalutamide also improve overall survival in castrate-resistant disease.

Docetaxel-based therapy improves median overall survival in patients with hormone-refractory metastatic prostate cancer.

Bisphosphonates (e.g., zoledronic acid) or denosumab reverse or prevent osteopenia due to hormonal therapy, inhibit tumor-mediated bone resorption, and decrease morbidity from bone fractures or bone pain. External-beam radiotherapy and bone-targeted radiopharmaceutical agents treat painful bone metastases. Radiation is most appropriate for a few painful metastatic sites and radium-223 is indicated for multiple painful sites.

◆ **DON'T BE TRICKED**

- Surgery or radiation therapy is not indicated for metastatic prostate cancer in the absence of local GU symptoms.

Testicular Cancer

Diagnosis

Primary testicular cancer, or germ-cell tumor, is the most common solid malignant tumor in men between the ages of 20 and 35 years. Characteristic findings in a young man include a testicular mass, testicular swelling and pain, weight loss, retroperitoneal lymphadenopathy, and metastatic pulmonary lesions. Cryptorchidism is a strong risk factor for testicular cancer.

The discovery of a testicular mass is followed by ultrasound imaging to confirm the presence of a solid mass. Diagnostic studies include obtaining tissue (inguinal orchiectomy, not needle biopsy) for histopathologic examination; chest x-ray; CT of the abdomen and pelvis; and measurement of the β-hCG and AFP levels.

- AFP is never elevated in a pure seminoma.
- An elevated serum AFP level always indicates the tumor has a nonseminomatous component.
- hCG may be present in seminomatous or nonseminomatous tumors.

Any testicular cancer that has a nonseminomatous component based on histologic examination or the presence of an elevated serum AFP level is considered a nonseminoma and is treated as such.

◆ **DON'T BE TRICKED**

- Do not order testicular biopsy.

Therapy

Semen cryopreservation is common for all men before they undergo therapy for testicular cancer. Inguinal orchiectomy is the initial step in treatment for all testicular tumors. Additional treatment modalities are determined by tumor histology and clinical stage.

Seminoma

- Low-risk, early-stage seminomas (stage I disease) are usually treated with radiation therapy to the para-aortic lymph nodes or with carboplatin chemotherapy. Observation is an option.
- Radiation therapy or cisplatin-based chemotherapy is recommended for patients with intermediate disease (stage IIA or IIB). Observation is not an option.
- Chemotherapy (cisplatin-based) is recommended for advanced disease (stage IIC or III).
- Chemotherapy (cisplatin-based) is recommended for nonpulmonary visceral metastases.

Nonseminoma

- Stage 1 disease can be managed with active surveillance, one cycle of cisplatin-based chemotherapy, or retroperitoneal lymph node dissection.
- For patients with bulky retroperitoneal lymphadenopathy identified on CT, cisplatin-based chemotherapy is recommended.

- Cisplatin-based chemotherapy is recommended for advanced disease (IIC or III).
- Patients with elevated serum tumor marker levels postoperatively but without radiographic evidence of disease also receive chemotherapy.

Residual retroperitoneal masses are common after chemotherapy. If tumor markers have normalized, consider surgical resection of residual masses for nonseminoma (masses may represent a teratoma) and follow up with CT without surgery for seminoma.

Patients with either seminoma or nonseminoma require frequent follow-up chest x-ray, serum tumor marker assays, and CT of the abdomen and pelvis because of the potential for cure even in patients with recurrent disease.

❖ Test Yourself

A 28-year-old man has weight loss and abdominal pain. Evaluation reveals para-aortic lymphadenopathy. Testicular examination is normal. A lymph node biopsy shows poorly differentiated CUP.

ANSWER: Measure the serum AFP and/or β-hCG levels.

Renal Cell Carcinoma

Diagnosis

Patients with renal cell carcinoma are often asymptomatic until they have advanced disease, but possible symptoms include:

- hematuria
- abdominal mass
- abdominal pain
- weight loss
- sudden onset of a varicocele

Renal cell carcinoma has been associated with various paraneoplastic syndromes, including erythrocytosis, AA amyloidosis, polymyalgia rheumatica, and hepatic dysfunction (unrelated to metastatic disease). The initial evaluation is a CT scan or ultrasound. Small lesions are biopsied whereas large lesions are removed without biopsy. Abdominal, pelvic, and chest CT scans are done to evaluate the local disease extent and assess for metastatic disease.

Therapy

Manage early-stage localized renal cancer with partial or radical nephrectomy. Targeted therapies include VEGF inhibitors and mTOR inhibitors.

- VEGF inhibitors include bevacizumab and various VEGF tyrosine kinase inhibitors, such as sunitinib, sorafenib, pazopanib, and axitinib.
- mTOR inhibitors include temsirolimus and everolimus.

Zoledronate decreases skeletal complications and delays progression of bone lesions.

❖ Test Yourself

A 48-year-old man has progressive, severe headaches. Physical examination is normal. Hemoglobin is 20.2 g/dL and urinalysis shows 30 to 50 erythrocytes/hpf. A chest x-ray shows multiple bilateral noncalcified nodules measuring 1 to 2 cm.

ANSWER: The probable diagnosis is renal cell carcinoma. Select an abdominal CT.

Thyroid Cancer

Diagnosis

The four main types of thyroid cancer are:

- papillary (75%)
- follicular (15%)
- medullary (5%)
- anaplastic (5%)

Characteristic findings are rapid nodule growth, a very firm nodule with fixation to adjacent structures, vocal cord paralysis, and enlarged regional lymph nodes.

Consider MEN type 2A or 2B and associated medullary thyroid cancer in a patient with:

- headache, sweating, palpitations, and hypertension (pheochromocytoma)
- kidney stones and hypercalcemia (hyperparathyroidism)
- marfanoid habitus and ganglioneuromas on the tongue, lips, and eyelids (MEN type 2B)
- elevated serum calcitonin level (nearly 100% sensitive and specific for medullary thyroid cancer)

FNAB is the diagnostic study for thyroid nodules >1 cm. The aspirate should be analyzed for the *BRAF* gene mutation when the diagnosis is indeterminate. The *BRAF* gene mutation is specific for papillary carcinoma and more aggressive forms of thyroid cancer. Inherited forms of medullary thyroid cancer are associated with germ-line mutations in the *RET* proto-oncogene. Screen family members for disease when a patient presents with a new diagnosis of medullary thyroid cancer.

Therapy

Treat papillary thyroid cancer and follicular thyroid cancer with total thyroidectomy followed by radioiodine therapy in most cases. Medullary thyroid cancer is treated with total thyroidectomy and varying degrees of neck dissection to remove involved lymph nodes.

◆ DON'T BE TRICKED

- Radioiodine is not taken up by C cells and is not a treatment option for medullary thyroid cancer.
- Chemotherapy does not prolong or improve the quality of life for patients with metastatic thyroid carcinoma.

✦ Test Yourself

A 37-year-old woman has a 2-cm right-sided thyroid nodule that is firm, nontender, and moves when she swallows. Serum TSH is 1.8 μU/mL and serum calcium is 11.8 mg/dL.

ANSWER: The probable diagnosis is medullary thyroid cancer. Order a serum calcitonin measurement.

Lymphoma

Patients with soft, small, freely moveable lymph nodes that are limited to one or two adjacent sites and who have no other significant history or physical examination findings can be followed over 6 to 8 weeks and require no other blood work or imaging.

Persistent or enlarging lymphadenopathy, particularly when associated with systemic symptoms requires further evaluation.

To establish a diagnosis of lymphoma, perform an excisional biopsy. Core needle biopsy can be used for deep lymph nodes, but fine-needle aspiration should be avoided.

After a diagnosis of lymphoma is made, a total-body CT scan with PET and an iliac crest bone marrow biopsy are done to complete staging.

Lymphomas are divided into Hodgkin and non-Hodgkin lymphomas. Lymphomas are further classified into three prognostic groups: indolent, aggressive, and highly aggressive.

Indolent lymphomas may not require therapy for decades but are difficult to cure. The most common indolent lymphomas are:

- follicular lymphoma
- MALT
- CLL
- hairy cell leukemia

Follicular Lymphoma

Most patients have lymphadenopathy but no other symptoms. Diagnosis is confirmed by cytogenetic analysis identifying a translocation [t(14:18)] that causes an overexpression of the *bcl-2* oncogene.

Therapy is withheld until patients become symptomatic. Localized symptoms can be treated with involved-field radiation combined with rituximab. Symptomatic, systemic disease is treated with rituximab plus multiagent chemotherapy. Allogeneic HSCT is curative therapy but is associated with significant morbidity and mortality.

Mucosa-associated Lymphoid Tissue Lymphoma

The clinical course of MALT lymphoma is usually indolent, and presentation is usually localized. Gastric MALT lymphoma occurs most commonly and is caused by chronic infection with *Helicobacter pylori*. Complete remissions are achieved in most patients after completion of antimicrobial therapy directed against *H. pylori* infection (e.g., clarithromycin, amoxicillin, and omeprazole) and concomitant PPI.

Chronic Lymphocytic Leukemia

Patients are usually asymptomatic and are identified by a relative lymphocytosis. Smudge cells may be seen on the peripheral blood smear. Diagnosis is confirmed by flow cytometry demonstrating cell surface antigens CD5 and CD23. Asymptomatic patients are observed without therapy. Combination therapy with rituximab and multiagent chemotherapy is used for symptomatic late stage disease.

Concomitant autoimmune disease, including immune thrombocytopenia and hemolytic anemia, is common among patients with CLL. Low serum IgG levels require replacement therapy to prevent infection. Patients are at increased risk for transformation from CLL to a large cell lymphoma (Richter transformation) requiring aggressive chemotherapy.

CLL "Smudge Cell": Peripheral blood smear showing a "smudge cell," which is a lymphocyte that appears flattened or distorted and is characteristic of CLL.

Hairy Cell Leukemia

Hairy cell leukemia is characterized by pancytopenia and progressing splenomegaly without lymphadenopathy. Typically, an attempt at bone marrow aspiration is unsuccessful. The cells have the classic appearance of thread-like projections emanating from the cell surface ("hairy" cells). Treatment with cladribine results in complete and durable remission in most patients.

Aggressive lymphomas require immediate therapy and often can be cured. The most common types of aggressive lymphomas are:

- DLBCL
- mantle cell lymphoma
- Hodgkin lymphoma

Hairy Cell Leukemia: Atypical lymphocytes with cytoplasmic projections characteristic of hairy cell leukemia.

Diffuse Large B-Cell Lymphoma

Most patients with DLBCL present with fever, night sweats, or weight loss ("B symptoms"), and experience rapid disease progression without therapy. Standard therapy for all patients with DLBCL, regardless of stage or prognosis, is R-CHOP. Involved-field radiation therapy is added for patients with bulky disease.

The most aggressive forms of large cell lymphoma are Burkitt lymphoma and lymphoblastic lymphoma. Onset of disease is acute, and patients usually present with life-threatening metabolic and structural abnormalities. Treatment is the same as that used to treat ALL; it is associated with high response rates and is curative in nearly 50% of patients.

Mantle Cell Lymphoma

Patients present with advanced disease characterized by lymphadenopathy, weight loss, and sometimes fever, and have diffuse sites of involvement, including the GI tract, bone marrow, and blood stream. Intensive chemotherapy and autologous HSCT have increased median survival rates. Allogeneic HSCT can produce long-term remissions but is associated with significant morbidity and mortality.

Hodgkin Lymphoma

Hodgkin lymphoma commonly presents locally, most typically with palpable, firm lymphadenopathy or a mediastinal mass on chest x-ray. Some patients may have B symptoms, splenomegaly, and hepatomegaly.

Hodgkin lymphoma is curable in most patients. The staging evaluation consists of PET scanning and a bone marrow biopsy.

Stage I and II disease in patients without B symptoms is treated with radiation alone, or more typically, radiation combined with a short course of chemotherapy.

Patients with advanced disease or those with B symptoms usually require a full course of chemotherapy.

Patients who have a negative PET scan after two to three cycles of chemotherapy have >90% likelihood of long-term disease response.

Patients with recurrent, chemotherapy-sensitive disease are candidates for autologous HSCT, whereas those with resistant disease can achieve long-term remissions with allogeneic HSCT.

Patients with Hodgkin lymphoma, including those cured by therapy, should be monitored for late reactivation of viruses. Patients are at risk for secondary cancers (breast, lung, skin) and MDS. For women, begin annual mammography. In certain high-risk women, the addition of MRI screening may be appropriate.

STUDY TABLE: Ann Arbor Staging System of Hodgkin Lymphoma

Stage	Description
Stage I	Involvement of a single lymph node region (I) or a single extralymphatic organ or site (I_E).
Stage II	Involvement of ≥2 lymph node regions on the same side of the diaphragm alone or limited involvement of contiguous extralymphatic organ or tissue (II_E).
Stage III	Involvement of lymph node regions on both sides of the diaphragm, which may include the spleen (III_S), or limited involvement of contiguous extralymphatic organ or site (III_E), or both (III_{ES}).
Stage IV	Multiple or disseminated foci of involvement of ≥1 extralymphatic organs or tissues, with or without lymphatic involvement.

All cases are subclassified to indicate the absence (A) or presence (B) of fever, night sweats, or weight loss.

The subscript "$_E$" refers to extranodal contiguous extension. The subscript "$_S$" refers to spleen involvement.

◆ **DON'T BE TRICKED**

- Evaluate all patients with chest pain after radiation therapy for CAD, regardless of age.

Cutaneous T-cell non-Hodgkin Lymphoma

Cutaneous T-cell lymphomas infiltrate skin and initially cause rash (mycosis fungoides), and occasionally circulate in the blood (Sézary syndrome). The large, CD4-expressing malignant T cells have classic cerebriform-appearing nuclei. Disease progression manifests with raised plaques, diffuse skin erythema, and skin ulcers. In the final stages of disease progression, organ infiltration and immunodeficiency cause recurrent bacterial infections, sepsis, and death.

Early-stage disease limited to skin is treated with topical glucocorticoids. Advanced-stage disease is often treated with electron-beam radiation therapy; photopheresis; and monoclonal antibodies. Allogeneic HSCT may be curative in young patients.

Carcinoma of Unknown Primary Origin

Diagnosis

Metastatic CUP accounts for as many as 3% to 5% of patients with solid tumors. The clinical evaluation in patients with CUP should not involve an exhaustive search for a primary site because finding an asymptomatic and occult primary site does not improve outcome. Diagnostic efforts should focus on identifying patients with CUP who have a more favorable prognosis and who can benefit from a specific treatment strategy.

Favorable subgroups include the following:

- isolated lymphadenopathy
- peritoneal carcinomatosis
- poorly differentiated nonadenocarcinoma

STUDY TABLE: Examples of Favorable Subgroups and Management

Axillary lymphadenopathy in women	Obtain breast MRI. If positive, treat according to stage. If negative, treat as if stage II breast cancer.
Isolated cervical lymphadenopathy	Obtain upper endoscopy, bronchoscopy, and laryngoscopy. If negative, treat with chemotherapy and radiation for head and neck cancer.
Isolated inguinal lymphadenopathy	Anorectal, perineal, and genital examination. If negative, lymph node resection or locoregional radiation.
Peritoneal carcinomatosis and ascites	Treat as ovarian carcinoma with cytoreductive surgery and chemotherapy.
Midline nonadenocarcinoma of mediastinum or retroperitoneum	Measure serum AFP and β-hCG, perform testicular exam and testicular ultrasound; treat with platinum-containing germ cell tumor regimens.

◆ DON'T BE TRICKED

- Do not select routine radiographic contrast studies of the GI tract.
- Do not measure CA-19-9, CA-15-3, and CA-125 since they are rarely helpful and virtually never diagnostic.
- Do not order PET scans because the findings are rarely definitive and do not improve long-term outcome.

❖ Test Yourself

A 45-year-old woman has an axillary lymph node that is positive for adenocarcinoma. Bilateral mammogram, breast MRI, and CT scans of the chest and abdomen are normal. She has never smoked.

ANSWER: The diagnosis is adenocarcinoma of unknown primary origin. Treat as if she had stage II breast cancer.

Effects of Cancer Therapy

STUDY TABLE: Short- and Long-Term Effects of Cancer Therapy	
Category	**Potential Complications**
Cardiac	Doxorubicin: dose-related HF (irreversible)
	Trastuzumab: non–dose-related HF (reversible)
	Mediastinal radiation: myocardial, valvular, pericardial fibrosis, and premature CAD
Pulmonary	Bleomycin: pulmonary toxicity, most commonly bleomycin-induced pneumonitis
	Radiation: radiation-induced pneumonitis
Reproductive	Chemotherapy: premature ovarian failure, male infertility
	Tamoxifen: endometrial cancer, VTE
Endocrine	Radiation therapy to head and neck: hypothyroidism
Musculoskeletal	Aromatase inhibitors: osteoporosis
	Leuprolide, goserelin, castration: osteoporosis
Cancer	Mantle radiation: breast, lung, and esophageal cancer
	Chemotherapy (breast cancer): MDS and acute leukemia
Kidney and bladder	Cisplatin and ifosfamide: renal tubular damage and CKD
	Cyclophosphamide and ifosfamide: hemorrhage cystitis

❖ Test yourself

A 44-year-old man is evaluated for cough and dyspnea 2 weeks after he completed his ABVD therapy for Hodgkin lymphoma. The chest x-ray shows bilateral interstitial infiltrates.

ANSWER: Bleomycin-induced lung injury.

Cancers of Infectious Origin

STUDY TABLE: Malignancies with Infectious Causes	
Cancer	**Associated Infection**
Cervical and anal cancers	HPV
	Increased incidence in HIV infection
	Risk proportional to number of sexual partners
Kaposi sarcoma	Human herpes virus 8
	Primarily in younger HIV-infected men who have sex with men
	May be mistaken for bacillary angiomatosis (bartonellosis)

(Continued on next page)

STUDY TABLE: Malignancies with Infectious Causes (*Continued*)	
Cancer	**Associated Infection**
Hodgkin lymphoma	EBV
Burkitt lymphoma	EBV t(8;14)-positive
	Increased incidence in HIV infection (AIDS-defining cancer)
	Presents as oral and nasopharyngeal cancer in China and Southeast Asia and as posttransplantation lymphoma in immunosuppressed patients
MALT lymphoma	*Helicobacter pylori*
	Usually involves the GI tract, particularly the stomach
	Treat early disease with antibiotics and PPIs (localized radiation therapy for *H. pylori*-negative disease)
HCC	Cirrhosis and hepatitis B infection are the most important risk factors
Non-Hodgkin lymphoma	Increased incidence in HIV infection (AIDS-defining cancer)
Head and neck (nasopharynx)	EBV
Head and neck (oropharynx)	HPV

Cancer Emergencies

Hypercalcemia

Characteristic findings are elevated serum calcium, low PTH, low or normal phosphorus, and low or normal 1,25-dihydroxy-vitamin D_3 levels. PTH-related protein can be a diagnostic aid in patients with hypercalcemia of unclear etiology. In these patients an elevated level would suggest tumor. All patients require immediate volume repletion with normal saline followed by forced diuresis with normal saline. Use bisphosphonates such as pamidronate and zoledronate or RANKL inhibitors (e.g., denosumab) for long-term control. Add glucocorticoids in steroid-sensitive malignancies such as myeloma and lymphoma.

Hyponatremia

See also Nephrology, Hyponatremia.

Initially treat asymptomatic or mildly symptomatic patients with SIADH with fluid restriction (500-1000 mL/d). Give 3% sodium chloride and furosemide to symptomatic patients with altered mental status or other neurologic findings to raise the serum sodium concentration by 1 to 2 mEq/L per hour to a total increase of 4 to 6 mEq/L within the first 6 hours (not to exceed 8 mEq in 24 h) until symptoms abate. An alternative treatment in hospitalized patients is use of the ADH receptor antagonist conivaptan (very expensive, with no evidence of improved outcomes).

Deep Venous Thrombosis

Begin long-term LMWH for initial treatment and secondary prevention of thromboembolic disease in patients with underlying cancer. Use an IVC filter if anticoagulation is contraindicated.

Metastatic Brain Tumor

See also Neurology, Metastatic Brain Tumors.

Characteristic findings:

- headache
- vomiting
- altered mental status
- focal neurologic deficits
- loss of consciousness

Obtain emergent assessment with CT or MRI.

Oral glucocorticoids are appropriate for minimally symptomatic disease whereas osmotic diuresis and IV glucocorticoids are used for more advanced disease. When intracranial pressure is controlled, an isolated brain metastasis can be treated with surgical excision followed by radiation. Multiple brain metastases are treated with radiation therapy and chemotherapy.

◆ DON'T BE TRICKED

- Do not treat an isolated brain mass in a young patient with HIV infection without first obtaining brain biopsy to confirm lymphoma.

Spinal Cord Compression

See also Neurology, Myelopathy.

Characteristic findings include:

- localized spinal or radicular pain
- sensory loss (especially perineal)
- muscle weakness
- change in bowel or bladder function
- autonomic dysfunction

The diagnosis is established by gadolinium-enhanced MRI of the entire spine (mulitple sites of compression is common).

◆ DON'T BE TRICKED

- Do not order plain x-rays or bone scans to diagnose spinal cord compression.

Treat immediately with glucocorticoids and decompressive surgery followed by radiation therapy. Systemic chemotherapy is useful in patients with highly chemosensitive tumors such as lymphoma or breast cancer. Prescribe opioid therapy as needed for pain.

Superior Vena Cava Syndrome

Characteristic findings are shortness of breath, cough, facial edema, plethora, swollen arms, jugular venous distention, stridor (tracheal obstruction), and prominent collateral veins on the anterior chest wall.

Mediastinal widening and pleural effusions are common radiographic findings. Tissue biopsy is essential for establishing a histologic diagnosis and guiding therapy for the specific cancer type. Mediastinoscopy is commonly used to obtain tissue and percutaneous transthoracic CT-guided needle biopsy is another acceptable approach. Diuretics and glucocorticoids can be used for symptomatic treatment pending definitive therapy.

◆ DON'T BE TRICKED

- Up to 16% of patients with SVC syndrome have a normal chest x-ray.

STUDY TABLE: Treatment for Superior Vena Cava Syndrome	
Situation	Response
Syndrome due to previously untreated SCLC, lymphoma, or germ cell tumor	Chemotherapy
Syndrome due to previously treated SCLC, lymphoma, germ cell tumor, or chemosensitive malignancies	Radiation therapy alone or in combination with chemotherapy

Superior Vena Cava Syndrome: The sudden appearance of dilated veins on the chest of this patient heralded the onset of the SVC syndrome.

Pericardial Tamponade

See also Cardiovascular Medicine, Pericardial Tamponade and Constriction.

Characteristic findings are:

- dyspnea, orthopnea, and clear lungs
- jugular venous distention and hepatic engorgement
- sinus tachycardia, hypotension, narrow pulse pressure, distant heart sounds, and pulsus paradoxus

Life-threatening hemodynamic compromise is treated with immediate drainage of fluid via pericardiocentesis or pericardiotomy.

Pleural Effusion

See also Pulmonary and Critical Care Medicine, Pleural Effusion.

Characteristic symptoms:

- dyspnea on exertion
- chest pain
- cough

Obtain chest x-ray or chest CT to establish a diagnosis then perform thoracentesis for diagnosis. To reduce the incidence of recurrence, standard therapies include chest tube placement, prolonged drainage (over the course of a few to several days), and pleurodesis. Placement of indwelling pleural catheters is an option.

Tumor Lysis Syndrome

Tumor lysis syndrome is the result of rapid breakdown of malignant cells, resulting in dangerous increases in serum urate, potassium, and phosphate concentrations. Symptoms may include:

- nausea, vomiting, and diarrhea
- lethargy
- HF
- seizures, tetany, and syncope
- sudden death

Typically, tumor lysis syndrome occurs within 1 to 5 days of treatment and develops most commonly in patients with hematologic malignancies or other rapidly dividing tumors, such as acute leukemia and high-grade lymphoma. Risk factors include bulky disease, a high leukocyte count, high pretreatment levels of LDH or urate, compromised kidney function, and use of nephrotoxic agents. Spontaneous (pretreatment) tumor lysis syndrome occurs commonly in patients with leukemia and Burkitt lymphoma.

Tumor lysis syndrome is prevented and managed by aggressive hydration and use of allopurinol or rasburicase. IV rasburicase is indicated for patients at high risk for tumor lysis syndrome or when rapid reduction of serum urate levels is indicated (e.g., emergently administered chemotherapy). Hyperkalemia is also aggressively treated. If acute kidney failure develops, hemodialysis may be indicated.

Febrile Neutropenia

Diagnosis

Fever is defined as a single oral temperature >38.5 °C (101.3 °F) or a temperature of >38.0 °C (100.4 °F) sustained over a 1-hour period. The first step in managing febrile neutropenia is identifying high- and low-risk patients.

- High risk is defined as neutropenia ≥7 days with an absolute neutrophil count ≤100/µL and/or significant comorbidities (e.g., hypotension, pneumonia, abdominal pain, neurologic changes).

- Low risk is defined as anticipated neutropenia <7 days and no or few comorbidities.

For all patients, obtain at least 2 sets of blood cultures drawn simultaneously from each central venous catheter lumen and peripheral site and culture any obvious source of infection. Signs and symptoms guide imaging; there are no routine imaging tests.

Therapy

Management of high-risk febrile neutropenia:

- admit all high-risk patients to the hospital for empiric IV antibiotics
- begin empiric monotherapy with an antipseudomonal β-lactam (e.g., cefepime), a carbapenem (e.g., imipenem-cilastin), or piperacillin-tazobactam

Management of low-risk febrile neutropenia:

- low-risk patients may be candidates for outpatient empiric antibiotic therapy
- begin oral or IV antibiotics in the clinic or hospital setting with transition to the outpatient setting if patients remain stable during a 4- to 24-hour period of observation
- begin oral ciprofloxacin plus amoxicillin-clavulanate except for patients already taking a fluoroquinolone

Modify the initial therapy for patients at high risk for antibiotic-resistant organisms (e.g., patient unstable, early suggestive blood culture results):

- add vancomycin, linezolid, or daptomycin for suspected MRSA infection
- add linezolid or daptomycin for suspected vancomycin-resistant enterococci
- begin empiric antifungal therapy for persistent fever despite 4 to 7 days of empiric antibiotics and anticipated neutropenia ≥7 days

Continue antibiotics until the absolute neutrophil count is ≥500/µL or longer depending on clinical circumstances.

◆ DON'T BE TRICKED

- Vancomycin is not recommended as standard initial therapy for febrile neutropenia.
- Do not use myeloid colony-stimulating factors for treatment of febrile neutropenia.
- Antiviral treatment is only indicated for clinical evidence of active viral infection.
- Typhlitis (necrotizing enterocolitis) should be suspected in patients with neutropenia and even minimal RLQ abdominal pain; obtain an abdominal CT scan.
- Diagnose angioinvasive aspergillosis in neutropenic leukemia patients on prolonged antibiotic therapy.

❖ Test Yourself

A 73-year-old man with AML develops febrile neutropenia on the eighth day of chemotherapy. Ceftazidime is begun, but after 5 days of therapy he remains febrile and neutropenic. Blood cultures are negative, and he has no localizing signs of infection.

ANSWER: Add amphotericin B or itraconazole.

Invasive Aspergillosis: CT scan showing a dense infiltrate surrounded by a ground glass-appearing halo ("halo sign") suggestive, but not diagnostic, of invasive aspergillosis.

Pulmonary and Critical Care Medicine

Pulmonary Function Tests

Indications

The four pulmonary function tests commonly used to measure static lung function are spirometry, flow-volume loops, lung volumes, and D_{LCO}.

Pulmonary function testing is indicated for patients with unexplained pulmonary symptoms, abnormal pulmonary findings (abnormal chest x-ray, hypoxemia, crackles), monitoring known pulmonary disease, and preoperative assessment for lung resection.

Key Tests and Patterns

Spirometry is used to diagnose airflow obstruction such as asthma, COPD, and bronchiectasis.

- FEV_1/FVC <0.7 indicates airflow obstruction.
- A ≥12% increase in either FEV_1 or FVC and an increase ≥200 mL from baseline in either parameter with bronchodilator therapy indicates reversible airway obstruction.
- Equal reductions in FEV_1 and FVC suggest restrictive lung disease.

Flow-volume loops can help localize anatomic sites of airway obstruction. Refer to the "Flow-Volume Loops" figures and consider the following factors:

- a "scooped-out" pattern with a decreased slope on the expiratory curve that does not improve with bronchodilation indicates COPD
- a "scooped-out" pattern with a decreased slope on the expiratory curve that improves with bronchodilation indicates reversible obstructive airway disease (asthma)
- "flattening" in both inspiratory and expiratory curves and decreased airflow indicates fixed obstruction (e.g., tracheal stenosis)
- following attainment of peak flow, the flow rate declines linearly and proportionally to volume, producing a relatively straight slope characteristic of a normal flow-volume loop

Lung volumes aid in confirming findings on spirometry:

- TLC <80% indicates restrictive lung disease (fibrosis, neuromuscular disease, skeletal abnormalities)
- decreased vital capacity with increased residual volume indicates airflow obstruction

D_{LCO} evaluates gas transport across the alveolar-capillary membrane.

STUDY TABLE: Interpreting D_{LCO}	
Finding	**Interpretation**
↓ D_{LCO} and reduced lung volumes	Pulmonary fibrosis
↓ D_{LCO} and normal lung volumes	Pulmonary vascular disease, anemia
↓ D_{LCO} and airflow obstruction	COPD, bronchiectasis
↑ or normal D_{LCO} and airflow obstruction	Asthma
↑ D_{LCO}	Pulmonary hemorrhage, left-to-right shunt, HF, polycythemia

◆ DON'T BE TRICKED

- In patients with low lung volumes, a normal DLCO suggests an extrapulmonary cause (e.g., obesity).

STUDY TABLE: Understanding Important Pulmonary Tests	
Tests	**Considerations**
Pulse oximetry	Measures percentage of oxyhemoglobin either at rest or during exercise
	Use co-oximetry when carboxyhemoglobin is suspected (e.g., smoke inhalation, carbon monoxide poisoning)
Bronchial challenge testing	Challenges include cold air, exercise, histamine, and methacholine
	Airflow is measured before and after challenge
	Methacholine is commonly used for patients with a history suggestive of bronchospastic disease but normal spirometry
Cardiopulmonary exercise testing	Performed for unexplained dyspnea, symptoms disproportionate to the measured pulmonary function abnormality, and other exercise-related symptoms
6-minute walk test	Useful to assess disability, need for supplemental oxygen, and prognosis in chronic lung conditions; simple oximetry and desaturation studies are performed at rest and with exertion
Exhaled nitric oxide test	Exhaled nitric oxide is increased in patients with airway inflammation, including asthma

◆ DON'T BE TRICKED

- Pulse oximetry is normal in patients with carbon monoxide and cyanide poisoning.
- Pulse oximetry may be falsely low in patients with shock.

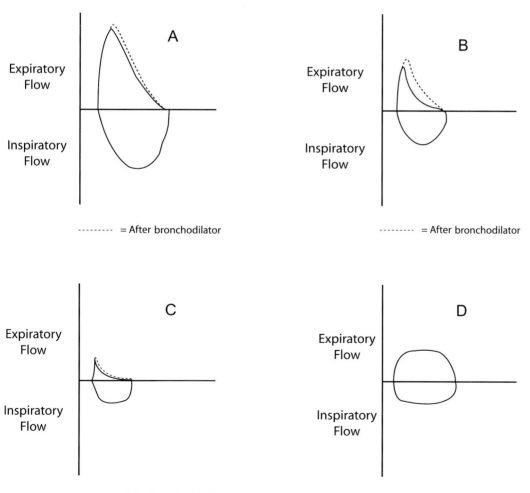

Flow-Volume Loops: Flow-volume loops plot flow (L/sec) as a function of volume.

Asthma

Diagnosis

The onset of asthma usually occurs during childhood but may begin at any age. Most patients with asthma are atopic; however, some patients, particularly those with adult-onset asthma, have no clear allergic basis for their disease. The cardinal features of asthma are reversible airway obstruction, inflammation, and airway hyperresponsiveness.

Characteristic findings are wheezing and dyspnea; consider any cough that is nocturnal, seasonal, or related to a workplace or activity as possible asthma. Look for nasal polyps and aspirin sensitivity.

Diagnostic studies include spirometry before and after bronchodilator administration. In patients with atypical features, perform PFTs. The presence of airflow irreversibility, restrictive patterns, and significantly reduced vital capacity suggest other diseases.

Bronchoprovocation testing with methacholine or histamine is indicated for patients with a suggestive clinical history for asthma but normal spirometry. Bronchoprovocation testing with exercise is indicated to diagnose exercise-induced asthma in patients who have dyspnea following exercise but normal spirometry.

◆ DON'T BE TRICKED

- Normal spirometry does not rule out asthma.
- A normal bronchoprovocation test rules out asthma; a positive test does not rule it in.
- Wheezing does not equal asthma; consider HF, COPD, vocal cord dysfunction, and upper airway obstruction.

STUDY TABLE: Differential Diagnosis of Asthma	
Disease	**Characteristics**
Chronic eosinophilic pneumonia	Chest x-ray shows "photographic-negative" pulmonary edema (peripheral pulmonary edema)
	Clinical findings: striking peripheral blood eosinophilia, fever, and weight loss in a long-term smoker
	Diagnose by bronchoscopy with biopsy or bronchoalveolar lavage showing a high eosinophil count
Allergic bronchopulmonary aspergillosis	Asthma manifests with eosinophilia, markedly high serum IgE levels, and intermittent pulmonary infiltrates
	Diagnose with positive skin test for *Aspergillus* and IgG and IgE antibodies to *Aspergillus*
	Often overlooked until onset of more advanced disease, including fixed obstruction and bronchiectasis; look for a patient with brown sputum
Eosinophilic granulomatosis with polyangiitis (formerly Churg-Strauss syndrome)	Upper airway and sinus disease precedes difficult-to-treat asthma; look for flares associated with use of leukotriene inhibitors and glucocorticoid tapers
	Serum p-ANCA may be elevated
	Hallmark diagnostic finding is eosinophilic tissue infiltrates

Consider alternative diagnoses when asthma is difficult to control. Additional studies in these cases may include chest x-ray and echocardiography. Obtaining flow-volume loops and direct visualization of the larynx during an acute episode may be helpful in diagnosing tracheal obstruction and vocal cord dysfunction. Asthma is an extraesophageal manifestation of GERD.

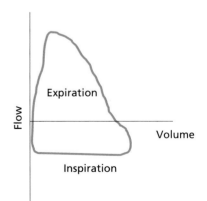

❖ Test Yourself

A 17-year-old man has difficult-to-control asthma associated with inspiratory tracheal sounds and minor wheezing. A flow-volume loop is shown.

ANSWER: Diagnosis is most likely vocal cord dysfunction characterized by flattening of the inspiratory portion of the flow-volume loop.

Therapy

If asthma is difficult to control, discontinue β-blockers (including ophthalmologic agents). If β-blockers must be continued, use selective β-blockers (metoprolol, atenolol). Also stop aspirin and NSAIDs if the patient is sensitive to these drugs.

Asthma must be classified correctly to select proper therapy. Severity is based on the worst feature present.

STUDY TABLE: Step Classification of Asthma		
Step Classification	**Symptoms**	**Nocturnal Symptoms**
Step 1: Intermittent	Symptoms ≤2 per week	≤2 per month
		Asymptomatic and normal PEF between exacerbations
Step 2: Mild persistent	Symptoms >2 per week but <1 per day	>2 per month
Step 3: Moderate persistent	Need for daily use of short-acting β-agonist	≥1 per week
		Acute exacerbations ≥2 per week
Step 4: Severe persistent	Continual symptoms that limit physical activity	Frequent

STUDY TABLE: Asthma Treatment	
Step Classification	**Treatment**
Step 1: Intermittent	Select a short-acting β-agonist, as needed
Step 2: Mild persistent	Add a low-dose inhaled glucocorticoid
Step 3: Moderate persistent	Add one of the following:
	1. Preferred treatment is low to medium doses of an inhaled glucocorticoid and a LABA (salmeterol or formoterol)
	2. Medium doses of an inhaled glucocorticoid
	3. Low to medium doses of an inhaled glucocorticoid and a single long-term controller medication (leukotriene modifier or theophylline)
Step 4: Severe persistent	Add high doses of an inhaled glucocorticoid plus a long-acting bronchodilator and possibly oral glucocorticoids

Allergy immunotherapy may be helpful in selected patients but the individual response is difficult to predict.

Omalizumab is a monoclonal antibody directed at IgE that can be administered subcutaneously in patients with moderate to severe persistent asthma with the following characteristics:

- inadequate control of symptoms with inhaled glucocorticoids
- evidence of allergies to perennial aeroallergen
- IgE levels between 300 and 700 kU/L

Peak flow meters can be used at home for serial measurement of lung function and to assess the relationship of lung function to symptoms. For all patients:

- annual influenza vaccination
- instruction about proper inhaler technique
- evaluate for thrush, hoarseness, and osteopenia caused by inhaled glucocorticoids
- calcium and vitamin D supplements for patients on chronic glucocorticoid treatment, and schedule early screening with DEXA

◆ DON'T BE TRICKED

- Do not administer theophylline with fluoroquinolones or macrolides (may result in theophylline toxicity).
- Do not use LABAs as single agents in asthma (increased mortality rate).

Treatment of exercise-induced asthma:

- for infrequent symptoms, treat with albuterol, cromolyn sodium, or nedocromil 15 to 30 minutes before exercise
- for symptoms more than twice weekly, treat with montelukast/zafirlukast, or use the Step Classification of Asthma Study Table (above).

Treatment of asthma in pregnancy:

- control GERD
- step-care therapy for chronic asthma is the same for pregnant and nonpregnant patients
- early addition of glucocorticoids is indicated for rapid reversal of airway obstruction during an exacerbation

Treatment of severe asthma exacerbation in the emergency department:

- administer repeated doses of albuterol by continuous flow nebulizer or metered-dose inhaler with a spacer
- early IV glucocorticoids should be given when inhaled albuterol is ineffective
- inhaled ipratropium may be helpful
- IV magnesium sulfate may be helpful for patients who have life-threatening exacerbations
- hospitalize patients who do not respond well after 4 to 6 hours
- intubate and mechanically ventilate patients with respiratory failure (see Invasive Mechanical Ventilation)
- patients discharged home should be given oral glucocorticoids, inhaled glucocorticoids, an asthma action plan, and follow-up instructions

◆ DON'T BE TRICKED

- A normal arterial P_{CO_2} in a patient with severe symptomatic asthma indicates impending respiratory failure.
- Consider vocal cord dysfunction for patients with "asthma" that improves immediately upon intubation.

✣ Test Yourself

A 35-year-old woman with asthma has daily coughing and shortness of breath. She uses triamcinolone, 4 puffs BID, and albuterol, 2 puffs BID as needed. Her sleep is disturbed nightly by coughing. The chest examination shows soft bilateral expiratory wheezing. PEF is 60% of predicted.

ANSWER: The diagnosis is severe persistent asthma. Add a long-acting bronchodilator. The short-term addition of an oral glucocorticoid to the inhaled glucocorticoid and a long-acting bronchodilator would also be correct.

Chronic Obstructive Pulmonary Disease

Screening

Screening asymptomatic patients for COPD is not recommended. No studies report improved outcomes for treating asymptomatic individuals with airflow obstruction.

Diagnosis

COPD is a heterogeneous disorder that includes emphysema, chronic bronchitis, obliterative bronchiolitis, and asthmatic bronchitis. Patients typically present with cough, sputum production, dyspnea, and decreased exercise tolerance and energy level. The features most predictive of COPD in a symptomatic patient are the combination of:

- smoking history
- wheezing on auscultation
- self-reported wheezing

Diagnose COPD when postbronchodilator spirometry shows an FEV_1/FVC ratio <0.70 associated with symptoms of chronic bronchitis, emphysema, or both. Test for AAT deficiency in the following situations:

- age ≤45 years
- no risk factors for COPD (smoking, occupational dust exposure)
- family history of AAT deficiency
- presence of basilar lung predominance of emphysema on imaging studies, unexplained liver disease, or necrotizing panniculitis

STUDY TABLE: Mimics of COPD	
Disease	**Characteristics**
Bronchiectasis	Often secondary to an inciting event, such as childhood pneumonia or TB; may be associated with foreign body, CF, immotile ciliary syndrome, nontuberculous mycobacteria and aspergillus infections
	Large-volume sputum production with purulent exacerbations
	Chest x-ray showing "tram lines"; diagnose with HRCT
Cystic fibrosis	Obstructive pulmonary disease is most common presentation in adult patients; other symptoms may include recurrent respiratory infections, infertility
	Positive sweat chloride test result
Adult bronchiolitis	Found in current or former smokers; may be idiopathic or associated with other diseases such as RA
	Poorly responsive to bronchodilators; responds to smoking cessation and glucocorticoids
Bronchiolitis obliterans	Presents with flulike illness and often mistaken for CAP and multiple courses of antibiotics; consider in patients after lung or stem cell transplantation
Upper airway obstruction	Stridor, which may be both inspiratory and expiratory
	Flow-volume loop shows expiratory or inspiratory flattening, or both

Therapy

Strong evidence-based recommendations:

- for symptomatic patients with COPD and FEV_1 <60% of predicted, monotherapy using either long-acting anticholinergic agents (LAMAs or LABAs) is recommended
- for symptomatic patients with an FEV_1 <50% of predicted, pulmonary rehabilitation is recommended
- for patients with COPD who have severe resting hypoxemia (arterial Po_2 <55 mm Hg or O_2 saturation <88%), continuous oxygen therapy is recommended

Weaker evidence-based recommendations:

- for stable patients with COPD with respiratory symptoms and FEV_1 between 60% and 80% of predicted, treatment with inhaled bronchodilators may be used
- for symptomatic patients with stable COPD and FEV_1 <60% of predicted, combination inhaled therapies (LAMAs, LABAs, or inhaled glucocorticoids) may be considered
- for symptomatic or exercise-limited patients with an FEV_1 >50% of predicted, pulmonary rehabilitation may be considered

Additional indications to consider long-term oxygen therapy:

- arterial blood Po_2 is 55 to 60 mm Hg with signs of tissue hypoxia (polycythemia, PH, right-sided HF)
- exercise arterial blood Po_2 is ≤55 mm Hg or O_2 saturation ≤88%

Other therapies for stable COPD

- smoking cessation (to slow loss of lung function)
- PDE-4 inhibitor (roflumilast) has been approved as add-on therapy for severe COPD

- nocturnal noninvasive mechanical ventilation to improve oxygenation, improve sleep, and decrease daytime somnolence
- palliative use of oral or parenteral opioids in patients with severe COPD and unremitting dyspnea at end of life
- annual influenza vaccination and pneumococcal vaccination according to current guidelines
- lung volume reduction surgery should be considered for patients with upper lobe emphysema (homogeneous disease) and low baseline exercise capacity to improve mortality, exercise capacity, and quality of life
- lung transplantation can increase quality of life and functional capacity in select patients
- augmentation therapy with IV human AAT is indicated for patients with homozygous AAT deficiency and decreased AAT activity levels

Antibiotics, glucocorticoids, oxygen supplementation, and noninvasive ventilation are indicated for exacerbations of COPD defined by increased sputum production, purulent sputum, and worsening dyspnea. Consider:

- tetracycline or trimethoprim-sulfamethoxazole for mild exacerbations
- β-lactam/β-lactamase inhibitor, extended-spectrum macrolides, second- or third-generation cephalosporins, or a fluoroquinolone for moderate or severe exacerbations
- IV or oral glucocorticoids
- short-acting bronchodilators (albuterol, ipratropium, or both)
- noninvasive ventilation (unless patient is obtunded, vomiting, or has excessive secretions)
- invasive mechanical ventilation if not responding or is not a candidate for noninvasive ventilation (See Invasive Mechanical Ventilation)
- pulmonary rehabilitation following hospital discharge

❖ **Test Yourself**

A 55-year-old man is evaluated for progressive dyspnea. He has a 40-pack year cigarette smoking history. On spirometry his FEV_1 is 54% of predicted. He is using an albuterol inhaler with increasing frequency. Therapy is prescribed.

ANSWER: Prescribe either a LAMA or LABA.

◆ **DON'T BE TRICKED**

- Do not use short-acting and long-acting anticholinergic agents together.
- Do not consider lung volume reduction surgery for patients with an FEV_1 ≤20% of predicted.
- Do not prescribe long-term prophylactic antibiotic therapy, antitussive drugs, or mucolytic drugs (*N*-acetylcysteine) for COPD.
- Short-term glucocorticoid use (<7 days) is as good as longer-term use.
- PDE-4 inhibitors are not indicated for acute bronchospasm.
- Clubbing is not a feature of COPD and suggests bronchiectasis, right-to-left cardiac shunts, or malignancy.

Cystic Fibrosis

Diagnosis

Chronic airway inflammation and bacterial infection characterize CF-related pulmonary disease. Most adults with CF present with pulmonary disease. Characteristic findings are recurrent or persistent respiratory infections with *Pseudomonas aeruginosa* or *Burkholderia cepacia*, bronchiectasis or hyperinflation, chronic sinusitis and nasal polyps, clubbing, steatorrhea, inability to gain weight, infertility, diabetes, and chronic or recurrent pancreatitis. The diagnosis is confirmed by a sweat chloride test followed by genetic testing.

◆ DON'T BE TRICKED

- In patients with CF and acute abdominal pain, consider intestinal intussusception.

Therapy

All patients should receive pneumococcal conjugate and polysaccharide vaccines and influenza vaccine.

Select:

- antipseudomonal antibiotics for acute pulmonary exacerbations
- aerosolized tobramycin for suppression of chronic pulmonary infections
- aerosolized recombinant human DNase (dornase alfa) or hypertonic saline for persistent airway secretions
- *CFTR* potentiator (oral ivacaftor), for patients age >6 years with at least one copy of the G551D mutation in the *CFTR* gene
- inhaled bronchodilators and glucocorticoids for airway obstruction
- nighttime noninvasive mechanical ventilation for nocturnal hypoxemia
- chest physiotherapy
- pancreatic enzyme replacement and fat soluble vitamin supplementation if indicated

Choose evaluation for transplantation for patients with advanced lung or liver disease.

❖ Test Yourself

A 34-year-old woman has had frequent episodes of bronchitis and three episodes of pneumonia in the past 5 years. Between episodes, she has a persistent cough producing yellow sputum. She also has been treated for multiple episodes of sinusitis. The patient is a lifelong nonsmoker. BMI is 18. The thorax is hyperresonant to percussion and has diminished air movement bilaterally. Digital clubbing is present.

ANSWER: The probable diagnosis is CF. Choose a sweat chloride test followed by genetic testing.

Diffuse Parenchymal Lung Disease

Diagnosis

In general, DPLDs are not infectious in origin, they most commonly present with dyspnea and cough, and imaging abnormalities are most often diffuse rather than focal.

The following steps should be used to diagnose DPLD:

- consider DPLD as a cause of subacute or chronic progressive dyspnea after infection and HF have been excluded
- obtain chest x-ray and look for interstitial reticular or nodular infiltrates
- obtain pulmonary function tests and look for restrictive or combined restrictive/obstructive findings

The diagnosis and differential of DPLD is aided by paying particular attention to the following:

- time course (typically months or years)
- active smoking history (suggests respiratory bronchiolitis–associated interstitial lung disease)
- occupation and environmental exposure history (e.g., automobile mechanics and ship builders and asbestos exposure)
- rheumatologic disease review of symptoms
- exposure to drugs and/or radiation

Obtain chest HRCT:

- the type and pattern of the infiltrate correlates well with underlying pathology on lung biopsy
- note presence of hilar lymphadenopathy (sarcoidosis), pleural effusion (connective tissue–related DPLD), and pleural plaques (asbestosis)

STUDY TABLE: Distinguishing Features of Select Forms of DPLD	
Known Causes	
Drug induced	Examples: amiodarone, methotrexate, nitrofurantoin, chemotherapeutic agents
Smoking related	"Smoker's" respiratory bronchiolitis characterized by gradual onset of persistent cough and dyspnea
	X-ray shows ground-glass opacities and thickened interstitium
	Desquamative interstitial pneumonitis and pulmonary Langerhans cell histiocytosis are other histopathological patterns associated with smoking and DPLD
Radiation	May occur 6 weeks to months following radiation therapy
Chronic aspiration	Aspiration is often subclinical
Pneumoconiosis	Asbestosis, silicosis, berylliosis
Connective tissue diseases	
Rheumatoid arthritis	May affect the pleura (pleuritis and pleural effusion), parenchyma, airways (bronchitis, bronchiectasis), and vasculature
	The parenchymal disease can range from nodules to organizing pneumonia to usual interstitial pneumonitis
Progressive SSc	Nonspecific interstitial pneumonia pathology is most common; antibody to Scl-70 or PH portends a poor prognosis
Polymyositis/dermatomyositis	Many different types of histology; poor prognosis
Hypersensitivity pneumonitis	Immune reaction to an inhaled low-molecular-weight antigen; may be acute, subacute, or chronic
	Noncaseating granulomas are seen
Unknown Causes	
Idiopathic interstitial pneumonias	
Idiopathic pulmonary fibrosis	Chronic, insidious onset of cough and dyspnea, usually in a patient age >50 y; usual interstitial pneumonia pathology (honeycombing, bibasilar infiltrates with fibrosis)
	Diagnosis of exclusion (see Idiopathic Pulmonary Fibrosis)
Acute interstitial pneumonia	Dense bilateral acute lung injury similar to ARDS; 50% mortality rate
Cryptogenic organizing pneumonia	May be preceded by flulike illness; x-ray shows focal areas of consolidation that may migrate from one location to another
Sarcoidosis	Variable clinical presentation (see Sarcoidosis)
Rare DPLD with Well-Defined Features	
LAM	Affects women in their 30s and 40s; associated with spontaneous pneumothorax and chylous effusions
	Chest CT shows cystic disease
Chronic eosinophilic pneumonia	Chest x-ray shows "radiographic negative" of HF, with peripheral alveolar infiltrates predominating
	Other findings may include peripheral blood eosinophilia and eosinophilia on bronchoalveolar lavage
Pulmonary alveolar proteinosis	Median age of 40 years, and males predominate among smokers but not in nonsmokers
	Diagnosed via bronchoalveolar lavage, which shows abundant protein in the airspaces; chest CT shows "crazy paving" pattern

◆ DON'T BE TRICKED

- Patients with dyspnea for days or weeks are more likely to have pneumonia or HF than DPLD.
- Plain radiography may be normal in 20% of patients with early DPLD; continue work-up if suspicion remains high.
- Consider DPLD in patients with dyspnea and pulmonary crackles but no other findings of HF.

Therapy

When possible, therapy is directed to the underlying cause (connective tissue disease), limiting exposure (drug discontinuation), and smoking cessation (respiratory bronchiolitis–associated interstitial lung disease). For most DPLD, the evidence for glucocorticoid efficacy is weak.

Idiopathic Pulmonary Fibrosis

Diagnosis

Idiopathic pulmonary fibrosis, the most common of the idiopathic interstitial pneumonias, is a fibrosing interstitial pneumonia. Characteristic findings are the gradual onset of a nonproductive cough and dyspnea over approximately 3 months in older adults. Physical examination findings include:

- normal temperature
- bibasilar crackles ("dry," end-inspiratory, and "Velcro-like" in quality)
- late-phase cor pulmonale
- clubbing (25% of patients)

Chest x-ray shows peripheral reticular opacities and honeycomb changes at the lung bases. HRCT scan reveals subpleural cystic changes and traction bronchiectasis. A restrictive pattern is found on pulmonary function tests.

Serum ANA, rheumatoid factor, c-ANCA, and p-ANCA levels are negative or low. Video-assisted thoracoscopic lung biopsy is indicated for patients with atypical presentations.

Diagnosis is based on clinical and radiographic findings, absence of exposure to substances or drugs that can cause interstitial lung disease, and negative evaluation for rheumatologic disease.

Therapy

No medical therapy can alter the natural history of IPF. Lung transplantation may improve survival and quality of life. Immunosuppressive therapies (glucocorticoids and cytotoxic agents) are the conventional approach to medical treatment, but only a few patients respond and therapy does not improve survival. Pirfenidone and nintedinib have demonstrated benefit for selected individuals. Oxygen therapy is indicated for patients with hypoxemia.

Idiopathic Pulmonary Fibrosis: High-resolution, thin-section chest CT scan showing extensive parenchymal involvement with fibrotic and honeycomb changes compatible with idiopathic pulmonary fibrosis.

◆ DON'T BE TRICKED

- Do not intubate and mechanically ventilate patients with IPF because it does not change the course of the disease.

Sarcoidosis

Diagnosis

Sarcoidosis is a multisystem granulomatous inflammatory disease of unknown cause. Ninety percent of patients with sarcoidosis have pulmonary involvement which may include a clinical presentation consistent with DPLD. Other common presenting manifestations include the lymphatic systems, eyes, and skin.

Characteristic findings include:

- fever, weight loss, and night sweats
- dry cough and dyspnea
- eye pain or burning and photosensitivity
- erythema nodosum
- violaceous or erythematous indurated papules, plaques, or nodules of the central face (lupus pernio); often associated with pulmonary disease
- a variety of papular, nodular, and plaque-like cutaneous lesions
- lymphadenopathy and hepatosplenomegaly
- asymmetric joint swelling
- Löfgren syndrome (fever, bilateral hilar lymphadenopathy, EN, and often ankle arthritis)
- uveoparotid fever (Heerfordt syndrome, featuring anterior uveitis, parotid gland enlargement, facial palsy, and fever)
- hypercalcemia (extrarenal production of calcitriol by granuloma cells) and kidney stones
- bilateral hilar lymphadenopathy, often with other enlarged mediastinal lymph nodes
- lymphadenopathy and lung parenchymal disease on chest x-ray

A definite diagnosis requires a compatible clinical picture, pathologic demonstration of noncaseating granulomas, and the exclusion of alternative explanations for the abnormalities (known causes of granulomatous inflammation such as infection). A diagnosis can be made without histologic studies in a patient with features of Löfgren or Heerfordt syndromes.

Diagnostic studies include:

- PFT (sarcoidosis may cause obstruction, restriction, or both)
- fiberoptic bronchoscopy with transbronchial biopsy and bronchoalveolar lavage for interstitial lung disease
- serum PTH level (low) for patients with hypercalcemia/hypercalciuria
- 1,25-dihydroxy vitamin D_3 level in patients with kidney stones and hypercalcemia
- biopsy of suspicious skin lesions
- slit-lamp examination for all patients
- ECG to rule out heart block or other cardiac abnormalities in all patients

Waxy Papular Lesions: Waxy papular lesions on the nose consistent with sarcoidosis.

◆ DON'T BE TRICKED

- **Always rule out TB and fungal infections by ordering appropriate stains and culture on tissue biopsy.**
- **Exposure to beryllium (often found in workers in light bulb or semiconductor factories) may cause a sarcoidosis-like clinical syndrome.**
- **Don't select a serum ACE level. It won't confirm the diagnosis or help in managing sarcoidosis.**

Therapy

Topical glucocorticoids are prescribed for skin lesions or anterior uveitis, and inhaled glucocorticoids are used for nasal polyps or airway disease. Oral glucocorticoids are indicated for progressive or symptomatic pulmonary sarcoidosis; hypercalcemia; or cardiac, ophthalmologic, or neurologic sarcoid. Patients with glucocorticoid-refractory disease are treated with immunosuppressive, cytotoxic, and antimalarial agents. Löfgren syndrome has a very high rate (80%) of spontaneous remission and resolution.

- Do not treat asymptomatic sarcoidosis.

❖ **Test Yourself**

A 66-year-old man is hospitalized because of azotemia and hypercalcemia. Laboratory studies show a normal serum PTH level and an elevated 1,25-dihydroxy vitamin D_3 level. A chest x-ray shows an interstitial infiltrate and an enlarged left paratracheal lymph node.

ANSWER: The probable diagnosis is sarcoidosis. Choose transbronchial lung biopsy.

Occupational Lung Disease

Sarcoidosis: X-ray shows bilateral hilar lymphadenopathy characteristic of sarcoidosis. Sarcoidosis can be associated with interstitial lung disease.

Diagnosis

Clinical manifestations may include rhinitis, asthma, COPD, constrictive bronchiolitis, and restrictive diseases. Symptom onset following exposure can be acute (reactive airways disease/small airways dysfunction as occurs in acute chlorine gas exposure) as well as prolonged or subacute with a significant latent period (as with asbestosis).

STUDY TABLE: Clues to Occupational Lung Disease
There is a temporal relationship to clinical symptoms and work:
Symptoms worsen during or after work
Symptoms abate or improve with time off or away from the workplace
Work-related changes in FEV_1 or PEF
Coworkers are affected with similar symptoms
There are known respiratory hazards at work (these can be identified by Material Safety Data Sheets from the workplace)
Failure to respond to initial therapy or symptoms that are further exacerbated upon returning to work
Onset of a respiratory disorder without typical risk factors
Clustering of disease in one geographic area

A positive response to a specific inhalation challenge test is the "gold standard" for diagnosis, but not always necessary.

Therapy

Overriding principle is discontinuing the exposure. Occupational asthma and reactive airways dysfunction syndrome are treated with inhaled glucocorticoids.

◆ **DON'T BE TRICKED**

- The incidence of TB is increased in those with silicosis and should be evaluated in patients with silicosis, fever, and cough.

❖ **Test Yourself**

A previously healthy 45-year-old man has a cough of 6 months' duration. He is a lifelong nonsmoker and works as an automobile spray painter. Physical examination discloses a few expiratory wheezes. FEV_1 is 0.65 and FEV_1/FVC ratio is 65% of predicted, and a 22% improvement occurs after bronchodilator administration.

ANSWER: Obtain spirometry or measure PEF before and after work (or during vacation) to confirm the diagnosis of occupational asthma.

Asbestos-Associated Lung Diseases

Diagnosis

The most important risk factor for development of asbestos-related lung disease is the cumulative exposure to the asbestos fiber. Occupations with the greatest exposure include those in the construction industry, the automotive servicing industry, and the shipbuilding and repair industry. The latent period for development of asbestosis and mesothelioma is 10 to 15 years. Cigarette smoking increases the risk of mesothelioma and lung cancer.

STUDY TABLE: Asbestos-Related Lung Syndromes	
Condition	**Characteristics**
Pleural plaques (localized, often partially calcified)	Often incidental finding; usually bilateral; most common manifestation of asbestos exposure
	Monitor patients for development of intrathoracic disease
Diffuse pleural thickening	Extensive pleural thickening extends into the visceral pleura and obliterates the costophrenic angles
	May cause hypercapnic respiratory failure secondary to impairment of ventilation
Rounded atelectasis	Presents as single or multiple masses due to infolding of thickened visceral pleura with collapse of the adjacent peripheral lung
	The classic radiographic finding is a "comet tail" on chest CT scan extending from the hilum toward the base of the lung and then sweeping into the inferior pole of the lesion
	Can cause ventilatory failure
Benign pleural effusion	Exudative hemorrhagic effusion; may be painful
Mesothelioma	Suggested by weight loss, fever, cough, dyspnea, chest pain, unilateral pleural abnormalities, and pleural effusion
	Tissue diagnosis required; cytological diagnosis can be established by thoracentesis or closed pleural biopsy
Asbestosis	Manifests with bilateral interstitial fibrosis of the lung parenchyma, bibasilar inspiratory crackles, clubbing, restrictive physiology, and low DLco
Lung cancer	Most asbestos-related cases occur in patients with asbestosis, but a diagnosis of asbestosis is not necessary to attribute lung cancer to asbestos exposure

Therapy

In patients with a history of asbestos exposure or asbestosis, the risk of lung cancer mortality can be decreased at any time with smoking cessation. Surgery is indicated for patients with localized mesothelioma, and radiation and chemotherapy are used to prevent recurrences. Most patients with mesothelioma have advanced disease and are treated symptomatically by controlling pleural effusions with thoracentesis.

Mesothelioma: Frontal chest x-ray showing multiple pleural-based nodular infiltrates at the right chest wall and pleural thickening consistent with mesothelioma.

Pleural Effusion

Diagnosis

Pleural fluid is characterized as transudative or exudative. Transudates form when hydrostatic pressures favor fluid formation exceeding clearance, whereas exudates form by means of increased vascular permeability. The vast majority of pleural effusions in the United States are due to HF, pneumonia, or malignancy. A thoracentesis is indicated for any new unexplained effusion; however, observation and therapy without thoracentesis is reasonable in the setting of known HF, small parapneumonic effusions, or following CABG surgery.

STUDY TABLE: Laboratory Tests for Identifying a Pleural Effusion as an Exudate	
Test	**Interpretation**
Pleural fluid protein–serum protein ratio	>0.5
Pleural fluid LDH	>200 U/L (or >2/3 the upper limit of normal)
Pleural fluid LDH–serum LDH ratio	>0.6

An effusion is considered an exudate if any 1 of the above criteria are met. However, treatment (diuretics for HF), a dual diagnosis (HF and a concomitant parapneumonic effusion), or some specific diagnoses (e.g., chylothorax) can result in discordant exudates (an exudate by either the protein or LDH criterion but a transudate by the other criteria). One of the more common causes of discordant findings is diuretic use. In the setting of ongoing diuresis, if the serum to pleural fluid albumin gradient is >1.2 g/dL, the fluid is most likely a transudate.

STUDY TABLE: Common Causes of Transudative and Exudative Pleural Effusions	
Transudative Pleural Effusions	**Exudative Pleural Effusions**
Increased hydrostatic pressure (HF, constrictive pericarditis, SVC obstruction)	Infection
Decreased oncotic pressure (hypoalbuminemia, nephrotic syndrome, cirrhosis, malnutrition)	Neoplasm
	Autoimmune diseases
	Pulmonary infarction
	Hemothorax
	Benign asbestos effusion
	Post-coronary bypass
	Pancreatitis
	Yellow-nail syndrome (lymphatic disorders)

Pleural fluid cell counts and chemistries can further narrow the differential diagnosis.

STUDY TABLE: Pleural Fluid Cell Counts and Chemistries	
If you see this...	**Think this...**
Bloody pleural fluid (RBC count 5000-10,000/μL)	Malignancy, pulmonary infarction, asbestos related
Nucleated cells >50,000/μL	Complicated parapneumonic effusions and empyema
Lymphocytosis >80%	TB, lymphoma, chronic rheumatoid pleuritis, sarcoidosis
pH <7.0	Complicated parapneumonic effusion, TB, rheumatoid and lupus pleuritis, esophageal rupture
Pleural fluid amylase to serum amylase ratio >1	Pancreatic disease, esophageal rupture, cancer
Glucose <60 mg/dL	Complicated parapneumonic effusion or empyema, cancer, TB, rheumatoid and lupus pleuritis, esophageal rupture

Other key points:

- pleural fluid adenosine deaminase is elevated in most TB effusions
- pleural biopsy is most likely to yield a positive TB culture
- the yield for positive malignant cytology is maximized after 2 samples
- thoracoscopy should be done for an undiagnosed exudative effusion (2 negative cytology examinations) when malignancy is suspected

Therapy

Parapneumonic pleural effusion requires chest tube drainage when the pH is <7.2 or the pleural fluid glucose level is <60 mg/dL.

Anaerobes are cultured in up to 72% of empyemas and empiric antibiotic therapy should include anaerobic coverage.

For patients with malignant effusions, indwelling pleural catheters provide symptom relief, and up to 70% of patients achieve spontaneous obliteration of the pleural space (pleurodesis) after 6 weeks. Chemical pleurodesis with talc has a 90% success rate.

Pleural Effusion: Chest x-ray showing a right-sided pleural effusion (*left panel*) that layers out along the right thorax in the right lateral decubitus view (*right panel*).

◆ DON'T BE TRICKED

- Always obtain thoracentesis for moderate to large effusions associated with pneumonia.
- Pleural effusions associated with nephrotic syndrome are common, but PE should be excluded in such patients because PE and renal vein thrombosis often occur in patients with nephrotic syndrome.
- Consider pulmonary LAM when chylothorax is diagnosed in a premenopausal woman.

❖ Test Yourself

A 65-year-old woman has a 2-week history of shortness of breath. A chest x-ray shows a large right-sided pleural effusion. Serum LDH is 190 U/L and total protein is 6.0 g/dL. Thoracentesis is performed; pleural fluid protein is 2.8 g/dL and pleural fluid LDH is 110 U/L.

ANSWER: The diagnosis is a transudative pleural effusion.

Pneumothorax

Diagnosis

Characteristic symptoms are chest pain and dyspnea. Spontaneous pneumothorax is considered to be primary when the lung is overtly normal. Tall men who smoke are at risk. Other risk factors include cocaine use and Marfan syndrome. Subpleural blebs and bullae are commonly detected on CT scan and predispose to primary pneumothorax.

Secondary pneumothorax is associated with lung disease. Consider:

- emphysema is the most common cause of secondary pneumothorax
- diagnose pulmonary LAM in premenopausal women presenting with a spontaneous pneumothorax and lung disease
- secondary pneumothorax is common in patients with HIV and *Pneumocystis jirovecii* pneumonia
- tension pneumothorax is suggested by falling BP and oxygen saturation, tracheal deviation, and no breath sounds in one hemithorax

Obtain an upright chest x-ray in patients with dyspnea, pleurisy, or both, even if the physical examination is normal.

◆ **DON'T BE TRICKED**

- Do not wait for chest radiography results before treating suspected tension pneumothorax with needle decompression.

Therapy

Treatment depends on the type of pneumothorax:

- observation and oxygen in asymptomatic patients with a small pneumothorax (rim of air <2 cm on chest x-ray)
- simple aspiration for symptomatic primary spontaneous pneumothorax of any size
- release of pressure with a large needle for tension pneumothorax followed by chest tube placement
- chest tube if a secondary pneumothorax measures >2 cm
- pleurodesis for a first primary spontaneous pneumothorax and after a second secondary spontaneous pneumothorax

Pulmonary Hypertension

Screening

Patients with SSc (scleroderma) should be screened with TTE. Also screen the following patients: liver transplantation candidates with portal hypertension, first-degree relatives of patients with familial PAH, and patients with congenital heart disease with systemic-to-pulmonary shunts.

Diagnosis

PH is defined by a resting mean pulmonary arterial pressure of ≥25 mm Hg. The current classification system subdivides PH into five groups.

- Group 1 is distinguished by disease localized to small pulmonary arterioles resulting in high pulmonary vascular resistance, and is referred to as PAH.
- Groups 2 through 5 refer to important secondary causes of PH and include left-sided heart disease, respiratory disorders (COPD, interstitial lung disease, portal hypertension, and sleep-disordered breathing), and chronic venous thromboembolic disease.

Characteristic findings of PH include:

- unexplained dyspnea
- decreased exercise tolerance
- syncope and near-syncope
- chest pain
- lower extremity edema

Other findings indicating RV failure may include an RV heave, right-sided S_3, widely split S_2, increased P_2, increased jugular venous distention with a large *a* wave, and a murmur of TR.

Look for use of fenfluramine, amphetamines, and cocaine and the presence of Raynaud phenomenon (suggesting SLE and SSc) and history of VTE. Typical evaluation of Group 1 pulmonary hypertension (PAH) includes:

- echocardiography as the initial study; a systolic pulmonary artery pressure >40 mm Hg is suggestive of PH
- bubble contrast echocardiography or TEE is indicated to evaluate for intracardiac shunts (e.g., ASD)
- right heart catheterization to confirm the diagnosis and quantify the degree of PH
- left heart catheterization and coronary angiography exclude LV dysfunction as a cause of PH

If the diagnosis of PAH is confirmed, the next step is a vasoreactivity test using vasodilating agents to measure changes in pulmonary artery pressure with a right heart catheter in place.

Additional recommended tests to rule out other causes of PH include pulmonary function tests, liver chemistry tests, polysomnography if clinically indicated, and serologic tests for HIV infection or connective tissue disease.

In some patients (<5%) following an acute PE, thromboemboli within the pulmonary arteries become remodeled into large occlusive scars, causing CTEPH and leads to right-sided HF.

Two diagnostic criteria for CTEPH:

- pulmonary arterial pressure ≥25 mm Hg in the absence of left-sided HF
- compatible imaging evidence of chronic thromboembolism by V/Q scanning

◆ DON'T BE TRICKED

- The vast majority of cases of PH are attributed to left-sided heart disease and hypoxic respiratory disorders.
- Do not select an HRCT scan to diagnose CTEPH. A V/Q scan is superior.

Therapy

Therapy for PH groups 2 through 5 is typically directed at the underlying condition.

For Group 1 PH (PAH), vascular-targeted treatments provide symptomatic relief but are not curative.

- Calcium channel blockers are used for patients demonstrating a vasodilator response on right heart catheterization.
- Oral agents (PDE-5 inhibitors, such as sildenafil or tadalafil, or endothelin receptor antagonists, such as bosentan or ambrisentan) are initial therapies for mild to moderate disease.
- A parenteral prostacyclin analogue such as epoprostenol, administered by a continuous central venous infusion, is first-line therapy for severe disease.
- Lung or heart-lung transplantation should be considered for patients in whom drug treatment is unsuccessful.
- Oxygen therapy is indicated for O_2 saturation ≤90%. PAH predisposes the patient to in-situ pulmonary vascular thrombosis and embolism; anticoagulation is recommended.

Life-long anticoagulant therapy is indicated in all patients with CTEPH. Pulmonary thromboendarterectomy is the only definitive therapy for CTEPH.

◆ **DON'T BE TRICKED**

- Do not select calcium channel blockers if pulmonary artery pressure is not decreased with a vasoreactivity test.

Pulmonary Arteriovenous Malformation

Diagnosis

Pulmonary AVMs consist of abnormal communications between pulmonary arteries and veins. They are included in the differential diagnosis of hypoxemia, pulmonary nodules, and hemoptysis. The following suggest a pulmonary AVM:

- hemoptysis
- mucocutaneous telangiectasias
- evidence of right-to-left pulmonary shunts (hypoxemia, polycythemia, clubbing, cyanosis, stroke, brain abscess)

Chest CT is the initial diagnostic test.

Therapy

Symptomatic or large pulmonary AVMs (>2 cm) are treated with either embolotherapy or surgery.

◆ **Test Yourself**

A 46-year-old man is evaluated for a TIA. Telangiectasias are present on the lips. The lungs are clear, and cardiovascular and neurovascular examinations are normal. Laboratory evaluation reveals polycythemia and an arterial P_{O_2} of 68 mm Hg. Chest x-ray shows a 2-cm SPN.

ANSWER: The diagnosis is pulmonary AVM.

Telangiectasia: Telangiectasias on the tongue in a patient with hereditary hemorrhagic telangiectasia.

Lung Cancer Screening

In high-risk populations, lung cancer screening results in a 20% lung cancer mortality reduction. Screen patients between the ages of 55 and 79 years who have a 30-pack-year history of smoking and who are currently smoking or quit within the last 15 years. Continue annual low-dose CT imaging until comorbidity limits survival or the patient reaches the age of 80 years. Stop screening in patients who have stopped smoking for 15 years.

◆ **DON'T BE TRICKED**

- The risks of screening outweigh the benefit in patients at low risk for lung cancer.

Hemoptysis

Diagnosis

Bronchitis, bronchogenic carcinoma, and bronchiectasis are the most common causes of hemoptysis, and diagnosis can be further narrowed by considering patient risk factors.

Common causes of hemoptysis:

- acute bronchitis (acute cough syndrome in an otherwise healthy patient with no other risk factors)
- lung cancer (older adult, smoking history)
- bronchiectasis (chronic history of cough, voluminous sputum production, and "tram lines" on chest x-ray)
- aspergilloma (fungus ball in lung cavity as shown in the Infectious Disease chapter; patient may have disease that causes pulmonary cavities or have allergic bronchopulmonary aspergillosis)
- TB (fever, night sweats, weight loss, prison stay, HIV, immigrant status)
- PE and infarction (pleural-based triangular opacity with a rounded apex [Hampton hump] or area of hyperlucency [Westermark sign] on chest x-ray)
- pulmonary-renal hemorrhage syndrome (hematuria and kidney disease)
- mitral stenosis (opening snap and rumbling diastolic murmur)
- HIV (bacterial infections, TB, and Kaposi sarcoma)

◆ DON'T BE TRICKED

- Confirm a patient has hemoptysis rather than epistaxis or GI bleeding, then check the platelet count and coagulation parameters.

STUDY TABLE: Diagnostic Tests for Hemoptysis	
Test	**Considerations**
Chest x-ray	Crucial initial study, but normal findings do not exclude lung cancer
Fiberoptic bronchoscopy	For patients at high risk for lung cancer, even if chest x-ray is normal
Chest CT	Alternative test when fiberoptic bronchoscopy is contraindicated or when bleeding persists despite normal bronchoscopic findings

Therapy

The cause of death from massive hemoptysis is asphyxiation from airway obstruction. If the bleeding site can be localized to one lung, position the patient with the bleeding lung dependent. Intubation and mechanical ventilation are required when adequate gas exchange is threatened. Angiography can localize and treat bronchial artery lesions.

Solitary Pulmonary Nodule

Diagnosis

A SPN is a lesion of the lung parenchyma measuring ≤3 cm in diameter that is not associated with other lesions or lymphadenopathy and is not invading other structures. Approximately 35% of SPNs are bronchogenic carcinomas.

The management of SPNs is dependent upon size and risk of malignancy. Solid SPN <8 mm are managed differently than larger nodules and "sub-solid" nodules. A sub-solid nodule is less dense than a solid nodule and normal lung structures such as blood vessels can be seen through the nodule. Risk models and surveillance recommendations exist for larger nodules but are unlikely subjects for the ABIM examination.

❖ Test Yourself

A 65-year-old man is incidentally found to have a 3 mm pulmonary nodule on chest x-rays obtained prior to an elective cholecystectomy. On follow-up chest CT, there are no other nodules or evidence of lymphadenopathy. He has a 50-pack year history of cigarette smoking.

ANSWER: Follow-up chest CT scan in 1 year.

STUDY TABLE: Criteria for Initial CT Imaging of Small Solitary Solid Pulmonary Nodules		
Nodule Size	**Nonsmoker**	**Smoker, Family History of Cancer**
≤4 mm	None	12 months
>4 to 6 mm	12 months	6 to 12 months
>6 to 8 mm	6 to 12 months	3 to 6 months

A pulmonary mass, defined as >3 cm in diameter, is highly suspicious for malignancy in a patient with risk factors. Biopsy for tissue diagnosis (in the absence of suspected metastases) or surgical resection (if no evidence of metastatic disease is found) is typically the first step in the evaluation.

STUDY TABLE: Diagnostic Tests for a Pulmonary Nodule	
Test	**Considerations**
Comparison with previous chest x-ray	Stability over time helps rule out malignancy
Contrast-enhanced CT	Most useful imaging method
Fiberoptic bronchoscopy with biopsy	Provides sufficient information in only 30% of lesions
Percutaneous transthoracic needle aspiration biopsy	Has a higher yield of malignant lesions but is not always diagnostic
PET scan	Positive in >90% of malignant solitary nodules >1 cm in diameter

◆ DON'T BE TRICKED

- Before ordering contrast CT, bronchoscopy, or PET scan, compare current image with previous image to determine stability over time.
- PET scans may be falsely negative in alveolar cell carcinoma or lesions <1 cm in diameter and falsely positive in various inflammatory lesions.
- A nonspecific negative result from fiberoptic bronchoscopy or transthoracic needle aspiration biopsy does not reliably exclude the presence of a malignant growth.

Pulmonary Metastases

Pulmonary metastases present as multiple, peripheral, or subpleural pulmonary nodules. The most common primary malignancies to metastasize to the lung are:

- carcinomas (colon, kidney, breast, testicle, and thyroid)
- sarcomas (bone)
- melanoma

Endobronchial metastases are rare and are most commonly associated with renal cell carcinoma.

Lymphangitic spread should be considered when a peripheral interstitial abnormality is identified on HRCT in a patient with one of these malignancies:

- adenocarcinoma (lung, breast, and GI tract)
- melanoma
- lymphoma
- leukemia

Mediastinal Masses

Diagnosis

The mediastinum can be divided into three separate compartments, which can help narrow the differential diagnosis of a mediastinal mass.

STUDY TABLE: Mediastinal Masses	
Origin of Mass	**Important Associations**
Anterior Mediastinum	
Thymus	Most common tumor of anterior mediastinum; 40% have MG
	Other syndromes include pure red cell aplasia and acquired hypogammaglobulinemia
Teratoma/germ cell	Teratomas may contain fat, fluid, and bone discernable on CT imaging
Lymphoma	Second most common anterior mediastinal tumor; Hodgkin disease is the most common lymphoma
Thyroid	Often causes compressive symptoms (dyspnea, dysphagia)
Middle Mediastinum	
Lymph nodes	Lymphadenopathy is the most common cause of middle mediastinal masses
Cysts	Include benign pericardial, bronchogenic, and esophageal cysts
Posterior Mediastinum	
Neurogenic tumors	Schwannomas are most common in adults

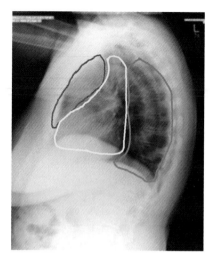

Mediastinum: A lateral chest x-ray demonstrates the anterior (red), middle (yellow), and posterior (blue) mediastinal compartments.

Obstructive Sleep Apnea

Diagnosis

An obstructive apnea is defined as the absence of airflow for at least 10 seconds despite persistence of respiratory effort. OSAs are typically accompanied by oxyhemoglobin desaturations and are terminated by an awakening from sleep. The severity of OSA can be classified based on the apnea-hypopnea index (AHI; number of apneas plus hypopneas per hour of sleep) as:

- mild (AHI 5-15)
- moderate (AHI 16-30)
- severe (AHI >30)

Characteristic findings of OSA include snoring, apnea, excessive daytime sleepiness, and obesity (determined by either BMI or neck circumference >17 in) and an enlarged and elongated soft palate (crowded pharynx).

Occasionally, OSA first presents following a surgical procedure involving general anesthesia and/or narcotic analgesia, where repeated apneas, acute respiratory failure, and even death occur. Screening questionnaires (STOP-Bang) are available to identify OSA during pre-anesthesia evaluation.

Patients with untreated OSA have a greater likelihood of developing CAD, acute MI during sleep, systemic and PAH, HF, recurrent AF, stroke, insulin resistance, mood disorders, and parasomnias.

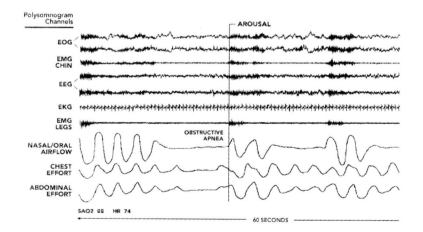

Obstructive Sleep Apnea: This polysomnogram shows obstructive apneas, indicated by the absence of flow and ongoing abdominal and rib cage effort that is terminated with evidence of an electroencephalographic arousal.

Diagnose OSA in patients with an AHI of >5/h during a sleep study. Other options include out-of-center sleep testing (OCST) that involves the use of portable equipment for home testing in the absence of a sleep technician. OCST performs comparably to polysomnography in patients without comorbid cardiopulmonary disease who have a high pretest probability of moderate to severe OSA.

◆ DON'T BE TRICKED

- Do not confuse obesity-hypoventilation syndrome with sleep apnea. Obesity-hypoventilation syndrome is usually associated with COPD and always with elevated arterial P_{CO_2} levels when awake.
- Obesity-hypoventilation syndrome may coexist with OSA.
- Overnight oximetry has not been validated as a screening tool for OSA.

Therapy

Lifestyle changes, including weight loss, avoiding alcohol and sedatives before bedtime, and sleeping in the lateral position are always indicated. CPAP is the treatment of choice. CPAP therapy has been shown to improve quality of life, cognitive function, and symptoms of daytime sleepiness.

BPAP therapy, in which inspiratory and expiratory pressures can be adjusted separately, may be useful in patients who do not tolerate CPAP, have concurrent central sleep apneas, or have persistent oxygen desaturation because of hypoventilation despite CPAP therapy. CPAP may help patients with daytime hypercapnia due to related obesity-hypoventilation syndrome. Therapy may be required for up to 4 weeks before ABGs improve.

Oral appliances are an alternative to CPAP therapy for mild to moderate OSA. They act by either: (1) advancement of the mandible by traction or (2) prevention of posterior displacement of the tongue by suction. Oral appliances are not as effective as CPAP in reducing AHI.

◆ DON'T BE TRICKED

- Supplemental oxygen is not recommended as a primary therapy for OSA.
- Upper airway surgery is not recommended as initial therapy for OSA.

High-Altitude Related Illness

Diagnosis

HAI encompasses a number of disorders that can occur when a person residing at low altitude ascends to higher elevation. HAI is more common at elevations ≥2500 meters (approximately 8200 feet).

STUDY TABLE: High-Altitude Illnesses		
Disorder	**Pathophysiology**	**Clinical Findings**
High-altitude periodic breathing (HAPB)	Hypoxia-induced hyperventilation lowers P_{CO_2} toward the apneic threshold, decreasing respiratory rate, which raises P_{CO_2} and results in recurrent hyperventilation	Repetitive arousals from sleep, often with paroxysms of dyspnea
Acute mountain sickness (AMS)	Hypoxia and hypocarbia-induced alterations in cerebral blood flow	Headache, fatigue, nausea, and vomiting, in addition to disturbed sleep related to HAPB
High-altitude cerebral edema (HACE)	Brain edema at altitudes typically above 10,000-13,000 feet	Confusion, irritability, ataxia, coma, and death
High-altitude pulmonary edema (HAPE)	PH and pulmonary edema	Cough, dyspnea at rest, pink frothy sputum, hemoptysis, and pulmonary crackles

Therapy

HAI can be prevented by gradually ascending. Acetazolamide accelerates the acclimatization. Acetazolamide, dexamethasone and supplemental oxygen are used to treat AMS. Definitive treatment for HACE is immediate descent from altitude; dexamethasone, supplemental oxygen, and hyperbaric therapy may also be used. HAPE treatment of choice is supplemental oxygen and rest. Salvage therapies include vasodilators such as nifedipine or PDE-5 inhibitors (sildenafil or tadalafil).

◆ DON'T BE TRICKED

- Do not treat HAPE with diuretics and nitrates.

Hypercapnic Respiratory (Ventilatory) Failure

Diagnosis

Hypercapnic respiratory (ventilatory) failure occurs when alveolar ventilation is inadequate and the level of CO_2 increases in the blood. Because oxygenation also depends on ventilation, patients are often hypoxic as well. However, hypoxia will often improve with supplemental oxygen. Chronic hypercapnic respiratory failure occurs most often in patients with:

- COPD
- neuromuscular disease (MG, ALS, MS)
- restrictive lung diseases (parenchymal lung disease, chest wall skeletal disorders, obesity)
- depressed respiratory drive (opioids and sedatives)

In patients with neuromuscular disease, pulmonary function tests show restriction on spirometry and lung volume measurement but normal diffusing capacity.

Patients with respiratory muscle weakness, obesity-hypoventilation syndrome, and disorders of ventilatory control first hypoventilate during REM sleep. Schedule polysomnography if nocturnal hypoventilation is suspected (daytime sleepiness, nocturnal awakenings, morning headaches).

❖ Test Yourself

A 36-year-old man with myotonic dystrophy awakens at night gasping for air and experiences increasing fatigue. Cardiopulmonary examination is normal. Neurologic examination shows 4+/5 strength in all muscle groups.

ANSWER: The probable diagnosis is nocturnal hypercapnic respiratory failure. Select polysomnography.

Acute Respiratory Distress Syndrome

Diagnosis

Hypoxic respiratory failure is due to V/Q mismatching. ARDS is a syndrome of hypoxemic respiratory failure due to alveolar damage and the leakage of fluid across the alveolar-capillary barrier (noncardiogenic pulmonary edema).

STUDY TABLE: Diagnosing and Classifying ARDS	
Features common to all cases of ARDS	Acute onset (<1 week) of respiratory symptoms and hypoxia
	Bilateral lung opacities on imaging not explained by other disease processes
	Respiratory failure not explained by HF or volume overload (although ARDS can coexist with HF or fluid overload states)
Mild ARDS	Arterial Po_2/Fio_2 ratio of 201-300 mm Hg, measured with PEEP ≥5 cm H_2O
Moderate ARDS	Arterial Po_2/Fio_2 ratio of 101-200 mm Hg, measured with PEEP ≥5 cm H_2O
Severe ARDS	Arterial Po_2/Fio_2 ratio of ≤100 mm Hg, measured with PEEP ≥5 cm H_2O

Precipitating causes of ARDS include pulmonary infection, hemorrhagic shock, pancreatitis, trauma, transfusions, and sepsis. Hemodynamic measurements by pulmonary artery catheterization are sometimes necessary to exclude cardiogenic pulmonary edema when clinical examination and bedside echocardiography are indeterminant. A PCWP ≥18 mm Hg favors cardiogenic pulmonary edema.

STUDY TABLE: Mimics of ARDS	
Disease	**Characteristics**
Cardiogenic pulmonary edema	History of cardiac disease, enlarged heart, S_3, chest x-ray showing an enlarged cardiac silhouette, pleural effusions, and Kerley B lines
	Rapid improvement with diuresis or afterload reduction
Diffuse alveolar hemorrhage	Kidney disease or other evidence of vasculitis present
	Associated with stem cell transplantation
	Hemosiderin-laden macrophages in bronchoalveolar lavage fluid
Acute eosinophilic pneumonia	Cough, fever, pleuritic chest pain, and myalgia; may be precipitated by initiation of smoking
	>15% eosinophils in bronchoalveolar lavage fluid
Acute PE	Occurs acutely, occasionally accompanied by severe hypoxemia that may be resistant to oxygen and by hypotension requiring vasopressors, mimicking ARDS with sepsis
	Patients typically have risk factors for acute PE and may not have common precipitating causes of ARDS
Hypersensitivity pneumonitis	Typically slower onset than ARDS (over weeks) with progressive course; however, may present in an advanced stage, mimicking ARDS
	Positive exposure history (farmers, bird fanciers, hot tub exposure)
Cryptogenic organizing pneumonia	May be precipitated by viral syndrome
	Slower onset than ARDS (>2 weeks) with progressive course; however, may present in an advanced stage, mimicking ARDS
Acute interstitial pneumonia	May be impossible to distinguish from ARDS
	Absence of typical inciting factors for ARDS
	May respond to glucocorticoid administration

Therapy

Optimal mechanical ventilation includes:

- lung-protective ventilation using volume-controlled ventilation with a tidal volume of ≤6 mL/kg of ideal body weight
- plateau (end-inspiratory) pressure <30 cm H_2O (even if this results in "permissive" hypercapnia and acidosis)
- PEEP

Limiting IV fluids and using diuretics to keep CVP at lower targets has been associated with a more rapid improvement in lung function, shorter duration of mechanical ventilation, and shorter ICU length of stay but no effect on mortality.

Use of prone positioning in the most severe forms of ARDS has a mortality benefit.

◆ DON'T BE TRICKED

- Glucocorticoids are not indicated for the acute treatment of ARDS.

❖ Test Yourself

A 55-year-old woman with acute pancreatitis has increasingly severe shortness of breath for 12 hours. She has no history of cardiac disease. Pulse rate is 116/min, respiration rate is 40/min, and arterial O_2 saturation is 86% (on supplemental oxygen). Diffuse bilateral crackles are heard. Chest x-ray shows diffuse airspace disease. She is intubated and mechanically ventilated. On an FIO_2 of 1.0, her arterial PO_2 is 150 mm Hg.

ANSWER: The diagnosis is moderate ARDS. Choose a tidal volume of 6 mL/kg of ideal body weight.

Noninvasive Positive-Pressure Ventilation

Indications

NPPV is the use of positive-pressure ventilation without the need for an invasive airway. NPPV may be used as the ventilatory mode of first choice in four conditions:

- COPD exacerbations (not stable COPD)
- cardiogenic pulmonary edema
- acute respiratory failure in immunosuppressed patients
- prevention of recurrent respiratory failure in recently extubated high-risk patients

The most common contraindications to NPPV include:

- respiratory arrest
- arterial blood pH <7.10
- medical instability
- inability to protect airway and/or excessive secretions
- uncooperative or agitated patient

Improvements in blood gas values and clinical condition should occur within 2 hours of starting NPPV. If not, intubation should be considered to avoid undue delay and prevent respiratory arrest.

Invasive Mechanical Ventilation

Indications

Patients may require invasive mechanical ventilatory support for hypoxic respiratory failure (low arterial P_{O_2}) or impaired alveolar ventilation (increased arterial P_{CO_2}). In general, if a patient cannot maintain an arterial P_{O_2} >60 mm Hg or an O_2 saturation >90% despite supplemental oxygen of 60% or higher, initiating mechanical ventilation is usually appropriate, regardless of the arterial P_{CO_2}.

Management

In volume-targeted ventilation, set tidal volume first:

- tidal volumes are based on the patient's weight
- the recommended range is 6 to 8 mL/kg of ideal body weight (≤6 mL/kg for ARDS)
- tidal volumes that are too high can result in barotrauma, respiratory alkalosis, and decreased cardiac output
- tidal volumes that are too low can result in atelectasis, hypoxemia, and hypoventilation

Set respiratory rate:

- the respiration rate is usually started at 8 to 14/min if the patient is otherwise clinically stable
- a respiratory rate that is too high can result in respiratory alkalosis and air trapping (auto-PEEP)
- a respiratory rate that is too low can result in hypoventilation, acidosis, hypoxemia, and patient discomfort

Set oxygen flow and PEEP to maintain arterial P_{O_2} >60 mm Hg.

Be alert for auto-PEEP:

- in the presence of increased airway resistance, a high demand for ventilation, or a short expiratory time, air flow may still occur at end exhalation, resulting in positive pressure in the alveoli at end exhalation
- suspect auto-PEEP if the flow tracing on the ventilator shows continuous expiratory flow until the start of inspiratory flow

Common causes of auto-PEEP include COPD or acute asthma, an endotracheal tube that is too narrow, long ventilator tubing, ARDS (increased flow resistance), and a high minute ventilation (>12-15 L/min). Characteristic findings are wheezing and marked expiratory prolongation, drop in BP, and patient restlessness. Strategies to minimize auto-PEEP:

- treat airway obstruction (e.g., bronchodilators in COPD or asthma)
- decrease the respiratory rate or tidal volume
- increase the peak inspiratory flow rate
- prolong the expiratory phase
- allow permissive hypercapnia
- sedate or paralyze the patient

STUDY TABLE: Ventilator Management

If you would like to...	...the intermediate step is...	... make the ventilator do this by:	Notes:
Improve respiratory acidosis	↓ Arterial P_{CO_2}	Increasing respiratory rate Increasing tidal volume: in volume control mode, directly choose the tidal volume; in pressure control modes, increase the inspiratory support pressure to increase tidal volume	Watch for auto-PEEP at high respiratory rates, which can cause hypotension by reducing preload Don't be tricked: If the patient has ARDS, respiratory acidosis (pH ~7.2) should generally be tolerated rather than raising the tidal volume >6 mL/kg
Improve respiratory alkalosis	↑ Arterial P_{CO_2}	Decreasing respiratory rate Decreasing tidal volume	If the patient is breathing faster than the set ventilator rate, this strategy won't work Determine why respiratory alkalosis is present (sepsis, PE, liver disease, pain)
Improve tissue oxygenation	↑ O_2 saturation, arterial P_{O_2}	Increasing F_{IO_2} Increasing PEEP	Occasionally, increasing PEEP will lower cardiac output by reducing preload; this can worsen oxygen delivery to tissues If no contraindications, attempt to increase preload with IV fluids

Difficult ventilation or complications of mechanical ventilation due to changes in airway resistance may first be manifested by an increase in the peak inspiratory pressure alone, resulting from:

- bronchospasm
- secretions in airways, endotracheal tube, or ventilator tubing
- obstructing mucus plug
- agitation with dyssynchrony with the ventilator

Difficult ventilation resulting from a change in lung compliance will be manifested by an increase in both peak inspiratory pressure and plateau pressure, resulting from:

- right mainstem intubation
- pneumothorax
- worsening airspace disease (ARDS, pneumonia, pulmonary edema)

Placing intubated patients in a semirecumbent position and selective decontamination of the oropharynx (using topical gentamicin, colistin, or vancomycin) reduces the risk of VAP.

When a patient can maintain an arterial O_2 saturation >90% on FIO_2 ≤0.5, PEEP <5 cm H_2O, and pH >7.30, it is reasonable to consider extubation. Paired daily spontaneous awakening trials (withdrawal of sedatives) with daily spontaneous breathing trials result in a reduction in mechanical ventilation time, ICU and hospital length of stay, and 1-year mortality rates.

◆ DON'T BE TRICKED

- Do not select synchronized intermittent mandatory ventilation as a weaning mode, because studies have demonstrated it actually takes longer to liberate patients from the ventilator.

❖ Test Yourself

A 73-year-old woman who weighs 56 kg (123 lb) is admitted to the ICU with an exacerbation of severe COPD. Intubation and mechanical ventilation are required: FIO_2 of 0.4, tidal volume of 700 mL, and respiration rate of 16/min. Thirty minutes later, her BP has dropped to 82/60 mm Hg. She is restless and has diffuse wheezing with prolonged expiration.

ANSWER: The diagnosis is auto-PEEP. Treat the airway obstruction or lower the tidal volume or respiration rate.

Sepsis

Diagnosis

Sepsis is a documented or presumed infection with some of the clinical and laboratory features of the SIRS. The sepsis response causes generalized vasodilation, increased microvascular permeability, and multiorgan dysfunction. Severe sepsis causes organ dysfunction, and septic shock refers to sepsis-related hypotension that persists despite fluid resuscitation.

STUDY TABLE: SIRS, Sepsis, Severe Sepsis, and Septic Shock	
Syndrome	**Definition**
SIRS	Two or more of the following:
	Temperature >38.0 °C (100.4 °F) or <36.0 °C (96.8 °F)
	HR >90/min
	Respiration rate >20/min or arterial PCO_2 <32 mm Hg
	Leukocyte count >12,000/µL or <4000/µL with 10% bands (in absence of other known causes of this condition)
Sepsis	Presence of a known or suspected infection (documented positive cultures are not required) and ≥2 criteria for SIRS
Severe sepsis	Organ dysfunction, hypoperfusion, or hypotension
	Hypoperfusion and hypotension abnormalities may include, but are not limited to, lactic acidosis, oliguria, or an acute alteration in mental status
Septic shock	Sepsis-induced hypotension and perfusion abnormalities develop despite adequate fluid resuscitation

Know the differential diagnosis of shock syndromes and their associated hemodynamic parameters.

STUDY TABLE: Shock Syndromes	
Condition	**Characteristics**
Cardiogenic shock	Low cardiac output, elevated PCWP, and high SVR
Hypovolemic shock	Low cardiac output, low PCWP, and high SVR
Obstructive shock	Low cardiac output, low PCWP, and high SVR
	Consider cardiac tamponade, PE, and tension pneumothorax
Anaphylactic shock	High cardiac output, normal PCWP, and low SVR
	Rash, urticaria, angioedema, and wheezing/stridor
Septic shock	High cardiac output (early) that can become depressed (late) and low SVR
	Fever and leukocytosis
SVR = systemic vascular resistance.	

Therapy

STUDY TABLE: Treatment of Sepsis and Septic Shock	
Treatment	**Application**
Fluid resuscitation	Normal saline or lactated Ringer solution
	500-1000 mL boluses
	2-4 L (30 mL/kg) in the first 6 h
Vasopressors	Norepinephrine
	Indicated for persistent hypotension unresponsive to fluids
	Target MAP ≥65 mm Hg
	Target lactic acid ↓ by 10-20% in first 6 h
Source identification and control	Blood cultures, cultures of potential sites of infection, chest x-ray, urinalysis
Antibiotic therapy	Initiate within 1 h of diagnosis
	Narrow coverage based on culture and sensitivity findings
	Reasonable choice for sepsis of unclear etiology and low *Pseudomonas* risk: vancomycin plus 1 anti-*Pseudomonas* drug (e.g., ceftriaxone or cefotaxime, or piperacillin-tazobactam, or imipenem)
	If high *Pseudomonas* risk: vancomycin plus 2 anti-*Pseudomonas* agents
Hydrocortisone	200 mg/d IV for persistent hypotension despite fluids and vasopressors
Glucose control	Insulin therapy to maintain glucose between 140-200 mg/dL
Mechanical ventilation	Tidal volume ≤6 mg/kg if ARDS present

◆ **DON'T BE TRICKED**

- Do not provide mineralocorticoid replacement.
- Do not perform cortisol stimulation testing.
- Do not use noninvasive ventilation.

Nutritional Support During Critical Illness

Diagnosis

Nutrition is an essential part of management for patients in the ICU and can be given enterally or parenterally, with the enteral route preferred. Total parenteral nutrition is associated with GI mucosal atrophy and translocation of gut bacteria into the bloodstream, which predisposes patients to infection.

Therapy

Initiation of enteral nutrition is recommended at 24 to 48 hours following admission if the patient is hemodynamically stable. The formula of 25 to 35 kcal/kg/d can be used to estimate caloric need in patients in the ICU. For patients who cannot tolerate enteral feeding, parenteral nutrition in the form of total parenteral nutrition should not be started before day 7 of an acute illness.

ICU-Acquired Weakness

Diagnosis

ICU-acquired weakness includes critical illness polyneuropathy (with axonal nerve degeneration) and critical illness myopathy (with muscle myosin loss), resulting in profound weakness. ICU-acquired weakness may be first recognized when a patient is unable to be weaned from mechanical ventilation. Risk factors include hyperglycemia, sepsis, multiple organ dysfunction, and SIRS. Exposure to glucocorticoids and neuromuscular blocking agents are not consistently associated with ICU-acquired weakness; however, limited use is recommended if these medications are required in the care of critically ill patients.

Therapy

Treatment is supportive and includes ongoing physical and occupational therapy.

❖ **Test Yourself**

A 65-year-old woman with type 2 diabetes cannot be weaned from mechanical ventilation. She has required prolonged respiratory support due to ARDS secondary to septic shock and bacterial pneumonia. Her course was complicated by an episode of AKI. During spontaneous weaning trials, her tidal volume is low and respiratory rate is elevated. She has weakness of her extremities and hyporeflexia.

ANSWER: ICU-acquired weakness. Treat with physical and occupational therapy.

Hyperthermic Emergencies

Severe hyperthermia is temperature ≥40.0 °C (104.0 °F) due to a failure of normal thermoregulation. Findings include loss of consciousness, muscle rigidity, seizures, and rhabdomyolysis with kidney failure, DIC, and ARDS.

STUDY TABLE: Severe Hyperthermia Causes and Therapy				
Diagnosis	**Suggestive History**	**Key Examination Findings**	**Treatment**	**Notes**
Heat stroke (exertional)	Young athlete or soldier with environmental exposure	Encephalopathy and fever	Ice water immersion	Rapid response supports diagnosis
Non-exertional heat stroke	Age ≥70 years Use of anticholinergic, sympathomimetic, and diuretic drugs	Encephalopathy and fever	Evaporative, external cooling	Avoid ice water immersion
Malignant hyperthermia	Exposure to volatile anesthetic (halothane isoflurane, succinylcholine, or decamethonium)	Masseter muscle rigidity; ↑ arterial P_{CO_2}	Stop inciting drug Dantrolene	Monitor and treat; ↑ K⁺ and ↑ arterial P_{CO_2}
Neuroleptic malignant syndrome	Haloperidol, olanzapine, quetiapine, and risperidone or withdrawal from L-dopa; onset over days to weeks	Altered mentation, severe rigidity, ↑ HR, ↑ BP, no clonus, ↓ reflexes	Stop the inciting drug Dantrolene Bromocriptine	Resolves over days to weeks
Severe serotonin syndromeᵃ	Onset within 24 h of initiation or increasing dose	Agitation, rigidity, clonus, ↑ reflexes,	Stop inciting drug Benzodiazepines Cyproheptadine	Resolves in 24 hours

ᵃNot routinely considered a cause of severe hyperthermia but commonly confused with neuroleptic malignant syndrome.

◆ **DON'T BE TRICKED**

- Neuroleptic malignant syndrome may occur in patients who have abruptly discontinued L-dopa for Parkinson disease.
- The serotonin syndrome is often caused by the use of SSRIs and the addition of a second drug that increases serotonin release or blocks its uptake or metabolism.

A 45-year-old woman undergoes open cholecystectomy. At the conclusion of the operative procedure, her temperature has abruptly increased to 39.2 °C (102.6 °F).

ANSWER: Diagnose malignant hyperthermia due to anesthesia. Begin dantrolene.

Hypertensive Emergency

Hospitalize a patient with hypertensive emergency (BP ≥180/120 mm Hg and symptoms or evidence of end organ damage).

STUDY TABLE: Treatment of Hypertensive Emergencies

Emergency	Target BP (mm Hg)	First-Line Agents	Notes
Hypertensive encephalopathy	↓ by 15%-20% or DBP to 100-110	Nicardipine Labetalol Nitroprusside	Risk of cyanide toxicity with nitroprusside
Ischemic stroke	Treat if SBP >220 or DBP >120; ↓ by 15%	Nicardipine Labetalol Nitroprusside	Target BP <185/110 mm Hg if a candidate for thrombolytics
Hemorrhagic stroke	BP 160/90 or mean BP 110	Nicardipine Labetalol	+/- intracranial pressure monitor to target BP
Aortic dissection	SBP 100-120	Esmolol or labetalol first, add nitroprusside as needed	Target HR <65/min
Myocardial infarct	MAP 60-100	Nitroglycerin β-Blocker	Avoid hydralazine
Acute left-sided HF	MAP 60-100	Nitroglycerin and/or nitroprusside	Caution with calcium and β-blockers, hydralazine
Acute kidney injury	↓ by 20%-25%	Fenoldopam Nicardipine β-Blocker	ACE if scleroderma renal crisis
Preeclampsia, eclampsia	SBP 130-150 DBP 80-100	Labetalol Hydralazine	Avoid ACE and nitroprusside Delivery = "cure"
Sympathomimetic drug use	↓ by 20%-25%	Nicardipine Nitroprusside	Benzodiazepine first Avoid β-blocker
Pheochromocytoma	↓ by 20%-25%	Phentolamine Nitroprusside	Avoid β-blocker

◆ **DON'T BE TRICKED**

- Do not select sublingual nifedipine for either hypertensive urgency or emergency.

Anaphylaxis

Diagnosis

Anaphylaxis is a life-threatening syndrome caused by the release of mediators from mast cells and basophils triggered by an IgE-allergen interaction (*anaphylactic reaction*) or by a non–antibody-antigen mechanism (*anaphylactoid reaction*). The most common causes are peanut/nut ingestion, insect stings, latex, and medications (penicillin, NSAIDs, aspirin).

Flushing, urticaria, conjunctival pruritus, bronchospasm, nausea, and vomiting usually develop within minutes to 1 hour if the antigen was injected or up to 2 hours if ingested.

Anaphylactic shock is caused by severe hypovolemia (fluid shifts owing to increased vascular permeability) and vasodilatation.

The diagnosis of anaphylaxis is made clinically. Death occurs from refractory bronchospasm, respiratory failure with upper airway obstruction, and cardiovascular collapse.

◆ DON'T BE TRICKED

- Consider latex allergy as cause of anaphylaxis during surgery or anaphylaxis in a woman during coitus.

Therapy

Epinephrine is first-line therapy even if the only presenting signs are hives or pruritus. Use inhaled bronchodilators for bronchospasm and IV saline for shock or hypotension.

β-Blockers may blunt the effect of epinephrine, but epinephrine remains the drug of first choice; reserve glucagon for epinephrine-refractory anaphylaxis.

Patients with diffuse rash or anaphylaxis from hymenoptera sting (bee, yellow jacket, and wasp) should undergo venom skin testing and immunotherapy.

◆ DON'T BE TRICKED

- IM or subcutaneous epinephrine (0.3-0.5 mg of 1:1000) is first-line treatment for classic anaphylaxis. IV epinephrine (1:10,000) is reserved for anaphylactic shock or refractory symptoms.

❖ Test Yourself

A 25-year-old woman has shortness of breath and wheezing after a bee sting 1 hour ago. Her BP is 80/50 mm Hg and HR is 110/min.

ANSWER: Treat anaphylaxis with epinephrine and IV fluids. Observe for at least 12 hours. Discharge with self-administered epinephrine.

Angioedema

Diagnosis

Angioedema is characterized by a sudden, temporary edema, usually of the lips, face, hands, feet, penis, or scrotum. Abdominal pain may be present owing to bowel wall edema.

Mast cell–mediated angioedema is often associated with urticaria, bronchospasm, or hypotension. This can be due to allergic reaction (peanuts, shrimp, latex, insect stings) or to direct mast cell stimulation (NSAIDs, radiocontrast media, opiates).

Bradykinin-mediated angioedema is NOT associated with urticaria. In the setting of angioedema without urticaria, the differential is very limited.

STUDY TABLE: Differential Diagnosis of Bradykinin-Mediated Angioedema		
Condition	**Historical Clues/Disease Associations**	**Laboratory Studies**
Hereditary angioedema	Family history of angioedema	Low C1 inhibitor and C4 levels
Acquired C1 inhibitor deficiency	Lymphoma, MGUS, or SLE	Low C1q levels (in addition to low C4 and C1 inhibitor levels)
ACE inhibitor effect	Medication history	Low C1 inhibitor and C4 levels

- In patients with urticaria and angioedema, diagnose food or drug allergy, food additive sensitivity, or urticarial vasculitis. Do not diagnose hereditary angioedema.

Therapy

Select epinephrine, antihistamines, and glucocorticoids for acute episodes of mast cell–mediated (allergic) angioedema with airway compromise or hypotension. Patients should carry an epinephrine autoinjector. Use antihistamines and glucocorticoids alone in cases of allergic angioedema that is not part of an anaphylaxis syndrome (absent airway compromise or hemodynamic instability).

Select C1 inhibitor concentrate for acute episodes of bradykinin-mediated angioedema (hereditary or acquired angioedema); use FFP in an emergency. For long-term management of hereditary angioedema, select danazol and stanozolol to elevate hepatic synthesis of C1 esterase inhibitor protein.

Angioedema: Angioedema differs from urticaria in that it covers a larger surface area and involves the dermis and subcutaneous tissues.

◆ **DON'T BE TRICKED**

- Epinephrine is not effective for hereditary angioedema.

❖ **Test Yourself**

A 40-year-old man has a 1-year history of cramping abdominal pain and 2- to 3-day episodes of face and hand swelling that have not responded completely to epinephrine and antihistamines. His mother died suddenly of "suffocation."

ANSWER: The patient has probable hereditary angioedema. Order serum C4 and C1 inhibitor levels (functional and antigenic). Treat severe acute episodes of swelling with C1 inhibitor concentrate.

Smoke Inhalation

Ensuring upper airway patency is the first priority:

- patients with a visibly damaged airway or stridor require immediate intubation
- in less severe cases, fiberoptic laryngoscopy can identify laryngeal edema that may warrant prophylactic intubation
- assess carbon monoxide level

◆ **DON'T BE TRICKED**

- Patients with inhalational injury involving the lower airways typically present with a clear chest x-ray; wheezing, cough, and dyspnea manifest 12 to 36 hours after exposure.
- A normal oxygen saturation does not exclude carbon monoxide poisoning.

Poisoning with Therapeutic Agents

Key Considerations

STUDY TABLE: Poisoning with Common Therapeutic Agents		
Toxin	**Clinical Syndrome**	**Antidote/Intervention**
Acetaminophen	Hepatotoxicity	*N*-acetylcysteine
Benzodiazepines	Sedative/hypnotic	Observation; flumazenil
β-Adrenergic blockers	Bradycardia, hypotension	Glucagon, calcium chloride, pacing
Calcium channel blockers	Bradycardia, hypotension	Atropine, calcium, glucagon, pacing
Digoxin	Dysrhythmia	Digoxin-immune fab
Heparin	Bleeding diathesis	Protamine sulfate
Narcotics	Narcotic effects	Naloxone
Salicylates	Metabolic acidosis/respiratory alkalosis	Urine alkalinization, hemodialysis
Tricyclic antidepressants	Anticholinergic effects	Blood alkalinization, α-agonist

Carbon Monoxide Poisoning

Diagnosis

Characteristic findings are unexplained flulike symptoms, frontal headache, lightheadedness, difficulty concentrating, confusion, delirium, coma, dyspnea, nausea, and chest pain that are often associated with use of a grill or burning heat source indoors. Order ABG studies and serum carboxyhemoglobin measurement for all patients with neurologic changes, dyspnea, chest pain, or smoke exposure. A carboxyhemoglobin level >25% in any patient is diagnostic of severe acute carbon monoxide poisoning.

◆ DON'T BE TRICKED

- Pulse oximetry data are unreliable because the oximeter is unable to differentiate carboxyhemoglobin from oxyhemoglobin.

Therapy

Normobaric oxygen therapy is the treatment of choice. Hyperbaric oxygen therapy is indicated for patients with severe carbon monoxide poisoning (characterized by loss of consciousness and persistent neurologic deficits), pregnant patients, or patients with evidence of cardiac ischemia.

❖ Test Yourself

A 39-year-old man is found unconscious by his family. He had not been seen since late the previous evening. The outside temperature was below freezing overnight. He is unresponsive and deeply cyanotic. The patient is intubated and ventilated with 100% oxygen. Although the O_2 saturation is 100%, he remains comatose.

ANSWER: The diagnosis is carbon monoxide poisoning. Measure the carboxyhemoglobin level.

Alcohol Poisoning

STUDY TABLE: Presentation and Treatment of Alcohol Poisoning

Alcohol	Common Sources	Major Findings	Anion Gap	Osmolar Gap[a]	Treatment
Ethanol	Alcoholic beverages	CNS depression	No	N/A	Supportive care
Isopropyl alcohol	Rubbing alcohol	CNS depression $\uparrow$ Ketones	No	Yes	Supportive care
Methanol	Windshield wiper fluid De-icing solutions	CNS depression Vision loss	Yes	Yes	Fomepizole Dialysis (if severe) Folic acid
Ethylene glycol	Antifreeze De-icing solutions	CNS depression Acute kidney injury	Yes	Yes	Fomepizole Dialysis (if severe)

[a]The serum osmolal gap represents the difference between the measured and calculated serum osmolality. The calculated osmolality = (2 × serum [Na]) + [glucose, in mg/dL]/18 + [BUN, in mg/dL]/2.8. Abnormal gap is >10.

Toxidromes

STUDY TABLE: Toxic Syndromes Manifestations and Treatments

Syndrome	Manifestations	Representative Drugs	Treatment
Sympathomimetic	Tachycardia Hypertension Diaphoresis Agitation Seizures Mydriasis	Cocaine Amphetamines Ephedrine Caffeine	Benzodiazepines for agitation Avoid β-blockers for hypertension Haloperidol may worsen hyperthermia
Cholinergic	"SLUDGE" Confusion Bronchorrhea Bradycardia Miosis	Organophosphates (insecticides, sarin) Carbamates Physostigmine Edrophonium Nicotine	Organophosphates poisoning requires external decontamination Atropine May require ventilatory support Add pralidoxime for CNS toxicity Benzodiazepines for convulsions
Anticholinergic	Hyperthermia Dry skin and mucous membranes Agitation, delirium Tachycardia, tachypnea Hypertension Mydriasis	Antihistamines Tricyclic antidepressants Antiparkinson agents Atropine Scopolamine	Physostigmine for those with peripheral and CNS symptoms Benzodiazepines for agitation May require ventilatory support
Opioids	Miosis Respiratory depression Lethargy, confusion Hypothermia Bradycardia Hypotension	Morphine and related drugs Heroin	Naloxone

SLUDGE = Salivation, Lacrimation, increased Urination and Defecation, Gastrointestinal upset, and Emesis.

Rheumatology

Approach to the Patient

Analyze joint disease using 3 parameters: acuity (acute or chronic), inflammation (inflammatory or noninflammatory), and number of joints involved (monoarticular, oligoarticular, or polyarticular).

STUDY TABLE: Features of Inflammatory Vs. Noninflammatory Pain

Feature	Inflammatory Pain	Noninflammatory Pain
Physical examination findings	Erythema; warmth; soft-tissue swelling	No soft-tissue swelling; minimal or no warmth; bony enlargement and joint effusions may occur in OA
Morning stiffness	>60 min	<30 min
Constitutional symptoms	Fever; fatigue; malaise	Generally absent
Synovial fluid	Leukocyte count >2000/µL, neutrophils in acute inflammation, monocytes in chronic inflammation	Leukocyte count between 200/µL and 2000/µL, predominantly monocytes
Other laboratory findings	Elevated ESR, CRP; anemia of chronic disease	Inflammatory markers usually normal or minimally elevated

Categorization of arthritis by number and distribution of involved joints narrows the differential diagnosis.

STUDY TABLE: Categories of Common Joint Disease

Acuity and Inflammation	Monoarticular	Oligoarticular (2-4 joints)	Polyarticular (≥5 joints)
Acute Inflammatory	Bacterial infection Crystal-induced	Disseminated gonococcal infection RF Lyme disease	Viral infections: hepatitis A and B, parvovirus, rubella, HIV
Chronic Inflammatory	Infections related to fungi, mycobacteria, spirochetes (syphilis and Lyme disease)	Spondyloarthropathies	RA, SLE, psoriatic arthritis, crystalline arthritis
Chronic Noninflammatory	OA	OA	OA

Serologic Studies in Rheumatologic Disorders

STUDY TABLE: Serologic Studies/Associations

Test	Association (does not establish diagnosis)
ANA	SLE, SSc, Sjögren syndrome; does not correlate with disease activity
Anti-Sm	SLE; most specific for SLE but does not correlate with disease activity
Anti–U1-RNP	MCTD
Anticentromere pattern of ANA	CREST syndrome; SSc and PH
Anti-dsDNA antibody	SLE; correlates with disease activity, especially kidney disease
Anti-smooth muscle antibody	Autoimmune hepatitis
Anti-La/SSB antibody	Sjögren syndrome (sicca syndrome); neonatal SLE

(Continued on next page)

STUDY TABLE: Serologic Studies/Associations (*Continued*)	
Test	**Association (does not establish diagnosis)**
Anti-Scl-70 antibody	SSc and pulmonary fibrosis/diffuse cutaneous SSc
Antihistone antibody	Drug-induced SLE
Anti-Ro/SSA antibody	Sjögren syndrome, neonatal heart block, subacute cutaneous lupus
c-ANCA (anti-PR3 antibody)	Granulomatosis with polyangiitis
p-ANCA (anti-MPO antibody)	Eosinophilic granulomatosis with polyangiitis (Churg-Strauss syndrome) and MPA
Anti-Jo-1 antibody	Polymyositis and antisynthetase syndrome
Anti-CCP antibody	Rheumatoid arthritis

CREST = calcinosis, Raynaud phenomenon, esophageal dysmotility, sclerodactyly, and telangiectasia.

◆ DON'T BE TRICKED

- Do not test for ANA sub-serologies if ANA is negative unless there is suspicion for subacute cutaneous lupus (anti-SSA) or polymyositis (anti-Jo-1)

Rheumatoid Arthritis

Diagnosis

RA is a symmetric inflammatory polyarthritis that primarily involves the small joints of the hands and feet. Characteristic findings include:

- morning stiffness lasting >1 hour
- seven classic sites of symmetric joint pain (PIP, MCP, wrist, elbow, knee, ankle, and MTP joints)
- synovitis characterized by soft-tissue swelling or effusion
- subcutaneous nodules over bony prominences or extensor surfaces

Laboratory findings include:

- positive rheumatoid factor (sensitivity 80%; specificity 87%)
- elevated ESR or CRP level
- normocytic anemia
- positive anti-CCP antibody assay (sensitivity 76%; specificity 96%)

More than half of patients with untreated RA develop erosions within the first 2 years of disease if not appropriately treated; baseline and subsequent x-rays aid in the diagnosis and follow-up of therapy. In addition to erosions, an x-ray can reveal peri-articular osteopenia and symmetric joint-space narrowing. Ultrasonography is more sensitive than x-ray for identification of synovitis and erosions. MRI lacks specificity for RA. However, MRI is useful to detect cervical spine subluxation or myelopathy.

◆ DON'T BE TRICKED

- Less than 10% of patients have an abrupt onset of disease over days, and it is rare for only a single joint to be initially involved (think infective or crystal-induced arthritis).
- Negative rheumatoid factor does not exclude RA; anti-CCP antibody assay may be positive.
- A positive rheumatoid factor alone is not diagnostic of RA.
- Fluctuations in rheumatoid factor do not mirror disease activity and serial testing is not indicated.
- Not all symmetric arthritis is RA.

STUDY TABLE: Rheumatoid Arthritis Mimics

If you see symmetric arthritis and...	Diagnose this...
Skin rash and leukopenia	SLE
Psoriasis or pitted nails	Psoriatic arthritis
Daycare worker or mother of small children	Parvovirus B19 infection (usually self-limited; 1 to 3 months)
2nd and/or 3rd MCP and PIP joint arthritis with hook-like osteophytes	Hemochromatosis
Raynaud phenomenon and sclerodactyly	SSc
Proximal muscle weakness	Polymyositis or dermatomyositis
Recent immunizations	Post-rubella immunization arthritis
Tophi	Chronic tophaceous gout may cause symmetric involvement of small joints of the hands and feet

◆ DON'T BE TRICKED

- Viral infections can cause short-lived inflammatory arthritis involving small joints, therefore joint inflammation should be present >6 weeks before diagnosing RA.

STUDY TABLE: Extra-articular Manifestations of Rheumatoid Arthritis

If you see this...	Think this...
Arm paresthesia and hyperreflexia	C1-C2 subluxation (increased risk of cord compression with tracheal intubation)
Cough, fever, pulmonary infiltrates	Bronchiolitis obliterans organizing pneumonia (BOOP)
Foot drop or wrist drop	Mononeuritis multiplex (vasculitis)
Hoarseness	Cricoarytenoid involvement
Multiple basilar pulmonary nodules	Caplan syndrome (pneumoconiosis related to occupational dust; characterized by rapid development of multiple basilar nodules and mild airflow obstruction)
Dry eyes and/or mouth	Sjögren syndrome
Pleural effusion with low plasma glucose (<30 mg/dL)	Rheumatoid pleuritis
Pulmonary fibrosis	Rheumatoid interstitial lung disease
Skin ulcers, peripheral neuropathy	Rheumatoid vasculitis
Splenomegaly and granulocytopenia	Felty syndrome
Red, painful eye	Scleritis, uveitis
HF	Rheumatoid disease or anti-TNF therapy

Other complications include increased risk of pulmonary infections, CAD, and osteoporosis.

◆ DON'T BE TRICKED

- All RA patients undergoing general anesthesia should have cervical spine x-rays to assess for atlantoaxial subluxation.

Hand X-ray, Rheumatoid Arthritis: Carpal, metacarpal, and PIP joints show periarticular osteopenia, joint-space narrowing, and marginal erosions, all characteristic of RA.

Therapy

Smoking cessation is important because continued smoking may impair the response to therapy and exacerbate rheumatoid lung disease.

Choose NSAIDs and low-dose oral and intra-articular glucocorticoids for quick symptomatic relief, but recognize these agents do not alter the course of the disease.

Methotrexate is the recommended initial DMARD for most patients with RA and should be instituted immediately in patients with erosive disease. It is continued indefinitely and can be used in combination with other nonbiologic and biologic DMARDs. Leflunomide may be used with or as a substitute for methotrexate.

Monotherapy with hydroxychloroquine or sulfasalazine or combination therapy with these agents is indicated to manage early, mild, and nonerosive disease.

Combination therapy with hydroxychloroquine, sulfasalazine, and methotrexate has been shown to be more effective than monotherapy with methotrexate or sulfasalazine plus hydroxychloroquine.

Initiate biologic therapy when adequate disease control is not achieved with oral DMARDs. The initial biologic therapy should be a TNF-α inhibitor:

- add a TNF-α inhibitor to baseline methotrexate therapy
- screen for TB before starting therapy
- treat for latent TB if TST or IGRA is positive before beginning any biologic therapy
- perform periodic TB screening while the patient continues to receive biologic therapy

The TNF inhibitors include etanercept (receptor antagonist) and the monoclonal antibodies infliximab, adalimumab, certolizumab, and golimumab). Tofacitinib is the first oral biologic agent that may be effective in patients not responding to methotrexate.

Common toxicities of TNF-α inhibitor therapy include pancytopenia, positive ANA formation associated with lupus-like syndromes, and demyelinating disorders. Combination therapy with multiple biologic therapies is not recommended.

Indications for surgical intervention include intractable pain or severe functional disability from joint destruction. Patients may also require surgical repair of ruptured tendons.

Manage bone disease, cardiovascular disease, and prevent infection:

- use DEXA scans to screen patients for osteoporosis
- prescribe calcium/vitamin D for all patients
- treat osteoporosis with a bisphosphonate
- screen for and treat standard cardiovascular risk factors
- give yearly influenza vaccination
- give pneumococcal vaccination

Also, begin adjuvant physical and occupational therapy.

◆ DON'T BE TRICKED

- Methotrexate and leflunomide are absolutely contraindicated in pregnancy and must be discontinued prior to conception.
- Hydroxychloroquine and sulfasalazine can be used during pregnancy.

❖ Test Yourself

A 46-year-old man has a 3-month history of swelling of the PIP and MCP joints and 90 minutes of morning stiffness. Rheumatoid factor is negative.

ANSWER: The probable diagnosis is RA. Select anti-CCP antibody assay.

Sjögren Syndrome

Diagnosis

Sjögren syndrome is an autoimmune disease characterized by:

- keratoconjunctivitis sicca
- xerostomia
- salivary gland enlargement

Salivary gland enlargement occurs in nearly half of patients during the course of the disease and is most obvious in the parotid glands.

Sjögren syndrome may occur as a primary disease process or may be associated with another autoimmune disease, most commonly RA and SLE.

A cardinal feature of Sjögren syndrome is the presence of antibodies to Ro/SSA and La/SSB. A positive ANA, rheumatoid factor, and hypergammaglobulinemia are also frequently found. In the presence of classic historical and physical findings, the presence of anti-Ro/SSA and anti-La/SSB antibodies is sufficient to diagnose Sjögren syndrome; in unclear cases, a lip biopsy demonstrating minor salivary gland inflammation is the gold standard for diagnosis.

Patients with Sjögren syndrome are up to 44 times more likely than the general population to have a B-cell lymphoma, large B-cell and MALT lymphomas being the most common. Careful follow-up is therefore required.

Be alert to the development of neonatal heart block in newborns of women with Sjögren syndrome due to the anti-Ro/SSA and anti-La/SSB antibodies.

Parotid Gland Enlargement: Bilateral parotid gland enlargement in a patient with Sjögren syndrome.

Therapy

Treatment is symptomatic. Choose artificial tear replacement and artificial saliva and mouth lubricants. Systemic immunosuppressive therapy is indicated only in patients with severe systemic manifestations.

Osteoarthritis

Diagnosis

Age is the most important risk factor for developing primary OA in women and men. Additional risk factors include genetics, obesity, and trauma-induced mechanical joint instability. OA most often affects the lower cervical and lumbar spine; hips; knees; DIP, PIP, and first carpometacarpal joints.

Characteristic findings include:

- morning joint stiffness lasting <30 minutes
- gelling (brief stiffness after inactivity)
- crepitus
- tenderness along the joint line
- reduced joint motion

- bony enlargement (including Heberden and Bouchard nodes)
- involvement of the first carpometacarpal joint results in "squaring" at the base of the thumb

Two important variants are erosive OA of the hand and DISH.

Erosive inflammatory OA is characterized by pain and palpable swelling of the soft tissue in the PIP and DIP joints. This condition also may be associated with disease flares during which these joints become more swollen and painful. Diagnosis is based on the presence of central erosions and collapse of the subchondral bone in the interphalangeal joints of the hands on plain x-ray. In contrast to RA, erosive OA is common in the DIP joints, does not typically affect the wrists or elbows, and is not associated with rheumatoid factor, anti–CCP antibodies, or an elevated ESR or CRP level.

DISH is an often asymptomatic form of OA that causes significant radiographic changes similar to those associated with degenerative spondylosis or ankylosing spondylitis. X-rays of the spine in patients with DISH reveal flowing ossification that develops along the anterolateral aspect of the vertebral bodies, particularly the anterior longitudinal ligament, in ≥4 contiguous vertebrae. However, neither disk-space narrowing nor syndesmophytes are visible in this setting, as they are in lumbar spondylosis or ankylosing spondylitis, respectively. Common complications attributable to DISH include dysphagia, unstable spinal fractures, spinal stenosis, and myelopathy.

Secondary OA results from previous joint injury or metabolic diseases such as hemochromatosis. Consider metabolic causes when OA develops in atypical joints (e.g., MCP joints, shoulder, wrist).

Be alert for an acutely painful calf mimicking a DVT, which represents a ruptured Baker cyst (herniation of fluid-filled synovium of the posterior knee) or ruptured gastrocnemius muscle.

In OA an individual joint in the hand may be swollen or erythematous, but the presence of multiple swollen joints suggests concomitant CPP deposition or RA. OA is the probable cause if the DIP joints are involved, whereas RA (or psoriatic) arthritis is more likely if there is involvement of the MCP joints, wrists, or elbows.

No pathognomonic laboratory tests are available for OA and in most cases, laboratory studies are not indicated. An x-ray is not helpful in the diagnosis of symptomatic hand OA (clinical examination is more specific) but is the "gold standard" for hip and knee OA. X-rays show joint-space narrowing, subchondral sclerosis, and osteophytes. Synovial fluid is usually noninflammatory, with a leukocyte count <2000/μL. Ultrasonography is useful in the diagnosis of a Baker cyst.

Hand Photograph, Osteoarthritis: Bony enlargement of the DIP joints and squaring of the first carpometacarpal joint characteristic of OA.

◆ DON'T BE TRICKED

Typical OA radiographic changes do not exclude other diagnoses. Be alert for:

- septic arthritis superimposed on OA
- trochanteric and anserine bursitis causing hip and knee pain
- de Quervain tenosynovitis mimicking carpometacarpal OA
- hemochromatosis, particularly if involving the 2nd and 3rd MCP joints and associated with hook-like osteophytes
- gout or CPPD disease

Therapy

Medical therapy includes:

- acetaminophen as first-line therapy for hip and knee OA
- NSAIDs in patients who do not respond to acetaminophen or as initial therapy for severe pain

- tramadol if NSAIDs are contraindicated or ineffective
- intra-articular glucocorticoids for acute exacerbations of knee OA
- patients with knee OA benefit from quadriceps-strengthening exercises
- weight loss is beneficial for hip and knee OA

Don't select NSAIDs for patients with CAD, HF, CKD, or ulcer disease. Joint arthroplasty of the hip or knee is indicated for pain that does not respond to nonsurgical treatment, especially when lifestyle or activities of daily living are affected.

◆ DON'T BE TRICKED

- Patients with signs of inflammation should not undergo intra-articular glucocorticoid therapy until synovial fluid analysis excludes infection.
- Do not select arthroscopic lavage, debridement, or closed lavage for knee OA.
- Do not select hyaluronan intra-articular injection or oral supplements with glucosamine or chondroitin.

Hand X-ray, Osteoarthritis: Joint-space narrowing, sclerosis, and osteophyte formation are shown. Prominent involvement of the PIP and DIP joints indicates OA.

Knee X-ray, Osteoarthritis: Medial compartment joint space-narrowing and subchondral sclerosis consistent with OA are shown.

Hypertrophic Osteoarthropathy

Diagnosis

Hypertrophic osteoarthropathy causes a proliferation of skin and osseous tissue at the distal parts of the extremities. Characteristic findings are:

- digital clubbing
- painful periostosis of long bones
- synovial effusions
- new periosteal bone formation

Pain is generally alleviated by elevating the affected limbs. Associated disorders include lung cancer, chronic pulmonary infections, and right-to-left cardiac shunts.

❖ **Test Yourself**

A 64-year-old man has a 1-month history of bilateral ankle pain. Elevating his feet alleviates the discomfort. On physical examination, his lower legs are warm. Pitting edema begins 6 cm above the malleoli; this area is very tender to palpation. An x-ray shows new periosteal bone formation of the tibia above the ankle joints.

ANSWER: The probable diagnosis is hypertrophic osteoarthropathy. Order a chest x-ray to determine the cause.

Hypertrophic Osteoarthropathy: Hypertrophic osteoarthropathy in this patient is characterized by clubbing of the toes (particularly the great toes), ankle effusions, and lower extremity edema.

Spondyloarthritis

Key Considerations

Spondyloarthritis comprises several systemic inflammatory joint disorders that share distinct clinical, radiographic, and genetic features. The spondyloarthritis disorders are:

- psoriatic arthritis
- reactive arthritis (formerly Reiter syndrome)
- ankylosing spondylitis
- IBD-associated arthritis

Common characteristics include:

- inflammatory spine and sacroiliac disease
- asymmetric inflammation in ≤4 peripheral joints (typically large joints)
- inflammation at the sites of ligament and tendon insertion (enthesitis)
- the presence of HLA-B27
- extra-articular conditions, such as uveitis, colitis, urethritis, aortitis, and psoriasis
- absent rheumatoid factor and anti-CCP antibodies

◆ **DON'T BE TRICKED**

- HLA-B27 testing may support, but cannot independently confirm or exclude, a diagnosis of ankylosing spondylitis or other forms of spondyloarthritis.

Psoriatic Arthritis

Characteristic findings are classic psoriasis (thick silvery scale on a well-demarcated red patch) and nail pitting in a patient with joint pain and stiffness. Skin involvement commonly precedes joint inflammation, although 15% of patients first develop joint inflammation.

The most common patterns of joint involvement are:

- asymmetric, lower extremity oligoarthritis (resembling reactive arthritis)
- symmetric polyarthritis (resembling RA) involving the DIP, PIP, and/or MCP joints

Less common presentations include:

- DIP involvement only
- chronic resorptive arthritis (arthritis mutilans) resulting in digital shortening with a "telescoping" appearance of the digits sometimes referred to as "pencil in a cup"
- spondylitis (spine or sacroiliac arthritis, usually asymmetric)

A sausage-shaped finger or toe (dactylitis) may be found and the DIP joints are often involved, which helps distinguishes psoriatic arthritis from RA.

Patients with psoriatic arthritis tend to be seronegative for rheumatoid factor, but at least 15% are seropositive, as are a similar percentage of patients with uncomplicated psoriasis. Serum urate levels may be elevated in patients with psoriatic arthritis because of rapid turnover of skin cells. Explosive onset or severe flare-up of psoriatic arthritis should prompt testing for HIV infection.

◆ DON'T BE TRICKED

- No relationship exists between the extent of skin and joint disease in patients with psoriatic arthritis.
- Do not make a diagnosis of gout based solely on joint pain and elevated serum urate levels.

Select NSAIDs as initial therapy. Select methotrexate for peripheral joint disease and enthesitis not responding to NSAID; methotrexate will treat skin disease as well. A TNF-α inhibitor is indicated for methotrexate-resistant peripheral disease and is beneficial for skin disease. Combination methotrexate and TNF-α inhibitor therapy is often more effective than either therapy alone.

NSAIDs, antimalarial drugs, and withdrawal from oral glucocorticoids may exacerbate psoriasis.

Dactylitis: Diffuse swelling of the left third and fourth toes and right fourth toe characteristic of dactylitis.

Psoriasis: Tiny pits scattered over the nail plate resulting from psoriatic involvement of the nail matrix.

Reactive Arthritis

Reactive arthritis is an acute aseptic inflammatory arthritis that occurs 1 to 3 weeks after an infectious event originating in the GU or GI tract. A high prevalence of HIV infection is found in patients with symptoms of reactive arthritis.

Characteristic findings include:

- monoarthritis or acute asymmetric oligoarthritis (usually in weight-bearing joints) is most common
- dactylitis
- enthesopathy (especially of Achilles tendon)
- sacroiliitis

Patients may also have keratoderma blennorrhagicum (a psoriasis-like skin lesion on the palms and soles) or circinate balanitis (shallow, moist, serpiginous ulcers with raised borders on the glans penis).

Patients with a presentation suggestive of reactive arthritis should be tested for HIV, GU infection (*Chlamydia*), and GI infection even in the absence of infectious symptoms.

If the causative organism can be isolated, begin specific therapy.

In the absence of an ongoing infection, reactive arthritis is usually self-limited, and symptoms resolve within 6 months; select symptomatic treatment with NSAIDs and glucocorticoid injections for these patients.

Keratoderma Blennorrhagicum: A papular and pustular rash of the palms and soles is associated with reactive arthritis.

♦ **DON'T BE TRICKED**

- The classic triad of arthritis, conjunctivitis, and urethritis (or cervicitis) is found in only one third of patients with reactive arthritis.
- Do not prescribe chronic antibiotic therapy for patients with reactive arthritis.

❖ **Test Yourself**

A 33-year-old man has a 3-month history of left shoulder and right ankle pain and a left inflamed second toe. He had 4 days of bloody diarrhea 3 months ago.

ANSWER: The diagnosis is reactive arthritis, consistent with an enteric infection.

Ankylosing Spondylitis

Ankylosing spondylitis primarily affects the spine and sacroiliac joints. It also may involve the shoulders and hips, although the small peripheral joints are not affected. Ankylosing spondylitis occurs most often in patients <40 years of age and presents as chronic inflammatory low back pain (more than 1 hour of morning stiffness). Characteristic findings are pain and stiffness that worsen at night and are relieved with physical activity or heat.

Physical examination findings include:

- decreased hyperextension, forward flexion, lateral flexion, and axial rotation
- diminished chest expansion
- asymmetric peripheral arthritis involving the large joints
- painful heels (enthesitis)

X-rays show subchondral bony sclerosis, vertebral body squaring, and bony ankylosis ("bamboo spine"). When radiographic findings are equivocal or absent, MRI can detect the early changes of sacroiliitis.

Extra-articular manifestations include acute anterior uveitis (most common), aortic valvular regurgitation, aortic aneurysm, cardiac conduction defects, apical pulmonary fibrosis and cavitation, and cauda equina syndrome.

A patient with ankylosing spondylitis with increased pain and mobility of the neck following a minor accident may have a fracture and requires an urgent CT of the cervical spine.

◆ DON'T BE TRICKED

- Ankylosing spondylitis occurs in both men and women.

An essential part of therapy is exercise to preserve range of motion and strengthen the spine extensor muscles to prevent kyphosis.

Drug therapy consists of:

- NSAIDs (not aspirin)–the mainstay of management
- glucocorticoid injections for recalcitrant enthesitis and persistent synovitis
- TNF-α inhibitors if inadequate response of axial (spine and SI joint) disease to NSAIDs
- methotrexate, sulfasalazine, and hydroxychloroquine for peripheral joint disease
- calcium and vitamin D supplements for all patients
- bisphosphonate for osteopenia or osteoporosis

X-rays, Ankylosing Spondylitis: Sclerosis and erosions of sacroiliac joints and bridging of the intervertebral disks by syndesmophytes are characteristic of ankylosing spondylitis.

◆ DON'T BE TRICKED

- Do not prescribe methotrexate, sulfasalazine, or hydroxychloroquine for patients with axial disease because they are ineffective. Select a TNF-α inhibitor.

❖ Test Yourself

A 40-year-old man has increasing neck pain after a fall from the second rung of a ladder 5 days ago. He has a long history of stiffness and pain in the neck and lower back and loss of lumbar spine flexion.

ANSWER: The probable diagnosis is ankylosing spondylitis with an acute cervical fracture. Select neck immobilization and emergent CT.

IBD-Associated Arthritis

Inflammatory arthritis can complicate Crohn disease and ulcerative colitis:

- polyarticular arthritis resembling RA
- asymmetric oligoarthritis predominantly of the lower extremities
- asymptomatic sacroiliac disease
- ankylosing spondylitis-like disease

Only the oligoarticular peripheral arthritis parallels IBD activity. The progression of spinal involvement is independent of the course of the bowel disease. NSAIDs may result in worsening bowel disease. Methotrexate and sulfasalazine help IBD-associated arthritis symptoms and also treat the underlying bowel disease but studies have not shown these drugs to prevent joint disease progression. Most TNF-α inhibitors are effective for IBD-associated arthritis.

◆ DON'T BE TRICKED

- Etanercept has not shown efficacy in treating IBD.

Systemic Lupus Erythematosus

Diagnosis

SLE is a chronic multisystem autoimmune disease with immune complex deposition of unknown cause. Diagnosis is based on characteristic clinical features and laboratory studies. Diagnose SLE when any four of the following are present:

- positive ANA
- malar ("butterfly") rash that spares the nasolabial folds and areas beneath the nose and lower lip
- discoid rash characterized by erythematous, raised patches with keratotic scaling and follicular plugging
- photosensitivity
- oral ulcers
- arthritis (joint pain is frequently the presenting symptom)
- serositis (pleural, pericardial, abdominal)
- kidney disorder (new-onset hypertension, proteinuria with or without hematuria)
- neurologic disorder (peripheral neuropathy, mononeuritis multiplex, cranial neuritis, transverse myelitis, aseptic meningitis, stroke, encephalitis, psychosis, seizures)
- hematologic disorder (autoimmune hemolytic anemia, leukopenia, lymphopenia, thrombocytopenia)
- immunologic disorder (APLA syndrome [venous and arterial thrombosis, recurrent fetal loss])

Additional SLE pearls:

- subacute cutaneous lupus erythematosus is frequently drug-induced (especially hydrochlorothiazide) and not related to systemic disease
- nonscarring alopecia is common in SLE
- periarticular inflammation can result in reducible subluxation of the digits, swan neck deformities, and ulnar deviation (Jaccoud arthropathy)
- pain or limitation of motion of the hips suggests osteonecrosis
- fibromyalgia can co-occur in 30% of patients with SLE
- kidney disease is most common in patients with anti-dsDNA antibodies
- nephritis and a rising serum creatinine is an indication for urgent kidney biopsy
- autoantibodies that assist in the diagnosis of neuropsychiatric SLE include antineuronal, anti-NMDA receptor, antiribosomal P, and APLA/LAC
- SLE parenchymal lung involvement is rare and lung infiltrates are more likely to be infectious
- diffuse alveolar hemorrhage presents as hypoxemia, diffuse alveolar infiltrates on chest x-ray, a dropping hematocrit, and a high DLCO
- shrinking lung syndrome is characterized by pleuritic chest pain, dyspnea, and progressive decrease in lung volumes
- patients with quiescent SLE can have mild cytopenias that do not require intervention
- clinical manifestations of APLA/LAC include venous and arterial thrombosis, miscarriage, livedo reticularis, cytopenias, and cardiac valve thickening/vegetations
- newborns of mothers who are positive for anti-Ro/SSA or anti-La/SSB antibodies are at risk for developing neonatal lupus erythematosus which may manifest as heart block

◆ DON'T BE TRICKED

- Do not diagnose SLE in a patient with a positive ANA and facial rash that involves the nasolabial folds; consider rosacea instead.

The ANA assay is sensitive but not specific for diagnosing SLE. Assays for anti-dsDNA and anti-Sm antibodies are highly specific. Anti-dsDNA antibodies correlate with disease activity.

Activation of the complement pathway, manifested by depressed serum C3 and C4 levels, often accompanies major flares of SLE.

Drug-induced lupus is most often caused by hydralazine, procainamide, isoniazid, or minocycline. Symptoms are usually limited to fever, serositis, and arthritis. ANA assays are positive, but anti-dsDNA and anti-Sm antibody assays are negative. Antihistone antibody assay may be positive. In contrast, TNF-α inhibitors appear to induce lupus-like disease with positive anti-dsDNA antibodies and rare kidney and CNS involvement.

◆ DON'T BE TRICKED

- An isolated low-titer ANA by immunofluorescence assay (1:40-1:80) is almost never associated with disease.
- Myalgia, arthralgia, and fatigue are insufficient reasons by themselves to check an ANA panel.
- Monitoring ANA titers is not warranted because these values do not reflect disease activity.

Systemic Lupus Erythematosus Rash: The discoid rash of lupus erythematosus consists of chronic, slowly progressive, scaly, infiltrative papules and plaques or atrophic red plaques on sun-exposed skin surfaces. Discoid lupus can be present in the absence of any other clinical feature of SLE.

Therapy

Major therapeutic points:

- reduce atherosclerosis risk factors in all patients
- prescribe vitamin D and calcium supplements for all patients and bisphosphonates for those with osteoporosis and osteopenia
- manage arthritis with NSAIDs and hydroxychloroquine
- manage photosensitive cutaneous lupus with sun block, topical glucocorticoids, and hydroxychloroquine
- hydroxychloroquine should be initiated and continued indefinitely in most patients to help prevent flares of SLE even in patients with quiescent disease
- prescribe IV cyclophosphamide (or mycophenolate mofetil) and high-dose glucocorticoids for proliferative GN
- manage any life-threatening disease such as lupus pneumonitis, inflammatory CNS disease, or severe cytopenia with high-dose glucocorticoids and (usually) cyclophosphamide or mycophenolate mofetil
- use belimumab for patients not responding to conventional therapy

◆ DON'T BE TRICKED

- Patients taking hydroxychloroquine require annual routine ophthalmologic examinations.
- Medications that can be used in pregnant patients with SLE include hydroxychloroquine and prednisone.

Malar Skin Rash: Bright red, sharply demarcated plaques in a butterfly pattern that spares the nasolabial folds and areas beneath the nose and lower lip are associated with SLE.

Systemic Sclerosis

Diagnosis

SSc is a disease of unknown cause characterized by microvascular injury and excessive connective tissue deposition. The presence of typical skin findings and one or more of the following features supports a diagnosis:

- sclerodactyly
- digital pitting
- interstitial lung disease
- Raynaud phenomenon
- PH
- GERD
- pseudo-obstruction (small bowel)
- malabsorption due to bacterial overgrowth

SSc is classified according to the degree of skin involvement.

STUDY TABLE: Differentiating Diffuse from Limited Cutaneous Systemic Sclerosis		
Findings	**Diffuse Cutaneous SSc**	**Limited Cutaneous SSc**
Skin findings	Skin thickening proximal to the elbows and knees, including chest and abdomen; may affect the face	Skin thickening distal to the elbows and knees; may affect the face
Antibodies	ANA and anti-Scl-70 antibodies	ANA and anticentromere antibodies
Pulmonary disease	Interstitial lung disease	PH
Scleroderma renal crisis	Present	Absent
CREST syndrome	Usually absent	Present
CREST = calcinosis, Raynaud phenomenon, esophageal dysmotility, sclerodactyly, and telangiectasia.		

◆ DON'T BE TRICKED

- **Inflammatory arthritis with palpable tenderness and joint swelling suggest an overlap syndrome with RA.**
- **Nailfold capillary destruction and dilated capillary loops distinguishes early SSc from primary Raynaud disease.**

Gastric antral vascular ectasia (GAVE or "watermelon stomach") can result in recurrent bleeding and chronic anemia.

Hydrogen breath test can diagnose small bowel bacterial overgrowth; response to empiric treatment is tried first.

Up to 50% of patients have mild proteinuria, elevation in the plasma creatinine concentration, and/or hypertension, but most do not progress to CKD.

Scleroderma renal crisis is characterized by:

- hypertension
- microangiopathy
- microangiopathic hemolytic anemia
- thrombocytopenia
- mild proteinuria, bland urine
- acute kidney failure

In addition, glucocorticoid therapy is a risk factor and may be associated with normotensive renal crisis (AKI in the absence of hypertension).

The primary cause of morbidity and mortality in patients with SSc is pulmonary disease. Screening tests include HRCT and pulmonary function tests (including D$_{LCO}$) for interstitial lung disease and echocardiography for PH. Baseline and annual monitoring of pulmonary artery hypertension is recommended in all patients with or without advanced interstitial lung disease.

STUDY TABLE: Scleroderma-like Conditions

Condition	Features	Considerations
Eosinophilic fasciitis	Edema of proximal extremities; sparing of hands and face; peripheral eosinophilia	Skin biopsy shows lymphocytes, plasma cells, and eosinophils Treat with glucocorticoids
Nephrogenic systemic fibrosis	Exposure to gadolinium in kidney disease; brawny, wood-like induration of extremities, sparing the digits	Changes in use and formulation of gadolinium have reduced incidence
Scleredema	Indurated plaques/patches on back, shoulder girdle, and neck	Seen in long-standing diabetes
Scleromyxedema	Waxy, yellow-red papules over thickened skin of face, upper trunk, neck, and arms	Associate with multiple myeloma or AL amyloidosis
Chronic GVHD	Lichen planus-like skin lesions or localized or generalized skin thickening	Occurs most commonly after HSCT
Diabetes mellitus	Chronic contractures of the hands without edema	Both in type 1 and 2 diabetes, typically poorly controlled and long duration

Sclerodactyly: Thickening and induration of the skin over the fingers and wrists is characteristic of scleroderma.

Raynaud Phenomenon: Areas of vasospastic skin blanching seen in a patient with Raynaud phenomenon.

◆ **DON'T BE TRICKED**

- Skin thickening or tightening without Raynaud phenomenon is not SSc but another scleroderma-like condition.

Therapy

Therapies are for organ-specific manifestations; no overall disease-modifying therapy is available.

Avoidance of cold exposure and avoiding smoking reduce the risk of Raynaud episodes. Use nifedipine, amlodipine, felodipine, sildenafil, and nitroglycerin paste to manage Raynaud phenomenon.

Prescribe PPIs for GERD and promotility agents (metoclopramide) for gastric and intestinal dysmotility.

Prescribe ACE inhibitors for scleroderma renal crisis regardless of the serum creatinine level and continue even in the setting of kidney failure.

Bacterial overgrowth manifests as diarrhea and is managed with broad-spectrum antibiotics. Manage overlap syndrome with RA similarly to RA.

Treat active alveolitis or rapidly progressive interstitial lung disease with cyclophosphamide.

Treat PAH similarly to idiopathic PAH (oxygen, anticoagulation, vasodilating agents).

◆ DON'T BE TRICKED

- **Scleroderma is not managed with glucocorticoids.**

✧ Test Yourself

A 59-year-old woman has accelerated hypertension and CKD. She has a history of Raynaud phenomenon. BP is 160/122 mm Hg. Her fingers appear tapered with very smooth skin and ulcers on the fingertips. Serum creatinine level is 5.4 mg/dL.

ANSWER: The patient is in scleroderma renal crisis. Prescribe an ACE inhibitor.

Mixed Connective Tissue Disease

MCTD is a specific overlap syndrome that includes features of SLE, SSc, and/or polymyositis in the presence of anti–U1-RNP antibodies.

Diagnosis

In addition to RNP antibodies, the diagnosis of MCTD requires the presence of ≥3 of the following:

- Raynaud phenomenon
- edema of the hands
- sclerodactyly
- synovitis
- myositis

The mortality of patients with MCTD is increased compared to those with SLE, with the difference largely attributable to PH.

◆ DON'T BE TRICKED

- **Positive anti-Sm or anti-dsDNA antibodies supports the diagnosis of SLE, not MCTD.**

Therapy

Glucocorticoids, azathioprine, and methotrexate can be used for arthritis and myositis; calcium channel blockers for Raynaud phenomenon; and PPIs for GERD.

Fibromyalgia

Diagnosis

Diagnostic clues include:

- widespread pain ("hurt all over")
- waking unrefreshed ("always tired and fatigued")

- cognitive fatigue (forgets words or loses track of conversation in mid-sentence)
- exercise intolerance ("if I overdo it, I pay for it for several days")
- lack of response to multiple medications and diffuse tenderness to palpation

Initial laboratory studies include a CBC, chemistry panel, TSH, and ESR or CRP.

Therapy

Nonpharmacologic therapy such as regular aerobic exercise and cognitive behavioral therapy is the cornerstone of treatment for fibromyalgia and should be initiated in all affected patients.

Three drugs are FDA approved for fibromyalgia: the anticonvulsant pregabalin and the dual serotonin/norepinephrine reuptake inhibitors duloxetine and milnacipran. Each provides a modest benefit over placebo. Off-label therapies that have provided benefit include the tricyclic antidepressants and, to a lesser extent, the SSRIs.

◆ DON'T BE TRICKED

- Do not obtain ANA, rheumatoid factor, or anti-CCP antibodies.
- Do not diagnose fibromyalgia in the presence of red flags such as fever, anemia, weight loss, and synovitis.
- Do not use opioids in the treatment of fibromyalgia.

Gout

Diagnosis

Gout is caused by the inflammatory reaction to monosodium urate crystal deposition in synovial tissue, bursae, and tendon sheaths. Gout is often precipitated by use of diuretics. Gout progresses through three stages:

- acute intermittent gout
- intercritical gout, the time between attacks of acute gout
- chronic recurrent and tophaceous gout, which is characterized by persistent synovitis and possible formation of tophi

Monosodium urate crystals (needle-shaped, negatively birefringent crystals) in the joint fluid and urate tophi are diagnostic. Crystals within synovial fluid neutrophils define acute gout and extracellular crystals confirm chronic gout. Other characteristic findings of acute intermittent gout include monoarticular arthritis (typically of the first MTP or tarsal joints), self-limited acute attacks, and hyperuricemia. If disease presents classically (acute onset of pain at night) at the first MTP joint (podagra), synovial fluid analysis is not required to make the diagnosis.

With time, attacks of gout may become more frequent and involve more joints. Patients may progress to have a chronic, smoldering arthritis. Tophi are yellowish nodular deposits of monosodium urate, sometimes with surrounding erythema, that develop on extensor surfaces of the extremities, on finger pads, and along tendons. Hydrochlorothiazide is a common drug-trigger of acute gout. Transplantation-associated gout is associated with the use of calcineurin antagonists (cyclosporine). Lead toxicity may present with gout, kidney disease, and abdominal pain.

X-rays show bone erosions with overhanging edges. The synovial fluid leukocyte count ranges from 2000 to 75,000/μL. Monosodium urate crystals may be visible on joint aspiration when an acute flare is not occurring. In all patients, Gram stain and cultures must be obtained to exclude infection.

◆ DON'T BE TRICKED

- An elevated serum urate level alone is not diagnostic of gout.
- A normal serum urate level at the time of an acute attack does not rule out gout.
- Gout-related soft-tissue inflammation can mimic cellulitis, tenosynovitis, or dactylitis.

- Leukocyte counts higher than 50,000/µL should raise suspicion for a concurrent bacterial joint infection, even when monosodium urate crystals have been identified.

Therapy

Dietary purine restriction, weight loss, and discontinuation of alcohol may help to decrease serum urate levels in patients with mild hyperuricemia and symptomatic gout. Medications that raise serum urate levels, such as thiazide diuretics (substitute losartan which lowers serum urate) and low-dose salicylates, should be discontinued. For an acute gouty flare, NSAIDs, colchicine, and glucocorticoids are first-line therapies. Use oral glucocorticoids when NSAIDs are unsafe (in older adult or postoperative patients, patients requiring anticoagulation, and those with CKD or PUD). Prescribe intra-articular glucocorticoids for a single joint if other interventions are ineffective or contraindicated.

Urate lowering therapy is indicated in patients with:

- ≥2 attacks of acute gout
- 1 attack of acute gout in the setting of stage 2 or worse CKD
- 1 attack of acute gout in the setting of previous nephrolithiasis
- tophi visible on examination or imaging

Treat most patients with allopurinol to achieve a serum urate level <6 mg/dL. More than 50% of patients require allopurinol, >300 mg/d, to reach this target serum urate level. Doses must be adjusted (lowered) for patients with kidney impairment. When starting allopurinol, also begin low-dose colchicine (or an NSAID) to prevent acute gout; colchicine (or NSAID) can be discontinued 3 to 6 months after the serum urate level stabilizes. Febuxostat is useful if patients cannot tolerate allopurinol and in patients with CKD. In chronic refractory gout or when standard urate-lowering therapy has been unsuccessful or not tolerated, select IV pegloticase. Pegloticase enzymatically converts urate to the more soluble compound allantoin.

Chronic Tophaceous Gout: Swollen interphalangeal joints and multiple tophi characteristic of chronic tophaceous gout.

Patients with kidney disease, especially those concomitantly taking hydrochlorothiazide, who are treated with allopurinol have an increased risk for a rare but potentially fatal hypersensitivity syndrome characterized by severe dermatitis, fever, eosinophilia, hepatic necrosis, and acute nephritis.

◆ DON'T BE TRICKED

- Do not select NSAIDs for patients with gout who also have CKD or PUD.
- Do not use allopurinol and azathioprine together, because azathioprine is metabolized through xanthine oxidase, which is inhibited by allopurinol.
- Do not begin allopurinol during an acute attack of gout; wait 1 or 2 weeks.
- Do not use uricosuric therapy (e.g., probenecid) in patients with a low estimated GFR who are at risk for nephrolithiasis or CKD.
- Do not prescribe colchicine for patients with kidney failure.

❖ Test Yourself

A 78-year-old man has a 6-hour history of an acutely painful and swollen left first MTP joint. Two days ago, he had an MI. His serum creatinine level is 1.7 mg/dL.

ANSWER: The diagnosis is gout. Aspirate the joint, and treat with an intra-articular glucocorticoid after infection is excluded.

Calcium Pyrophosphate Deposition

Diagnosis

The four clinical presentations of CPPD are:

- cartilage calcification (also known as chondrocalcinosis)
- acute CPP crystal arthritis (also known as pseudogout)
- chronic CPP crystal inflammatory arthritis
- OA with CPPD

Characteristic findings in acute CPP crystal arthritis (pseudogout) are:

- inflammation localized to one joint, affecting the knee, wrist, shoulder, or ankle
- acute onset of several painful joints following trauma or surgery
- rhomboid-shaped and positively birefringent synovial fluid crystals

Characteristic findings in pyrophosphate arthropathy include:

- two distinct patterns: chronic inflammatory arthritis and OA with CPPD
- chronic inflammatory arthritis resembles RA
- OA with CPPD exhibits OA findings in atypical locations including wrist, MCP, or shoulder joints

Characteristic findings in cartilage calcification are (patients are typically asymptomatic):

- triangular fibrocartilage of the wrist joint (space between the carpal bones and distal ulna)
- menisci of the knee joint (appearing as a line in the cartilage)
- symphysis pubis

CPPD may be associated with underlying metabolic disorders. Screen patients with CPPD who are <50 years of age for:

- hemochromatosis
- hyperparathyroidism
- hypothyroidism
- hypomagnesemia

The definitive diagnosis of CPPD requires both the presence of positively birefringent, rhomboid-shaped crystals and typical cartilage or joint capsule calcification on x-ray.

X-ray of Knees, Chondrocalcinosis: Linear calcifications of the meniscus and articular cartilage are characteristic of CPPD.

◆ DON'T BE TRICKED

- The absence of chondrocalcinosis on x-ray does not rule out CPPD.

Therapy

NSAIDs are appropriate as initial therapy for most patients. Prescribe colchicine for patients with any variant of CPPD deposition disease that does not respond to NSAIDs. Intra-articular glucocorticoids are indicated for acute pain after infection is ruled out. This is always the correct treatment for a patient with noninfectious inflammatory monoarticular arthritis who cannot take NSAIDs because of an elevated serum creatinine level.

Infectious Arthritis

Diagnosis

Infectious arthritis should be considered in any patient who presents with:

- sudden onset of monoarthritis
- acute worsening of chronic joint disease
- previously painless joint prosthesis that is now painful
- radiographic loosening or migration of a cemented prosthetic device

The risk for infection is increased in persons with previously damaged joints (e.g., patients with RA), in older adults, and in immunosuppressed patients. In patients with underlying rheumatologic disorders, a sudden joint flare that is not accompanied by other features of the preexisting disorder and is unresponsive to usual therapy suggests a diagnosis of infectious arthritis.

The hallmark of an infected joint is pain on passive range of motion in the absence of trauma, and an infected joint typically appears swollen and warm with overlying erythema.

Gram-positive organisms are the most common causes of infectious arthritis in adults. *Staphylococcus aureus* is the most common offending organism, regardless of age or underlying risk factors.

Gonococcal arthritis is the most common form of bacterial arthritis in young sexually active persons in the United States. Disseminated gonococcal infection can produce two distinct syndromes:

- tenosynovitis, polyarthralgia, and dermatitis syndrome
- purulent gonococcal arthritis

Patients with the tenosynovitis, polyarthralgia, and dermatitis syndrome have cutaneous lesions that progress from papules or macules to pustules that are sterile on culture. Fever and chills are common. Patients with purulent gonococcal arthritis do not have systemic features (fevers, chills) or dermatitis. Blood cultures for *Neisseria gonorrhoeae* are positive in 50% of infected patients. Obtaining culture specimens from the pharynx, GU system, and rectum, in addition to synovial fluid cultures, increases the diagnostic yield. Evaluate for deficiencies in terminal complement components for patients with recurrent episodes of disseminated gonococcal infection.

Other less common causes of infectious arthritis:

- Gram-negative infections are more common in older, immunosuppressed, and postoperative patients, and those with IV catheters.
- Tuberculous arthritis typically is an indolent, monoarticular arthritis involving the hip or knee; it does not cause systemic features, and is not associated with positive TST; synovial fluid is Gram stain and culture negative. Diagnosis is made by synovial biopsy.
- Fungal arthritis typically manifests as subacute monoarthritis in patients with a systemic fungal infection.

STUDY TABLE: Synovial Fluid Characteristics				
Characteristic	**Normal**	**Group Iª (Noninflammatory)**	**Group IIᵇ (Inflammatory)**	**Group IIIᶜ (Septic)**
Leukocytes/μL	200	200-2000	2000-100,000	>50,000 (usually >100,000)
PMN cells (%)	<25	<25	>50	>75

ᵃExamples: OA, osteonecrosis, hemochromatosis, sickle cell disease.

ᵇExamples: crystalline arthritis, RA, spondyloarthropathy, SLE.

ᶜInfectious arthritis, including staphylococcal, gonococcal, and tuberculous.

A synovial fluid leukocyte count >50,000/μL is specific but not sensitive for infectious or crystalline arthropathy. For example, disseminated gonococcal infection may present with synovial fluid leukocyte counts <25,000/μL.

◆ **DON'T BE TRICKED**

- Always select arthrocentesis with Gram stain, polarized microscopy for crystals, cell count, and differential for all acutely swollen, painful joints.
- Infectious arthritis can develop in patients with gout or pseudogout, and the presence of crystals in synovial fluid does not exclude a concomitant infection.
- X-rays are not helpful in the early diagnosis of acute native joint infection.

Therapy

Begin immediate empiric antibiotic therapy for suspected bacterial arthritis even if culture results are pending or negative.

STUDY TABLE: Empiric and Definitive Antibiotic Treatment for Septic Native Joint Arthritis			
Gram Stain Results	**Likely or Identified Pathogen**	**First-Line Therapy**	**Second-Line Therapy**
Gram-positive cocci	*S. aureus*, other staphylococcal species	Oxacillin/nafcillin or cefazolin	–
	If MRSA is a concern (risk factors or known MRSA carrier)	Vancomycin or linezolid	Clindamycin, daptomycin
Gram-negative cocci	*N. gonorrhoeae*	Ceftriaxone	Fluoroquinolones (only if known to be sensitive)
Gram-negative bacilli	Enteric gram-negative bacilli	Ceftriaxone or cefotaxime	Fluoroquinolones
	Pseudomonas aeruginosa	Ceftazidime (plus gentamicin if proven)	Carbapenems, cefepime, piperacillin-tazobactam, fluoroquinolones
Gram stain unavailable	Consider MRSA and gram-negative organism if immunocompromised, at risk for gonococcal infection, or with joint trauma	Vancomycin or vancomycin plus ceftazidime	–
	Borrelia burgdorferi	Doxycycline or amoxicillin	–
	Mycobacterium tuberculosis	3-4 drug treatment (e.g., isoniazid, pyrazinamide, rifampin, ethambutol, streptomycin)	–
	Fungal infections	Amphotericin B, azoles	–

Use needle aspiration to drain reaccumulated purulent joint fluid. If this procedure fails or is too difficult to complete, perform arthroscopy/arthrotomy drainage. Manage infected prosthetic joints with surgery plus antibiotics, usually for 6 weeks.

◆ **DON'T BE TRICKED**

- Suspect tubercular infectious arthritis if the appropriate empiric antimicrobial therapy is unsuccessful.

❖ **Test Yourself**

A 28-year-old woman has a 9-day history of arthritis, fever, and chills followed by pain and swelling of the second and third MCP joints. As swelling resolves, the right wrist becomes inflamed. As the wrist improves, the right knee becomes inflamed. She also has a 5-mm vesicle surrounded by red skin on the forearm.

ANSWER: The diagnosis is disseminated gonorrhea. Prescribe ceftriaxone and doxycycline for empiric treatment of chlamydia.

Idiopathic Inflammatory Myopathies

Diagnosis

The idiopathic inflammatory myopathies are heterogeneous immune-mediated disorders; the major types are polymyositis, dermatomyositis, and inclusion body myositis.

The characteristic finding in polymyositis and dermatomyositis is the gradual onset of painless proximal muscle (cannot comb hair, rise up from chair, or climb stairs), pharyngeal, and respiratory muscle weakness.

Photosensitivity rashes are commonly associated with dermatomyositis. The presence of Gottron papules (scaly, purplish papules and plaques over the metacarpal and interphalangeal joints) and heliotrope rash (edematous lilac discoloration of periorbital tissue) is virtually diagnostic of dermatomyositis. "Mechanic's hands" (scaly, rough, dry, cracked horizontal lines on the palmar and lateral aspects of the fingers) may occur in either polymyositis or dermatomyositis.

ANA is present in 80% of patients with polymyositis or dermatomyositis. Autoantibodies to aminoacyl-transfer (t)RNA synthetase enzymes (e.g., anti–Jo-1 antibodies) are found in 20% of patients with myositis and are associated with an antisynthetase syndrome characterized by:

- interstitial lung disease
- inflammatory polyarthritis
- fever
- Raynaud phenomenon
- mechanic's hands
- increased risk of premature death

Diagnostic tests for inflammatory myositis include measurement of serum CK and aldolase levels and EMG. The characteristic triad of EMG findings are:

- short duration small, low-amplitude polyphasic potentials
- fibrillation potentials at rest
- bizarre, high frequency, repetitive discharges

Muscle biopsy is the definitive study. MRI of the proximal musculature, particularly the thighs, may assess the degree of muscle inflammation and damage and may be helpful when other diagnostic studies are equivocal or to identify the most promising biopsy site.

The onset of symptoms in inclusion body myositis is insidious and involves proximal and distal muscles, frequently with an asymmetric distribution. Quadriceps, wrist, and finger flexor muscle weakness is common. ANA is found in <20% of patients with inclusion body myositis.

Certain medications (glucocorticoids, statins) or alcohol may also cause a toxic myopathy.

◆ DON'T BE TRICKED

- Serum AST and ALT levels may be elevated in myositis, mimicking liver disease.
- Muscle pain in patients with an inflammatory myopathy is atypical and, if present, is generally mild.

STUDY TABLE: Mimics of Polymyositis	
If you see this...	**Diagnose this...**
Muscle fasciculations	ALS
Oculomotor weakness with ptosis	Myasthenia gravis
Proximal muscle tenderness	Polymyalgia rheumatica
Muscle atrophy, hyporeflexia	Peripheral neuropathy
Goiter, delayed reflexes, weight gain	Hypothyroidism
Treatment with a statin	Statin myopathy

If myositis is unresponsive to treatment, consider a diagnosis of inclusion body myositis.

When ≥2 connective tissue diseases are present, diagnose an overlap syndrome.

When ≥2 connective tissue diseases are associated with high titers of anti-RNP antibodies, diagnose MCTD.

The association between malignancy and the inflammatory myopathies is well established. The types of malignancies correlate with those that develop in an age-matched population, except that ovarian cancer is more common. No guidelines exist for the evaluation of malignancy in patients with inflammatory myositis. Minimally, follow such patients with sex- and age-appropriate cancer screening.

Therapy

High-dose oral glucocorticoid therapy is first-line treatment for polymyositis and dermatomyositis. Adding methotrexate and/or azathioprine may be indicated if disease is refractory to high-dose glucocorticoid therapy or if patients develop intolerable glucocorticoid-related side effects. Use IV immune globulin in patients with refractory disease. Hydroxychloroquine may help to treat cutaneous manifestations of dermatomyositis. Baseline bone mineral density testing is indicated in patients who undergo long-term high-dose glucocorticoid therapy. Begin prophylactic therapy for osteoporosis with calcium and vitamin D supplementation and bisphosphonates.

Heliotrope Rash: Heliotrope rash on edematous eyelids characteristic of dermatomyositis.

◆ DON'T BE TRICKED

- Suspect glucocorticoid-induced myopathy in patients with continued or new-onset worsening of proximal muscle weakness despite normalization of muscle enzyme levels.

- CK elevation may occur several years before clinical manifestations of hypothyroidism. Always check TSH levels when evaluating myopathy.

Gottron Papules: Red patches and plaques over the knuckles (Gottron papules) characteristic of dermatomyositis.

❖ Test Yourself

A 34-year-old man has a 3-month history of pain and swelling of his hands, wrists, and ankles. He also has difficulty climbing stairs and reaching over his head; this weakness is not associated with pain. Anti-RNP antibody is positive.

ANSWER: The diagnosis is an overlap syndrome with elements of polymyositis and arthritis.

Vasculitis

Diagnosis

Vasculitis is an inflammation of blood vessels that causes stenosis, obstruction, or attenuation with subsequent tissue ischemia, aneurysms, or hemorrhage. This condition may be secondary to an underlying process or occur as a primary disease of unknown cause. Primary vasculitides may be categorized based on the size of the blood vessel that is predominantly involved, the pattern of organ involvement, and the histopathology.

Large-vessel vasculitis:

- Giant cell arteritis → older adults with fever, headaches, scalp tenderness, jaw claudication, and visual symptoms. Obtain an ESR (>50 mm/h) and temporal artery biopsy.

- Polymyalgia rheumatica → older adults with aching and morning stiffness in the proximal muscles of the shoulder and hip girdle; muscle strength and muscle enzymes are normal; may also develop in patients with giant cell arteritis or as a primary condition. Obtain an ESR (>50 mm/h).

- Takayasu arteritis → young women with fever, malaise, weight loss, and arthralgia preceding arm/leg claudication, pulse deficits, vascular bruits, and asymmetric arm BP readings. Obtain aortography.

Medium-vessel vasculitis:

- Polyarteritis nodosa → nonglomerular kidney disease, hypertension, mononeuritis multiplex, and skin lesions (nodules, livedo reticularis, palpable purpura). Obtain hepatitis B serologic studies, biopsy of involved tissue (usually skin or testicle), and mesenteric or renal angiography (aneurysms and stenoses).
- Primary angiitis of the CNS → recurrent headaches, stroke, TIA, and progressive encephalopathy; select LP, MRI, cerebral angiography, and brain biopsy (granulomatous vasculitis).

Small-vessel vasculitis:

- Granulomatosis with polyangiitis → recurrent middle ear infections, destructive rhinitis or sinusitis, saddle-nose deformity, tracheal collapse, pulmonary infiltrates/cavities/hemoptysis, and pauci-immune GN. Obtain c-ANCA and anti-PR3 antibody assay; biopsy often required to make diagnosis.
- Microscopic polyangiitis → pulmonary infiltrates, palpable purpura, and rapidly progressive pauci-immune GN. Obtain p-ANCA and anti-MPO antibody assay. Biopsy skin, lung, or kidney.
- Eosinophilic granulomatosis with polyangiitis (formerly known as Churg-Strauss syndrome) → asthma, eosinophilia, elevated IgG, and pulmonary infiltrates/hemoptysis. Obtain p-ANCA and anti-MPO antibody assay and biopsy.
- Henoch-Schönlein purpura → palpable purpura, joint, and gut involvement (abdominal pain), and GN. Obtain skin biopsy (IgA immune complex deposition) or kidney biopsy (IgA nephropathy).
- Hypersensitivity vasculitis (leukocytoclastic vasculitis) → palpable purpura (lower legs), cutaneous vesicles, pustules, maculopapular lesions, urticaria, recent viral infection, drug exposure, or diagnosis of malignancy. Obtain skin biopsy.
- Cryoglobulinemic vasculitis → skin lesions (red macules, palpable purpura, nodules, or ulcers), GN, mononeuritis multiplex, and elevated serum aminotransferase levels. Obtain serum cryoglobulins and hepatitis C serologic studies.
- Behçet syndrome → oral and genital ulcers; uveitis; pathergy, and nonerosive, asymmetric oligoarthritis. This is a clinical diagnosis.

◆ DON'T BE TRICKED

- Aortic aneurysm and aortic dissection are potential complications of giant cell arteritis as is aortic dissection which may occur with or without preceding aneurysm formation.
- Include Takayasu arteritis in the differential diagnosis of aortic coarctation, aortic aneurysm, and aortic value regurgitation in young women.
- Polyarteritis nodosa kidney disease does not involve the glomerulus (no urine erythrocytes, casts, or proteinuria).
- Lung biopsy most reliably provides the characteristic histopathologic findings associated with granulomatosis with polyangiitis.
- Do not make a diagnosis of eosinophilic granulomatosis with polyangiitis in the absence of eosinophilia.

Therapy

STUDY TABLE: Treatment of Large-Vessel Vasculitis	
Disease	**Treatment**
Giant cell arteritis	Prednisone and low-dose aspirin; treat immediately to prevent blindness and obtain biopsy in <2 weeks
Polymyalgia rheumatica	Low-dose prednisone; relapse common and prolonged courses typical (1-3 years)
Takayasu arteritis	Prednisone

STUDY TABLE: Treatment of Medium-Vessel Vasculitis

Disease	Treatment
Polyarteritis nodosa	Prednisone and cyclophosphamide; treat concomitant HBV infection
Primary angiitis of the CNS	Prednisone and cyclophosphamide

STUDY TABLE: Treatment of Small-Vessel Vasculitis

Disease	Treatment
Granulomatosis with polyangiitis	Prednisone and cyclophosphamide
Microscopic polyangiitis	Prednisone and cyclophosphamide
Eosinophilic granulomatosis with polyangiitis	Prednisone; cyclophosphamide added for severe, multiorgan disease
Henoch-Schönlein purpura	Typically self-limited; glucocorticoids for severe GN
Hypersensitivity vasculitis	NSAIDs, antihistamines, colchicine, dapsone, prednisone; if drug-associated, withdraw offending drug
HCV-associated cryoglobulinemic vasculitis	Treat underlying HCV infection
	If organ dysfunction is severe, also treat with prednisone, cyclophosphamide, and plasmapheresis
Behçet syndrome	Low-dose prednisone or colchicine

❖ **Test Yourself**

A 72-year-old woman has had a left temporal headache for the past 8 days with blurred and double vision that lasted 15 minutes this morning.

ANSWER: The diagnosis is giant cell arteritis. Select immediate prednisone, and arrange for temporal artery biopsy.

A 32-year-old woman has a 6-month history of fever, myalgia, arthralgia, and weight loss. She is of Korean descent. Two days ago, she developed achy pain in her arms when working with her arms above her head.

ANSWER: The diagnosis is Takayasu arteritis. When ethnicity is identified, it is an essential key to the diagnosis.

Relapsing Polychondritis

Diagnosis

Relapsing polychondritis is a systemic inflammatory connective tissue disease characterized by inflammation and destruction of cartilaginous structures. Auricular pain and swelling are the most common presenting features. Characteristic findings are:

- red, hot, painful ears
- respiratory stridor caused by tracheal collapse
- saddle nose deformity

Relapsing polychondritis is often a clinical diagnosis, and biopsy of affected cartilage is confirmatory. Saddle nose deformity can also occur in syphilis, cocaine use, leprosy, and granulomatosis with polyangiitis.

Therapy

Glucocorticoids are indicated for acute flares and NSAIDs for chronic disease management.

Polychondritis: Recurrent episodes of polychondritis involving the ear can permanently alter the structure of cartilage, resulting in a "cauliflower" appearance.

Familial Mediterranean Fever

Diagnosis

FMF occurs most often in persons from the Eastern Mediterranean basin. Characteristic findings are:

- recurrent, self-limited attacks of fever
- serositis (abdominal or pleuritic pain)
- arthritis
- rashes that last 3 to 4 days

Laboratory findings include an elevated ESR and serum CRP concentration, positive serum amyloid A (AA) protein, proteinuria, and the Mediterranean fever (*MEFV*) gene.

Therapy

Begin colchicine for confirmed or suspected FMF to prevent symptomatic attacks and development of AA amyloidosis.

❖ **Test Yourself**

> A 23-year-old woman has episodic fever and abdominal pain every 1 to 2 months, lasting 2 to 3 days per episode. She is well between episodes. She is of Ashkenazi Jewish descent. Physical examination and imaging studies are normal.
>
> **ANSWER:** The diagnosis is FMF.

Adult-Onset Still Disease

Diagnosis

The clinical features of AOSD include:

- quotidian fever in which the temperature usually spikes once daily and then returns to subnormal
- fatigue, malaise, arthralgia, and myalgia
- proteinuria
- serositis
- evanescent pink rash
- joint manifestations include an nonerosive inflammatory arthritis

Ferritin levels are elevated in AOSD, and serum levels >2500 ng/mL are highly specific for this condition and reflect disease activity.

Rarely patients may develop the hemophagocytic syndrome, a life-threatening process characterized by fever, splenomegaly, cytopenias, elevated ferritin, and evidence of hemophagocytosis on bone marrow biopsy.

Therapy

NSAIDs are generally used as first-line agents in management, but glucocorticoids may be helpful in patients whose disease is refractory to NSAIDs. In patients with refractory disease, therapy with methotrexate, a TNF-α inhibitor, or the interleukin-1 receptor antagonist anakinra may be helpful.

Complex Regional Pain Syndrome

Diagnosis

Complex regional pain syndrome is characterized by pain, swelling, limited range of motion, vasomotor instability, skin changes, and patchy bone demineralization of the extremities. It typically follows an injury, surgery, MI, or stroke. Look for onset of pain after injury, persistence of pain, and at least two associated symptoms or signs, including:

- neuropathic pain (allodynia, hyperalgesia, hyperpathia)
- autonomic dysfunction of the affected extremity (edema, color changes, sweating)
- swelling
- dystrophy (hair loss, skin thinning, ulcers)
- movement disorder (difficulty initiating movement, dystonia, tremor, weakness)

No tests are needed for the diagnosis but usually are required to exclude underlying pathology. The finding of abnormal bone metabolism and osteoporosis by bone scan, bone densitometry, MRI, or plain x-ray supports the diagnosis.

Therapy

Physical therapy is essential to preserve joint mobility and prevent contractures and osteoporosis. Glucocorticoids may abort the syndrome if started soon after symptom development. Early sympathetic blockade is effective. Gabapentin and tricyclic antidepressants are adjuvants for pain control. Bisphosphonates are effective treatment for pain even in the absence of osteoporosis.

Abbreviations

3f-PCC	3-factor prothrombin complex concentrate		aPTT	activated partial thromboplastin time
4f-PCC	4-factor prothrombin complex concentrate		AR	aortic regurgitation; absolute risk
5-ASA	5-aminosalicylic acid		ARB	angiotensin receptor blocker
5-FU	5-fluorouracil		ARDS	acute respiratory distress syndrome
5-HIAA	5-hydroxyindoleacetic acid		ARR	absolute risk reduction
6-MP	6-mercaptopurine		ART	antiretroviral therapy
A-a	alveolar-arterial oxygen gradient		AS	aortic stenosis
AA	amyloid A		ASCVD	atherosclerotic cardiovascular disease
AAA	abdominal aortic aneurysm		ASD	atrial septal defect
AAT	α_1-antitrypsin		ASH	alcoholic steatohepatitis
ABG	arterial blood gas		AST	aspartate aminotransferase
ABI	ankle-brachial index		ATN	acute tubular necrosis
ABIM	American Board of Internal Medicine		ATRA	all-*trans*-retinoic acid
ABVD	doxorubicin (Adriamycin), bleomycin, vinblastine, dacarbazine		AUDIT-C	Alcohol Use Disorders Identification Test
ACC	American College of Cardiology		AV	atrioventricular
ACE	angiotensin-converting enzyme		AVM	arteriovenous malformation
ACS	acute coronary syndrome		AVNRT	atrioventricular nodal reentrant tachycardia
ACTH	adrenocorticotropic hormone		AVP	arginine vasopressin
ADH	antidiuretic hormone		AVRT	atrioventricular reciprocating tachycardia
ADHD	attention-deficit/hyperactivity disorder		β-hCG	beta–human chorionic gonadotropin
ADPKD	autosomal dominant polycystic kidney disease		β_2-GPI	beta-2 glycoprotein I
ADT	androgen deprivation therapy		BCC	basal cell carcinoma
AED	antiepileptic drug		BE	Barrett esophagus
AF	atrial fibrillation		BID	twice daily
AFLP	acute fatty liver of pregnancy		BMI	body mass index
AFP	α-fetoprotein		BNP	B-type natriuretic peptide
AGEP	acute generalized exanthematous pustulosis		BP	blood pressure
AH	alcoholic hepatitis		BPAP	bilevel positive airway pressure
AHA	American Heart Association		BPH	benign prostatic hyperplasia
AHI	apnea-hypopnea index		*BRCA*	breast cancer susceptibility gene
AIDS	acquired immunodeficiency syndrome		BUN	blood urea nitrogen
AIN	acute interstitial nephritis		CA	cancer antigen
AIP	autoimmune pancreatitis		CABG	coronary artery bypass graft
AKI	acute kidney injury		CAD	coronary artery disease
ALL	acute lymphoblastic leukemia		c-ANCA	cytoplasmic antineutrophil cytoplasmic antibody
ALS	amyotrophic lateral sclerosis		CAP	community-acquired pneumonia
ALT	alanine aminotransferase		CAPOX	capecitabine plus oxaliplatin
AMD	age-related macular degeneration		CAUTI	catheter-associated urinary tract infection
AMI	acute mesenteric ischemia		CBC	complete blood count
AML	acute myeloblastic leukemia		CEA	carcinoembryonic antigen
AMS	acute mountain sickness		CF	cystic fibrosis
ANA	antinuclear antibody		CH_{50}	total hemolytic complement
ANCA	antineutrophil cytoplasmic antibody		CI	confidence interval
anti-CCP	anti-cyclic citrullinated peptide		CK	creatine kinase
anti-DNase	anti-deoxyribonuclease		CKD	chronic kidney disease
anti-dsDNA	anti-double-stranded DNA		CLL	chronic lymphocytic leukemia
anti-HBc	antibodies to hepatitis B core antigen		CML	chronic myeloid leukemia
anti-HBe	antibodies to hepatitis B e antigen		CMR	cardiac magnetic resonance (imaging)
anti-HBs	antibodies to hepatitis B surface antigen		CMV	cytomegalovirus
anti-MPO	anti-myeloperoxidase		CNS	central nervous system
anti-NMDA	anti-N-methyl-D-aspartate		COPD	chronic obstructive pulmonary disease
anti-RNP	antiribonucleoprotein		CPAP	continuous positive airway pressure
anti-Sm	anti-Smith		CPP	calcium pyrophosphate
anti-TNF	anti–tumor necrosis factor		CPPD	calcium pyrophosphate deposition
AOSD	adult-onset Still disease		CRAO	central retinal arterial occlusion
APLA	antiphospholipid antibody		CRP	C-reactive protein
			CRVO	central retinal vein occlusion

CSF	cerebrospinal fluid
CT	computed tomography
CTA	computed tomography angiography
CTEPH	chronic thromboembolic pulmonary hypertension
CUP	carcinoma of unknown primary
CVA	cerebrovascular accident
CVI	common variable immunodeficiency
CVP	central venous pressure
DASH	Dietary Approaches to Stop Hypertension
DBP	diastolic blood pressure
DCIS	ductal carcinoma in situ
DDAVP	1-deamino-8-D-arginine vasopressin
DEXA	dual energy x-ray absorptiometry
DHEAS	dehydroepiandrosterone sulfate
DI	diabetes insipidus
DIC	disseminated intravascular coagulation
DIP	distal interphalangeal
DISH	diffuse idiopathic skeletal hyperostosis
DKA	diabetic ketoacidosis
DLBCL	diffuse large B-cell lymphoma
D_{LCO}	diffusing capacity of lung for carbon monoxide
DMARD	disease-modifying antirheumatic drug
DNA	deoxyribonucleic acid
DPLD	diffuse parenchymal lung disease
DRESS	drug reaction with eosinophilia and systemic symptoms
DVT	deep venous thrombosis
EBV	Epstein-Barr virus
ECG	electrocardiogram
EDTA	ethylenediaminetetraacetic acid
EE	eosinophilic esophagitis
EEG	electroencephalogram
EF	ejection fraction
EGD	esophagogastroduodenoscopy
EGFR	epidermal growth factor receptor
eGFR	estimated glomerular filtration rate
EHEC	enterohemorrhagic *Escherichia coli* O157:H7
EIA	enzyme immunoassay
ELISA	enzyme-linked immunosorbent assay
EM	erythema multiforme
EMG	electromyography
EN	erythema nodosum
ENT	ear, nose, and throat
ERCP	endoscopic retrograde cholangiopancreatography
ESR	erythrocyte sedimentation rate
FDA	Food and Drug Administration
FE_{Na}	fractional excretion of sodium
FEPO4	fractional excretion of filtered phosphate
FE_{Urea}	fractional excretion of urea
FEV_1	forced expiratory volume exhaled in 1 second
FiO_2	fraction of inspired oxygen
FFP	fresh frozen plasma
FMF	familial Mediterranean fever
FNAB	fine-needle aspiration biopsy
FOBT	fecal occult blood testing
FOLFIRI	5-fluorouracil, leucovorin, and irinotecan
FOLFIRINOX	5-fluorouracil, leucovorin, irinotecan, and oxaliplatin
FOLFOX	5-fluorouracil, leucovorin, and oxaliplatin
FSH	follicle-stimulating hormone
FTA-ABS	fluorescent treponemal antibody absorption test
FVC	forced vital capacity
G6PD	glucose 6-phosphate dehydrogenase
GAD65	glutamate decarboxylase antibody

GBM	glomerular basement membrane
GE	gastroesophageal
GERD	gastroesophageal reflux disease
GFR	glomerular filtration rate
GH	growth hormone
GI	gastrointestinal
GLP-1	glucagon-like peptide 1
GN	glomerulonephritis
GnRH	gonadotropin-releasing hormone
GP	glycoprotein
GU	genitourinary
GVHD	graft-versus-host disease
HACE	high-altitude cerebral edema
HAI	high-altitude illness
HAP	hospital-acquired pneumonia
HAPB	high-altitude periodic breathing
HAPE	high-altitude pulmonary edema
HAV	hepatitis A virus
HBeAg	hepatitis B e antigen
HBIG	hepatitis B immune globulin
HBsAg	hepatitis B surface antigen
HBV	hepatitis B virus
hCG	human chorionic gonadotropin
HCC	hepatocellular carcinoma
HCM	hypertrophic cardiomyopathy
HCV	hepatitis C virus
HDL	high-density lipoprotein
HELLP	hemolysis, elevated liver enzyme levels, and a low platelet count
HES	hypereosinophilic syndromes
HF	heart failure
HFpEF	heart failure with preserved ejection fraction
HFrEF	heart failure with reduced ejection fraction
HGA	human granulocytic anaplasmosis
HIDA	hepatobiliary iminodiacetic acid
HIPAA	Health Insurance Portability and Accountability Act
HIT	heparin-induced thrombocytopenia
HITT	heparin-induced thrombocytopenia with thrombosis
HIV	human immunodeficiency virus
HLA	human leukocyte antigens
HME	human monocytic ehrlichiosis
HNPCC	hereditary nonpolyposis colorectal cancer
HPA	human platelet antigen
HPV	human papillomavirus
HR	hazard ratio; heart rate
HRCT	high-resolution computed tomography
HSCT	hematopoietic stem cell transplantation
HSV	herpes simplex virus
HUS	hemolytic uremic syndrome
IA-2	islet antigen-2 antibody
IBD	inflammatory bowel disease
IBS	irritable bowel syndrome
IBS-C	irritable bowel syndrome with constipation
IBS-D	irritable bowel syndrome with diarrhea
IBS-M	mixed irritable bowel syndrome
ICD	implantable cardioverter defibrillator
ICH	intracerebral hemorrhage
ICU	intensive care unit
IE	infective endocarditis
IGF-1	insulin-like growth factor-1
IgM anti-HAV	IgM antibodies to hepatitis A virus
IGRA	interferon-γ release assay
IM	intramuscular

INR	international normalized ratio	N/A	not applicable
IPF	idiopathic pulmonary fibrosis	NAAT	nucleic acid amplification testing
IPSS-R	revised International Prognostic Scoring System	NAFLD	nonalcoholic fatty liver disease
IRIS	immune reconstitution inflammatory syndrome	NASH	nonalcoholic steatohepatitis
ITP	immune thrombocytopenic purpura	NCCN	National Comprehensive Cancer Network
IV	intravenous	NET	neuroendocrine tumor
IVC	inferior vena cava	NMO	neuromyelitis optica
JNC 8	Eighth Joint National Committee	NNH	number needed to harm
KOH	potassium hydroxide	NNT	number needed to treat
LABA	long-acting β_2-agonist	NPH	intermediate-acting insulin or Lente
LAC	lupus anticoagulant	NPPV	noninvasive positive-pressure ventilation
LAM	lymphanogioleiomyomatosis	NSAIDs	nonsteroidal anti-inflammatory drugs
LAMA	long-acting muscarinic agent (also called long-acting anticholinergic agent)	NSCLC	non–small cell lung cancer
		NSTEMI	non–ST-elevation myocardial infarction
LBBB	left bundle branch block	NYHA	New York Heart Association
LDH	lactate dehydrogenase	OA	osteoarthritis
LDL	low-density lipoprotein	OGTT	oral glucose tolerance test
LES	lower esophageal sphincter	OSA	obstructive sleep apnea
LFT	liver function test	PAD	peripheral arterial disease
LGI	lower gastrointestinal	PAH	pulmonary arterial hypertension
LH	luteinizing hormone	p-ANCA	perinuclear antineutrophil cytoplasmic antibodies
LKM	liver-kidney microsome	PCI	percutaneous coronary intervention
LLQ	left lower quadrant	PCNSL	primary central nervous system lymphoma
LMWH	low-molecular-weight heparin	P_{CO_2}	partial pressure of carbon dioxide
LN	lupus nephritis	PCOS	polycystic ovary syndrome
LP	lumbar puncture	PCR	polymerase chain reaction
LR	likelihood ratio	PCV13	pneumococcal conjugate vaccine
LTBI	latent tuberculosis infection	PCWP	pulmonary capillary wedge pressure
LV	left ventricular	PDA	patent ductus arteriosus
LVEF	left ventricular ejection fraction	PDE-4	phosphodiesterase type 4
LVH	left ventricular hypertrophy	PDE-5	phosphodiesterase type 5
MAC	*Mycobacterium avium* complex	PE	pulmonary embolism
MAOI	monoamine oxidase inhibitor	PEEP	positive end-expiratory pressure
MALT	mucosa-associated lymphoid tissue	PEF	peak expiratory flow
MAP	mean arterial pressure	PEG	polyethylene glycol
MAT	multifocal atrial tachycardia	PET	positron emission tomography
MCI	mild cognitive impairment	PF4	platelet factor 4
MCP	metacarpophalangeal	PFO	patent foramen ovale
MCTD	mixed connective tissue disease	PH	pulmonary hypertension
MCV	mean corpuscular volume	PID	pelvic inflammatory disease
MDS	myelodysplastic syndromes	PIP	proximal interphalangeal
MEN1	multiple endocrine neoplasia type 1	PMDD	premenstrual dysphoric disorder
MEN2	multiple endocrine neoplasia type 2	PMN	polymorphonuclear
MET	metabolic equivalent	PMS	premenstrual syndrome
MG	myasthenia gravis	PNES	psychogenic nonepileptic seizures
MGUS	monoclonal gammopathy of undetermined significance	PNH	paroxysmal nocturnal hemoglobinuria
		PO	by mouth
MHA-TP	microhemagglutination assay for *Treponema pallidum*	P_{O_2}	partial pressure of oxygen
		PPD	purified protein derivative
MI	myocardial infarction	PPI	proton pump inhibitor
MIBG	metaiodobenzylguanidine	PPSV23	pneumococcal polysaccharide vaccine
MMR	measles, mumps, rubella	PR3	proteinase 3
MPA	microscopic polyangiitis	PSA	prostate-specific antigen
MPN	myeloproliferative neoplasm	PSC	primary sclerosing cholangitis
MPO	myeloperoxidase	PT	prothrombin time
MR	mitral regurgitation	PTH	parathyroid hormone
MRA	magnetic resonance angiography	PTSD	posttraumatic stress disorder
MRCP	magnetic resonance cholangiopancreatography	PUD	peptic ulcer disease
MRI	magnetic resonance imaging	PV	polycythemia vera
MRSA	methicillin-resistant *Staphylococcus aureus*	PVC	premature ventricular complex
MS	multiple sclerosis	RA	rheumatoid arthritis
MSSA	methicillin-sensitive *Staphylococcus aureus*	RANKL	receptor activator of nuclear factor κB ligand
mTOR	mammalian target of rapamycin	RAST	radioallergosorbent test
MTP	metatarsophalangeal	RBBB	right bundle branch block
MVP	mitral valve prolapse	RBC	red blood cell

R-CHOP	rituximab, cyclophosphamide, doxorubicin, vincristine, prednisolone		TBI	traumatic brain injury
RCT	randomized controlled trial		TBW	total body weight
REM	rapid eye movement		Tdap	diphtheria and reduced tetanus toxoids and acellular pertussis vaccine
RF	rheumatic fever		TEE	transesophageal echocardiography
rfVIIa	recombinant factor VIIa		TEN	toxic epidermal necrolysis
RLQ	right lower quadrant		TIA	transient ischemic attack
RNA	ribonucleic acid		TIBC	total iron-binding capacity
RNP	ribonucleic protein		TIMI	Thrombolysis in Myocardial Infarction (risk score)
ROC	receiver operating characteristic		TIPS	transjugular intrahepatic portosystemic shunt
RPR	rapid plasma reagin		TLC	total lung capacity
RR	relative risk		TNF	tumor necrosis factor
RRR	relative risk reduction		TR	tricuspid regurgitation
RTA	renal tubular acidosis		TSH	thyroid-stimulating hormone
rtPA	recombinant tissue plasminogen activator		TST	tuberculin skin testing
RUQ	right upper quadrant		TTE	transthoracic echocardiography
RV	right ventricular		tTG	tissue transglutaminase
SAAG	serum-ascites albumin gradient		TTP	thrombotic thrombocytopenic purpura
SAH	subarachnoid hemorrhage		UACS	upper airways cough syndrome
SBP	systolic blood pressure		UAG	urine anion gap
SCC	squamous cell carcinoma		UFH	unfractionated heparin
SCLC	small cell lung cancer		UGI	upper gastrointestinal
SEID	systemic exertion intolerance disease		UPEP	urine protein electrophoresis
SGLT2	sodium-glucose transporter-2		URI	upper respiratory infection
SIADH	syndrome of inappropriate antidiuretic hormone secretion		USPSTF	United States Preventive Services Task Force
SIRS	systemic inflammatory response syndrome		UTI	urinary tract infection
SJS	Stevens-Johnson syndrome		VAP	ventilator-associated pneumonia
SLE	systemic lupus erythematosus		VDRL	venereal disease research laboratory
SNRI	serotonin-norepinephrine reuptake inhibitor		VEGF	vascular endothelial growth factor
SPEP	serum protein electrophoresis		VF	ventricular fibrillation
SPN	solitary pulmonary nodule		VKA	vitamin K antagonist
SSA	sulfosalicylic acid		V/Q	ventilation/perfusion ratio
SSc	systemic sclerosis		VSD	ventricular septal defect
SSRI	selective serotonin reuptake inhibitor		VT	ventricular tachycardia
STEMI	ST-elevation myocardial infarction		VTE	venous thromboembolism
STI	sexually transmitted infection		vWD	von Willebrand disease
SVC	superior vena cava		vWF	von Willebrand factor
SVT	supraventricular tachycardia		WBC	white blood cell
T_4	free thyroxine		WNND	West Nile neuroinvasive disease
TB	tuberculosis		WNV	West Nile virus
			WPW	Wolff-Parkinson-White